The
Spiritual
Life
of
Children

PRIVILEGED ONES:
The Well-off and the Rich in America
(Volume V of Children of Crisis)

A FESTERING SWEETNESS (*poems*)

THE LAST AND FIRST ESKIMOS (with Alex Harris)

WOMEN OF CRISIS, I:
Lives of Struggle and Hope (with Jane Coles)

WALKER PERCY: *An American Search*

FLANNERY O'CONNOR'S SOUTH

WOMEN OF CRISIS, II:
Lives of Work and Dreams (with Jane Coles)

DOROTHEA LANGE

THE DOCTOR STORIES OF
WILLIAM CARLOS WILLIAMS (ed.)

AGEE (with Ross Spears)

THE AMERICAN TEENAGER

THE MORAL LIFE OF CHILDREN

THE POLITICAL LIFE OF CHILDREN

SIMONE WEIL: *A Modern Pilgrimage*

DOROTHY DAY: *A Radical Devotion*

IN THE STREETS (with Helen Levitt)

TIMES OF SURRENDER: *Selected Essays*

HARVARD DIARY: *Reflections on the Sacred and the Secular*

THAT RED WHEELBARROW: *Selected Literary Essays*

THE CHILD IN OUR TIMES:
Studies in the Development of Resiliency
(ed. with Timothy Dugan)

THE CALL OF STORIES: *Teaching and the Moral Imagination*

The
Spiritual
Life
of
Children

✺✺✺

Robert Coles

A Peter Davison Book

HOUGHTON MIFFLIN COMPANY

BOSTON

For information about permission to reproduce selections from
this book, write to Permissions, Houghton Mifflin Company,
2 Park Street, Boston, Massachusetts 02108.

Library of Congress Cataloging-in-Publication Data

Coles, Robert.
The spiritual life of children / Robert Coles.
p.   cm.
"A Peter Davison book."
Includes bibliographical references and index.
ISBN 0-395-55999-5
ISBN 0-395-59923-7 (pbk.)
Children — Religious life.   I. Title.
BL625.C64   1990   90-40097
291.4'083 — dc20   CIP

Printed in the United States of America

BP 18 17 16 15 14 13 12 11 10 9

To Jane

To our sons, Bob, Danny, Mike

and

In memory of Walker Percy

Contents

List of Figures

(following page 154)

Introduction

This book brings to an end thirty years of writing about children in various regions of the United States and in many parts of the world. In 1960, having served in Mississippi as an Air Force physician for two years and witnessing there the developing racial struggle in the deep South, I began a study of school desegregation in New Orleans. I had been trained in pediatrics and child psychiatry in Boston[1] and was getting a psychoanalytic education in New Orleans when that old cosmopolitan port city, overnight it seemed, became a place of serious social unrest. History had knocked on the city's door — a city whose people were frightened and divided.

Had I not been right there, driving by the mobs that heckled six-year-old Ruby Bridges, a black first-grader, as she tried to attend the Frantz School, I might have pursued a different life. I had planned until then to enter the profession of psychoanalytic child psychiatry. Instead, I became a "field-worker," learning to talk with children going through their everyday lives amid substantial social and educational stress.[2] In time, I extended the work I was doing in New Orleans to other Southern cities and got involved with the sit-in movement. By 1967, after eight years of Southern work, our family was back in the North, living in a Boston suburb, but I chose to continue being a field-worker. I had learned to talk with children who were not "patients" but had their own difficulties: they were black in a time and place that made that racial heritage a hard one to bear; or, as the children of migrant farm workers and sharecroppers, they were extremely poor and vulnerable; or they were white, yet from families with little money and few social and educational prospects. It was such children whom I sought to meet, to get to know, and later to describe — first in articles for medical, psychiatric, and psychoanalytic journals, and eventually in a series of books for the general public.[3] In the late 1960s and early 1970s I worked in Appalachia, and then in Boston, as it, too, went through a serious school desegregation struggle. By 1973 our family was living in Albuquerque, New Mexico; I got to know Pueblo children and Spanish-speaking children and, in Arizona, Hopi children. I also worked in Alaska, where young Eskimos helped me understand a lot about their lives in small, isolated Arctic communities.[4]

By 1975 we had returned to Boston, where I tried to see American life from the vantage point of the children whose families are most likely to be rather familiar with doctors like me: the well-to-do and well-educated. Actually, I had met these families all along as I did my work — lawyers figure prominently in school desegregation struggles, growers hire and house migrant farm workers, coal mine owners and operators make decisions that deeply affect most Appalachian people, and, in our Western states, agribusiness officials, oil company executives, and big ranchers all exert their authority over Chicanos and Native Americans. The privileged sons and daughters have their own distinctive ways of looking at the world, I soon discovered.

By the late 1970s I had finished my American travels. The five volumes of *Children of Crisis* had been published, and my wife and I were left with many hundreds of children's drawings and paintings, a large collection of tapes, the notebooks we kept, lots of photographs of children, and, not least, memories of the good and not so good days we had as we did our work. I had by then gotten to know Erik H. Erikson rather well: I had studied with him and helped teach the course he gave at Harvard. I also came to know, luckily, Anna Freud, first by correspondence and later through meetings in both the United States and England.[5] Those two veteran child psychoanalysts, both wise, thoughtful human beings, were of enormous help to Jane and me as we tried to make sense of what we'd done and tried as well to figure out where we might next go. In 1978 Anna Freud made a suggestion: "It would be of interest if you went over your earlier work and looked for what you might have missed back then," she said. I remember being somewhat perplexed and amused at the time. I got no leads from her as to what we might discover if we followed her advice; it was her manner as she made the suggestion which was especially persuasive: a mix of wry detachment and warm-spirited interest. Meanwhile, Erik Erikson had been sharing with Jane and me his experiences in South Africa, where he had gone to deliver an address at the University of Cape Town.[6] "You might want to compare what you've seen in the South with what is happening over there," he remarked one day as the three of us were having lunch. Years later, as we worked in South Africa with black and "colored" and white children, we often remembered that moment.

During the last two years of the 1970s and the first half of the 1980s, Jane and our three sons, by then in adolescence, and I conducted interviews in Northern Ireland, Poland, Nicaragua, South Africa, Brazil, and our native New England and nearby Canada. We wanted to learn how children obtain their values, their sense of right and wrong, and we wanted to explore the meaning for them of citizenship. In *The Moral Life of Children* and *The Political Life of Children* we explored those matters. During our regular encounters with children we couldn't help but be impressed with the constant mention of religious matters. Who, after all, can talk with people in Belfast or Warsaw or Managua and not hear about "Prods" and "Papists," about "the Polish Pope," about "the Cardinal" who resists the Sandinistas? The better I knew the children, the more closely I listened to them, the more drawings and paintings of theirs I collected and tried to comprehend, the more evident it became that in many of them religion and nationalism, combined in various and idiosyncratic ways, gave constant shape to their sense of how one might (or ought not) live a life.

Over time, and especially as I was working on the actual writing of both *The Moral Life of Children* and *The Political Life of Children*, I began to remember certain long-ago moments with children: a remark, a picture drawn, a daytime reverie shared, a dream or nightmare reported — all of them in some fashion having a religious or spiritual theme. It was then that Anna Freud's comment came back to mind, and so my wife and I began a review of old transcripts of tapes and hundreds of drawings and paintings. We were surprised indeed, both by what we uncovered and by what we'd managed to avoid examining in all those years. In *A Study of Courage and Fear,* the first volume of *Children of Crisis,* a chapter called "When I Draw the Lord He'll Be a Real Big Man" offered a discussion of how children put their personal life — its assumptions, experiences, possibilities, and constraints — into the drawings and paintings they make. At the very end of the chapter a black Mississippi girl is quoted (after she had drawn a picture of herself) as saying, "That's me, and the Lord made me. When I grow up my momma says I may not like how He made me, but I must always remember that He did it, and it's His idea. So when I draw the Lord He'll be a real big man. He has to be to explain the way things are."

Those words end the chapter. It's a pity, I now realize, that I didn't explore with that girl in 1965 what ideas she held about God, His nature, His purposes, as the daughter of parents who spent long stretches of time fervently praying to God that He "smile" on them. This child knew well how marginal and vulnerable her parents' lives, and their parents' lives, had always been. No wonder, then, the ironic if not sardonic side to her comment about the Lord. How *will* He explain all this, my young friend was wondering, politely but firmly. With any encouragement, I suspect, she'd have gone on to wonder aloud exactly what He had in mind when He made us.[7]

But I never pursued that line of inquiry, never picked up her strong hint. I heard similar hints from other children over the years. Many migrant children, for instance, asked aloud of God when they would stop traveling, when they would find a stable home and school life. Many of the children who lived way up in the hills of eastern Kentucky and West Virginia looked even higher, to the sky, to the Lord they believed to be "up there, somewhere way, way up there," for guidance, of course, but also, as a boy once put it to me, "for a little boost, so we can do better hereabouts." In the midst of that vernacular expression of need, I also heard an outburst of gloom and anger as the boy tried desperately to survive a terrible blow to his community — a mine cave-in, with over two dozen men killed "below," one of them his father: "Why does He sit back and let that happen — and those operators and owners, they won't even apologize, and God must know they won't?" I might have let that boy reflect upon religion, his sense of it — but other interests, psychological and sociological, held my attention then. Chicano children and Native American children, Hopis in particular, also gave me any number of chances, even invitations, to talk about "the land we have here and the One who created it," to quote a Hopi girl in 1973. Among Eskimo youngsters questions about creation, about "the God of the tundra" and His relentlessly fierce "breathing" (the wind that howls across miles of bare and desolate land), offered more invitations. And I did not follow, finally, the leads of the well-to-do children I described in *Privileged Ones,* the fifth volume of *Children of Crisis.* Many of those young people craved not only moral understanding but also, in the words of a boy I described at great length in that book, "a talk about God, what He's like." A shrug of my shoulders (a thought to myself: who will ever know?) and a remark of mine that moved us into quite another realm of discourse — such are the fateful turns in what later gets called "research."

By 1985, as I was finishing the writing of *The Moral Life of Children,* I was more than ready to follow Anna Freud's suggestion: I wanted to look back at research already done and look forward to what might be attempted with it — a study of the religious and spiritual life that children in a number of places, following a number of traditions, will own to having. To start, my wife and I reviewed the work we had done and compiled a long list of those lost opportunities, those hints not pursued. As we looked at old notes, listened to old tapes, we were reminded yet again how even the most unselfconscious and freewheeling conversations can end up being directed when all sorts of avenues of possible exploration are shut off. A black youth I was interviewing with relentless insistence in 1962, the year he pioneered school desegregation in Atlanta, said, "You've been asking me about how it feels, how it feels to be a Negro in that school, but a lot of the time I just don't think about it, and the only time I really do is on Sunday, when I talk to God, and He reminds me of what He went through, and so I've got company for the week, thinking of Him." Another missed chance.

Before I could let children begin to teach me a few lessons, I had to look inward and examine my own assumptions about religion as a psychological phenomenon and as a social and historical force.[8] Trained in the world of psychoanalytic psychiatry and child psychiatry, I had to take up one more time the vexing matter Freud posed so provocatively in *The Future of an Illusion* — how religious practices and beliefs should be regarded. I had been struggling with that question since my medical school days, when I started studying with psychoanalysts while also working in a Catholic Worker soup kitchen and taking courses at Union Theological Seminary. During my psychiatric residency years, during the years of personal psychoanalysis and courses in a psychoanalytic institute, I kept trying to address that same question — and now, about to ask children about God and His nature and purposes, I once more stopped and wondered what in the world I myself felt and thought on that score. In the first chapter of this book I try to come to tentative terms with the question of faith in the light of twentieth-century psychoanalytic knowledge. During my third visit with Anna Freud, I had discussed the question of religion both abstractly and personally. She, of course, had listened carefully. Eventually she had suggested a direction: "Let the children help you with their ideas on the subject." At the time I was rather put off — I thought she was telling me that close attention to boys and girls as they talked about religious issues would bring me closer to the way my own thinking, some of it childish, made use of religious interests. But years later, as I looked back at some of our early talks (which I'd tape-recorded), I realized that she meant precisely what she said; she had in mind no condescension or accusation of psychopathology.

By late 1985 I did start letting a wide range of children help me. This research project took many years to complete; it was pursued in the United States, Central and South America, Europe, the Middle East, and Africa; and it brought me close to three great world religions, Christianity, Islam, and Judaism. It is a project that prompted me to take a careful look at those who live in the secular precincts of my own country and other countries. It is a project that, finally, helped me see children as seekers, as young pilgrims well aware that life is a finite journey and as anxious to make sense of it as those of us who are farther along in the time allotted us.

A reviewer once described the work my wife and sons and I
do as "a cottage industry." At no other time has that description
been more appropriate. For years, when our sons were boys of,
say, six to ten, my wife took them every week to an Episcopal
Sunday school, even though I got weary of (sometimes really
annoyed by) some of the pieties the children brought home.
They got quite immersed in that formal religious life — but one
of our sons, on a Palm Sunday afternoon, made me forever a
fan of such educational experience, because out of it, with wonderful irony, came this considered assertion: "There's religion
and there's the spirit." Whence *that* idea? Our ten-year-old answered, "St. Paul talked about 'the letter and the spirit,' the
difference, and the teacher said you can go to church all the
time and obey every [church] law, and you're not really right in
what you do, you're not spiritual." We asked him how we could
know if we were being spiritual, not just religious, and he
promptly said, "It's up to God to decide, not us."
    Moments like that one gave shape to this work, an investigation
of the ways in which children sift and sort spiritual matters. To
be sure, we talked with a lot of children whose specific religious
customs and beliefs came under discussion; but we also talked
with children whose interest in God, in the supernatural, in the
ultimate meaning of life, in the sacred side of things, was not by
any means mediated by visits to churches, mosques, or synagogues. Some were the sons and daughters of professed agnostics or atheists; others belonged to "religious" families but
asked spiritual questions that were not at all in keeping with the
tenets of their religion. Such children have often echoed the
sentiment my son brought back from his Sunday school teacher;
they have expressed visionary thoughts, thoughts sharply critical
of organized religion. There is a natural overlap between the
moral life and the religious life of children, as is the case with
grownups. There is certainly an overlap for many children between their religious life and their spiritual life — even for young
people who have never set foot in any religious institution or
received any religious instruction whatsoever. "I wonder about
God, who He is, and whether He's just someone who got made
up a long time ago by people — and if He's real, what He thinks
we should be like," a twelve-year-old girl from a Boston suburb
told me. The emphasis in this book is not so much on children

as students or practitioners of this or that religion, but on children as soulful in ways they themselves reveal: young human beings profane as can be one minute, but the next, spiritual.

I could not have done the research that preceded the writing of this book without the generous help of the Lilly Endowment and the Ford Foundation. It was harder by far for me to obtain support for this research than for other work I'd done. From foundation executives I kept hearing, "We are not involved in religion." One foundation executive who wrote those words, a friend, followed them up with a phone call and an earnest, friendly question: "We were wondering what someone like you hopes to do with a subject like that." I have tried in this book to provide a somewhat satisfactory answer.

Thanks go, as in the past, to Peter Davison, a good friend and a vigorous, knowing editor. Thanks go to Jay Woodruff, for continual help in our Harvard office, in the teaching we do together — he is another good, good friend. Thanks go to my wife, Jane, for long ago prodding me to recognize the ideological underpinnings of much secular thought, and for making me aware of a good deal that I chose for a long time not to recognize. She was the one who noticed, early in our Southern work, spiritual interests and yearnings among children not conventionally religious, and she kept challenging me to press on toward the years of research we eventually did.

Our sons, Bob, Danny, and Mike, did yeoman work all over the world — as colleagues. Even as their mother read every interview, looked at and commented on every picture drawn or painted, they sought out children in various countries for talks and thus learned what characterizes the spiritual life of children, both the devout and those who, as Dorothy Day once put it, "reach out to eternity" in their private and often passionate ways. My son Bob, with the help of his friend Ian Helfant, worked in Sweden, Hungary, and Tunisia; and in the United States he talked with a number of Seventh-Day Adventist children (in Tennessee) as well as Catholic, Protestant, and Jewish children in the South. Bob also worked with me and my good friend Bruce Diker in Israel. We were helped by Bruce's intimate knowledge of Israel. My sons Danny and Mike got to know a number of Pakistani children in London, and they also helped me in my work in Nicaragua, where, additionally, a student of mine, James Himes, spent a summer talking with children about their religious and spiritual concerns. Wayne Arnold, another student and in the past a great help in the office, ventured to Japan, where a particular kind of Christianity and some variants of Buddhist and Shinto thinking and belief impressed themselves on him as he talked with children. As the reader will notice, I did not work long enough and closely enough with children of the Buddhist tradition to justify a discussion of them and their faith, though at times when I have talked with Hopi children, or, for that matter, certain children of secular background, those Buddhist and Shinto children have come to mind.

Three final acknowledgments: my parents, who gave me much early encouragement to call on spiritually alert novelists, such as Tolstoy and George Eliot; Perry Miller, who spent his life studying and writing about the New England Puritans, in all their great and sometimes frenzied complexity, and who, as my undergraduate tutor, inspired me to study religious and spiritual matters in spite of the powerful agnosticism I met with in post–World War II medicine and psychoanalysis; and my friend Walker Percy, whose novels and philosophical essays have meant so much to so many readers — his life an enormous gift to all of us.

The
Spiritual
Life
of
Children

※ ※ ※

1

Psychoanalysis and Religion

STILL RELATIVELY UNKNOWN and living in a strongly Catholic city, Freud dared take on belief in God at a meeting in early March 1907 of the Vienna Psychoanalytical Society. He presented a paper with the title "Obsessive Actions and Religious Practices." Most of the observations were clinical; a brilliant physician was fitting instances from his practice into a narrative presentation meant to convey a theoretical point of view. But at the end, when Freud mentioned "the sphere of religious life," a morally argumentative strain began to appear. "Complete backslidings into Sin are more common among pious people than among neurotics" was an incautious generalization even then (despite the inhibitions Freud had noticed among "his" neurotics) and a quaintly unsupportable one now.

When Freud discusses "religious practices," he is intelligent and helpful to the kind of scholar who is interested not in debunking but rather in understanding man's churchgoing history. The "petty ceremonials" of a given religion can, he points out, become tyrannical; they manage to "push aside the underlying thoughts." He suggests that historically various religious "reforms" have been intended to redress "the original balance" — rescue beliefs from arid pietism. But in his concluding paragraphs Freud again makes a sweeping generalization, tries to join an analysis of psychopathology to social criticism: "One might venture to regard obsessional neurosis as a pathological formation of a religion, and to describe that neurosis as an individual religiosity and religion as a universal obsessional neurosis."

This is the kind of naive and gratuitous reductionism we have seen relentlessly pursued these days in the name of psychoanalysis. Freud himself was often more careful. In the well-known essay "Dostoievski and Patricide" he acknowledged the futility of a psychoanalytic "explanation" of a writer's talent, as opposed to any psychological difficulties the writer may happen to share with millions of other human beings. When he risked social and political speculation (in the exchange of letters with Einstein or in *The New Introductory Lectures*), he could be guarded about using his ideas to interpret culture. Sometimes, even when writing about religious matters, as in *Totem and Taboo* or *Moses and Monotheism,* he was frank about being conjectural. His first draft, completed in 1934, of a book on the origins of monotheism was titled *The Man Moses: A Historical Novel.*

But religion clearly excited him to truculence, nowhere more evidently than in *The Future of an Illusion* (1927). He starts out warning himself to be objective, to summon a long-range historical view, to be modest, restrained. Yet he quickly connects religious ideas to man's obvious helplessness in the face of life's mysteries. He then connects *that* condition to the child's predicament — "an infantile prototype." After pointing out that there is no conclusive "proof," in the word's modern scientific sense, of God's existence, he refers to "the fairy tales of religion" and indicates with a rising vehemence that religion is a mere illusion, "derived from human wishes." His tone here is distinctly different from that of his other sociological writing. He contrasts his line of argument ("correct thinking") to another ("lame excuse"). "Ignorance is ignorance," he reminds us, and adds immediately that we have "no right to believe anything can be derived from it." And then: "In other matters [than religion] no sensible person will behave so irresponsibly or rest content with such feeble grounds for his opinions." He declares that "the effect of religious thinking may be likened to that of a narcotic," and that religion, "like the obsessional neurosis" he had described so vividly years earlier, arises "out of the Oedipus complex, out of the relation to the father."

To his credit, he then pulls back and acknowledges that "the pathology of the individual" does not provide a fully accurate analogy to the nature of religious faith, but he is soon referring to faith as "the consolation of religious illusion" and expressing the hope that at some future time, when human beings have been "sensibly brought up," they will not have this "neurosis," will "need no intoxicant to deaden it." Then, at the end, he embraces "our God, Logos," insists yet again that "religion is comparable to a childhood neurosis," and makes an invidious distinction between his stoic adherence to science and the faith of the religious in God: "My illusions are not, like religious ones, incapable of correction. They have not the character of delusion."

Philip Rieff, whose essays and books have been among the most learned and suggestive responses to Freud's writings, has been harsh about *The Future of an Illusion* and the kindred writing that preceded it.[1] Rieff refers to Freud's "genetic disparagements of the religious spirit" and finds his reasoning tautological: "He will admit as religious only feelings of submission and dependence; others are dismissed as intellectual delusions or displacements of the primary infantile sentiment." It is, Rieff says, "scientific name-calling," though in the service of a sincerely held modern rationalism.

Most Freudian psychologists have not challenged Freud's views. But in 1979 Ana-Maria Rizzuto, who teaches at the Psychoanalytic Institute of New England, published a major study of the relation between psychiatry and faith, *The Birth of the Living God*.[2] "The cultural stance of contemporary psychoanalysis," she begins, "is that of Freud: religion is a neurosis based on wishes. Freud has been quoted over and over again without considering his statements in a critical light." Examining her own experience as a psychoanalyst, she finds herself rejecting Freud's assertion that "God really *is* the father"; she also rejects his insistence that religion is a kind of oedipal offshoot — a "sublimation," a means by which erotic and aggressive feelings toward a particular man, the father, are given expression. Such an explanation, she argues, takes an extremely complicated and continuing emotional and intellectual process and "reduces it to a representational fossil, freezing it at one exclusive level of development." And such sublimation, incidentally, denies mothers, grandparents, brothers, and sisters any substantial involvement in the emotional events that affect religious belief. Extremely preoccupied with "the father-son relationship" in his analysis of the psychology of religion, "Freud does not concern himself with religion or God in women." The British psychoanalysts D. W. Winnicott, Charles Rycroft, and Harry Guntrip have obviously influenced the American Rizzuto. Like them, she puts strong emphasis on the texture of "object relations," seeing the mind as constantly responding to and reflecting involvements with a range of human beings, rather than as a battlefield in which certain "agencies" fight things out. She seems especially influenced by Winnicott's revisions of Freud as a result of his work as a pediatrician and child psychoanalyst.[3] He emphasized the significance of early months and years, when babies begin to distinguish themselves — the mother is there, and I am here — and begin to show the distinctively human characteristic of symbolization. The first instance of that lifelong habit is known to most parents — the adoption of those "transitional objects" that mean so much to young children: a part of a blanket, a teddy bear, a doll, a spoon, an article of clothing, and, later on, a song or story or scene. To be sure, even in the nursery, history, culture, and class determine what "materials" are available; but Winnicott's work casts a new light on infants' mental complexity and variability. Anywhere, anytime, infants discover their very own world of word and thought, symbol and memory.

Winnicott did not find that adult ideas or inclinations were similar to a baby's mental stratagems. His point is that, early on, all children learn to carry with themselves ideas and feelings connected to persons, places, and things, and that these mental "representations" attest to nothing less or more than powerful human capacities. It would be foolish to equate a baby's attachment to a part of a blanket with a poet's use of synecdoche or a supplicant's attachment to rosary beads, but there *is* a connection, like the connection between incipient and full-fledged humanity rather than between early and later psychopathology. What such analysts as Winnicott and Rizzuto aim to document is a beginning effort at self-definition through our thoughts and interests, likes and dislikes, fantasies and dreams, affections and involvements.

Dr. Rizzuto calls one of these efforts "God representation," referring to the notion about God that most of us in the West acquire early in life from what we hear at home, at school, in church, in the neighborhood. Even agnostics and atheists, she finds, have had ideas about God, given Him some private form — a mental picture, some words, a sound. In the lives of children God joins company with kings, superheroes, witches, monsters, friends, brothers and sisters, parents, teachers, police, firefighters, and on and on. Dr. Rizzuto offers histories of His presence in the minds of people who firmly call themselves nonbelievers. She points out that God may be rejected, denied, or ridiculed as well as embraced or relied upon, and that each of those psychological attitudes can be connected to the constraints and opportunities (and good luck and bad luck) of a given life. Rather than making categorical judgments and looking for psychopathology, she is writing as a phenomenological psychologist, someone who wants to describe and understand the world.

Freud continually returned to the idea of God; he wrote about His origin in the minds of others, devoted numerous articles and three books to Him. Why? Like Winnicott, Rizzuto sees religious ideas as part of our cultural life, like music, art, literature, or, for that matter, formal intellectual reasoning and scientific speculation. They are all instrumental in helping us to place ourselves in space and time, to figure out where we come from and what we are and where we're going. In a touching statement at the end of her book Rizzuto arrives at the point where her "departure from Freud is inevitable":

> Freud considers God and religion a wishful childish illusion. He wrote asking mankind to renounce it. I must disagree. Reality and illusion are not contradictory terms. Psychic reality — whose depth Freud so brilliantly unveiled — cannot occur without that specifically human transitional space for play and illusion . . . Asking a mature, functioning individual to renounce his God would be like asking Freud to renounce his own creation, psychoanalysis, and the "illusory" promise of what scientific knowledge can do. This is, in fact, the point. Men cannot be men without illusions. The type of illusion we select — science, religion, or something else — reveals our personal history — the transitional space each of us has created between his objects and himself to find a "resting place" to live in.

In Rizzuto's view, it is in the nature of human beings, from early childhood until the last breath, to sift and sort, and to play, first with toys and games and teddy bears and animals, then with ideas and words and images and sounds and notions. We never stop trying to settle upon some satisfying idea of who and what we ourselves are, to build a world that is ours — with blocks or bricks or iron, with money and signatures of ownership, with acts of affirmation and loyalty and affiliation, with outbursts of meanness and rancor, with mental images, and, not least, with theories about how the life we live should go. One wonders, though, how we ought to evaluate the different "illusions" Dr. Rizzuto refers to. The history of science is in large part the demonstration of illusion; and if "reality and illusion are not contradictory terms," they are not identical, either.

In trying to demonstrate the universality of an element of mental function, Dr. Rizzuto claimed perhaps too much of a link between "reality" and "illusion." It seems to me that she did so, actually, because Freud had repeatedly thrown down that either/ or gauntlet — emphasized the polarity between the two — to his readers and followers. What she means she states better when she refers to a "capacity" each of us has "to symbolize, fantasize and create super-human beings"; or when she describes the role that fantasy has in people's lives: a means by which they (meaning, again, every single one of us) "moderate their longings for objects, their fears, their poignant disappointment with their limitations." A baby uses its eyes with the "longings" Dr. Rizzuto mentions, and we adults, babes in the woods of a universe whose enormity and mystery and frustrations are only too obvious, do likewise. The word "theory" is derived from θεωρία, which refers to the act of looking and seeing — what the spectator does at a religious ceremony, or the augur in examining portents, or the soothsayer scanning the sky to figure out what will happen next. Theorists assemble facts to help us look with a little less anguish at enigmas often enough impenetrable: "The objects we so indispensably need are never themselves alone, they combine the mystery of their reality and our fantasy."

What does Dr. Rizzuto mean by that crucial statement? Facts may be stated independently, as in a chemical equation, a physics formula, a finding by a psychologist about rat behavior in a maze, an observation by a psychoanalyst that people who do X have had, to a significant degree, a Y kind of childhood — but the matter cannot be left to rest there. B. F. Skinner takes his behaviorist laboratory findings and uses them to construct stories, to make recommendations on childrearing, to imagine utopias — to suggest how we should live our lives. And Steven Weinberg, in a lovely book, *The First Three Minutes*, uses his work in theoretical physics to give us "a modern view of the origin of the universe." Wonderfully, he starts with an old Norse myth about that origin, yet ends up with his own candid surmise, his own effort to deal with the "uncertainties" he keeps on mentioning. "It is almost irresistible," he tells us, "for humans to believe that we have some special relation to the universe, that human life is not just a more-or-less farcical outcome of a chain of accidents reaching back to the first three minutes." A little later on he observes that "the more the universe seems comprehensible, the more it also seems pointless."

Dr. Rizzuto knows, from her work with children, that they, too, struggle with just such a sense of things, and can be heard saying so again and again. Witches emerge from children's desire to understand life's cruel arbitrariness. It is not necessarily "neurotic" for a child to talk of witches, nor is it necessarily "immature" or, again, "neurotic" for a religious grownup to summon Satan or for Freud to talk of a "primal horde" or a "totem" or of Thanatos — examples of *his* move from fact-finding to the kind of rumination Dr. Rizzuto refers to: an exploratory play of the mind characteristic of all of us, though of course it varies in symbolic complexity and content, and in clarity or pretentiousness. From Plato's *Timaeus* to Professor Weinberg's essay, from Egyptian stories to the modern-day notion of black holes, our cosmological yearnings have found in various facts, or in ancient geometry or contemporary physics, a means for — what? Not illusion, maybe, strictly defined, but a little help in knowing what this life is about. The issue is not, though, a "regressive" tendency; the issue is the nature of our predicament as human beings, young or old — *and* the way our minds deal with that predicament, from the earliest years to the final breath.

That is why it is particularly ironic and dismaying to find both Freudian and Marxist thought so arrogantly abusive when the subject of religion comes up. True, religious thought, like every-thing else, has lent itself to tyranny and exploitation of people. But so has Marxist thought, Freudian thought. The writings of Marx the economist and historian, for all their original clarity, become the futurist "fantasies" of a supposedly (one day) "with-ering" entity called "the dictatorship of the proletariat." The writings of Freud the clinician and historian of lives turn into the "movement" called psychoanalysis, with a few anointed ones, with sectarian argument, with "schools" and splits and expul-sions, with references by analysts themselves to "punitive ortho-doxy." A century that has seen Lenin's mausoleum, pictures of Karl Marx waved before the leaders of the Gulag, Freud fainting in the arms of Jung and postponing for years a trip to Rome, even as he immersed himself in accounts of Hannibal's life and turned heatedly on one colleague after another, cannot be ob-livious to what Dr. Rizzuto has described: among the most bril-liant and decent of individuals, those most determined to explore "reality," one or another fantasy, even illusion, will take deep root.

Both Winnicott and Rizzuto connect our religious thinking to the kind of thinking we do, from the time of childhood to the time of old age, as the aware creatures who hunger for an answer to the well-known question: What is the meaning of life? The history of philosophy and theology is, to a significant degree, the history of proposed answers to that question.

Winnicott and Rizzuto, not to mention the philosophical nov-elist Walker Percy, would add something like this: we are the creatures who recognize ourselves as "adrift" or as "trapped" or as "stranded" or as being in some precarious relationship to this world; and as users of language, we are the ones who not only take in the world's "objects" but build them up in our minds, and use them (through thoughts and fantasies) to keep from feeling alone, and to gain for ourselves a sense of where we came from and where we are and where we're going.

Kierkegaard says that a genius and an apostle are "qualitatively different." The former is pursuing an intellectual or aesthetic inquiry with the greatest distinction. The latter is on an errand: "No genius has an *in order that*; the Apostle has, absolutely and paradoxically, an *in order that*." Here is how Kierkegaard dis-cusses the matter:

That is how the errors of science and learning have confused Christianity. The confusion has spread from learning to the religious discourse, with the result that one not infrequently hears priests, bona fide, in all learned simplicity, prostituting Christianity. They talk in exalted terms of St. Paul's brilliance and profundity, of his beautiful similes and so on — that is mere aestheticism. If St. Paul is to be regarded as a genius, then things look black for him, and only clerical ignorance would ever dream of praising him in terms of aesthetics, because it has no standard, but argues that all is well so long as one says something good about him.

For Kierkegaard, the God of Faith is not available to us through factual analysis or presentation, however gifted the genius making the attempt. For Rizzuto, the "difference" Kierkegaard mentions is not so absolute; we successfully see larger and larger elements of the world (by means of rationality, logic, the work of various "geniuses"); but we also embark on quite other (subjective, existential, teleologically or cosmologically speculative) lines of mental activity. In any event, speaking of "aestheticism," one can imagine the contempt Kierkegaard would feel for some of the stupid talk and dreary banalities that have become the proud property of twentieth-century "psychological man" — a contempt, one suspects, not unlike Philip Rieff's, and perhaps a contempt Freud himself would feel, were he given a chance to take a look at what has happened to his name.

The seventeenth-century physicist and mathematician Blaise Pascal struggled hard and knowingly with the issue of science and religion. Freud's *The Future of an Illusion* can be read as a footnote to Pascal's *Pensées* and *Provincial Letters*. What Pascal made preeminently clear is the difference between, on the one hand, a consideration of humankind and nature (scientific inquiry) and, on the other hand, a consideration of God. Pascal sees the latter inquiry as being accomplished intellectually, through theology, but also through the various mental motions of a life — not just the awareness of prayers or the commitment of energy to rituals of church attendance, but a day-to-day attentiveness (including the fantasies and reveries, the symbolic work, that Rizzuto and Winnicott describe) that touches all spheres of activity. Pascal puts it in this matter-of-fact way: "Those to whom

God has imparted religion by intuition are very fortunate, and justly convinced. But to those who do not have it, we can give it only by reasoning, waiting for God to give them spiritual insight, without which faith is only human, and useless for salvation."

This comment (part of the 282nd *pensée*) is a recognition that for some men and women there comes a point at which the issue is really what Pascal calls "spiritual insight," a quite distinct kind of psychology, put in the service of a particular exertion of love; it could perhaps be called, in Dr. Rizzuto's words, a love for "a living God" — for, that is, a particular "representation" which (Who) rescues us, we fervently hope and pray, from our otherwise absurd condition. Dr. Rizzuto, one suspects, would find Pascal's *Pensées* congenial; they would be, for her, yet additional examples of the kind of rapt and suggestive contemplation she has seen repeatedly in the lives she has studied — lives of particular boys and girls, men and women, who are all on a decidedly perplexing journey and are trying to sort out, as Pascal has tried to do, the various requirements of the head and heart.

On a more personal note, I couldn't even have begun the research that this book describes had I not considered these theoretical issues at some length. I was trained to work with children medically and psychiatrically in the 1950s, at the height of the psychoanalytic orthodoxy that Erik H. Erikson has described in his memorable epilogue to *Childhood and Society*. The people I met in hospitals and clinics were all too often turned into a reductive putty by my mind, which had become quite tamely subservient to an intensely hierarchical structure of authority. Even today I recall with sadness and remorse some of the thoughts I had, the words I used, as I worked with children who had their own moral concerns, their philosophical interests, their religious convictions. I tended to focus on their "psychodynamics" unrelievedly, to the point that they and I became caricatures: the stuff shrewd ironists like Mike Nichols and Elaine May in the late 1950s and Woody Allen in the 1970s would start offering their listeners and viewers.

In particular, I remember a girl of eight whom I treated at the Children's Hospital in Boston for two years, a girl whom I suspect Dr. Rizzuto would have found a helpful colleague in her religious and psychoanalytic explorations. This girl, Connie, was utterly accepting of the Catholic Church. But what Connie lacked, I certainly at the time felt pressure to share — a sharply fault-finding, even disparaging attitude toward the kind of involvement she had with her parish. "The Church saves me," she once told me, and I dutifully wrote down the assertion and, naturally, asked for details: how does it do so, and what is thereby "saved"? She told me, too. She sensed in herself "bad habits," and they were confronted successfully, she claimed, only by prayers in church, by talks with a priest who was a great friend of her parents. When I first heard the expression "bad habits" I had a hunch it was a smokescreen for the sexual feelings I presumed she had and possibly acted upon. As for my supervisor, he wondered about the thin remnant of doubt I still seemed to retain, and said to me, "In a while she will talk with you about her sexual life, and all this religion talk will go away."

I wasn't about to disagree. On the contrary, I kept trying to press for just such an outcome, asking questions and picking up on her comments in such a way as to take both her and me closer to the kind of "resolution" my supervisor had envisioned. Gradually I began to realize that in this child a concrete struggle of viewpoints was taking place. She had been referred to us in the child psychiatry unit at the hospital because she was unruly at school — fresh and surly with certain classmates and then also with a teacher, who called her a "tense girl." A school psychologist had talked with her and suggested she would become "antisocial" or "delinquent" when she got older if she were not "treated" before then. Moreover, during an initial workup, the girl, as mentioned, agreed: she did have "bad habits." Soon, however, the girl was far from willing to convert to our way of regarding her. Not that we spelled out with her what we surmised, had discussed among ourselves. Rather, she took note of the way we kept asking for more information, more "thoughts," while we ignored lots of thoughts she most emphatically did make known to us. Yet, at some moment in therapy, she'd be "ready" — so I hoped, and my supervisors with me — to look at things as we did.

This devoutly Catholic girl had seen a rerun of the movie *Song of Bernadette* with her parents, and wanted very much to talk with me about it — a film about the woman Bernadette of Lourdes, who would ultimately be sanctified by the Catholic Church. I did not, of course, stop Connie from talking about the movie, so full of Catholic piety, but I also evinced no interest in her remarks, at least no interest in their substance. For me, such discussion was essentially "defensive" — a case of a girl hiding behind religious interests as a means of not coming to terms with her sexual impulses and her aggressive ones. But for young Connie the movie was an important event in her life that required reflection, as was the matter of her "bad habits." I thought I was at least being civil, courteous, as I waited her out — listened patiently to both her religious speculations and her religious judgments upon herself. But one day she became forthright with me and critical toward me in a surprising way never before shown. First, she asked me if I was "an atheist or a believer." Astonished, I quickly threw the question back at her (was I not "trained"?), all the while wondering what had been the occasion for a question both personal and by implication negative in tone. When I asked her why she asked, she said, "Because," and then fell silent. I was about to inquire why she had used that conjunctive word in such a solitary fashion when she let me know. Doctor, I was told, you're not interested in my religion, only my "problems." But without my religion I'd be much worse off, don't you see? How about *encouraging* me to talk about that movie, about what I experience when I go to church, instead of sitting there, bored, waiting for God to pass from this conversation? How about trying to learn what I've learned as a child at home, at church, at Sunday school, so that you will be able to respond to *me* rather than to some paradigm, of which my mind and its workings seem to be for you a mere illustrative instance?

I need not add that Connie put the matter in her own blunt, earthy, child's language. Some things she didn't so much say as convey with a look. ("Our patients can tell us everything with a glance, and let us add the words," Anna Freud once observed.) Some she condensed into the skeptical question about my status, atheist or believer. Some she spoke loud and clear: "I'd like to be like Bernadette was in the movie, but you don't believe me!" How well I still recall that moment, both confessional and accusatory in nature! She was dead wrong, actually: I *did* "believe" her — in the sense that I knew she meant what she said, or she *thought* she did. That is, of course, the heart of the matter for me and my psychiatric kind, our conviction that there is an ultimate or bedrock psychological reality to whose depths and contours we are specially privy. Sometimes we have good reason for our claims. But conquistadors (Freud called himself one) have a way of becoming wanton imperialists at times. I wasn't letting Connie tell me about an important part of her life (I would eventually realize) because in my mind and in my manner I was pressing her to hurry up, let me get (with her cooperation) to what was far more important, the "truth" underneath, "disguised" in this child's life by a Catholic fastidiousness that had already broken down in school and put her in our clinic.

Thank God (if I may use so colloquial an expression) for Erik H. Erikson's *Young Man Luther*, which had just come out, and for one of my supervisors who had been analyzed by Erikson. She suggested I read the book, which gave me permission to connect psychoanalysis to religion, as Erikson had done in his biographical effort at understanding part of Luther's life. Even though she was not supervising my work with Connie, I felt free to speculate with her on what was happening with the child, and I received suggestions: Take her religious life seriously, and see where you both go doing so. What have you got to lose? That question, word for word, gave me strength, as did the smile and shrug that came with it. A shrewd and relaxed clinician was telling a novice to ramble a bit, let the path meander.

No miracles (of the secular kind) happened as Connie's therapy progressed, but she did keep coming, and we began to have fairly earnest and extended conversations, some about her "bad habits," some about her interest in Bernadette of Lourdes and other Catholic saints whose lives she had heard celebrated at home and in Sunday school. She told me her "bad habits" were those of "pride." I wondered aloud if she (a mere child of eight!) might explain herself further. Yes, most assuredly: "pride" is "the sin of sins," and it has to do with being "stuck on yourself." I was surprised and intrigued by this way of putting things. Even today, as I look over the notes I took on her (and used when I "presented" her at a "grand rounds"), I am reminded of how idiosyncratic this child was, how thoroughly she had integrated a body of religious imagery and various spiritual assumptions into her young life, her vocabulary. She did not want to become "a religious," she told me one afternoon, and she saw that the word had me puzzled. She explained, first, her use of that word — it is a way some Catholics refer to a person who becomes a priest or a nun. Then she told me why a nunnery would not be suitable for her: she did not want to miss out on a good time in life. Some people, she declared, even children her age, were "more religious than the priests and nuns." I wanted examples. She gave one — in her phrase, a "too nice person." She had already made her break with that ideal. She had spoken a bit freshly to a nun, and at the public elementary school she attended, she was "picture perfect" one day, "a real troublemaker" the next.

All this about Connie, with her help, I now began to understand both psychologically and religiously. She let me know that the rebellious side of Jesus had not escaped her notice, and that in Bernadette of Lourdes and Joan of Arc she admired young Catholic women whose virtues, whose important spiritual lives, were not at all acceptable to established Catholic authorities. Most important, she let me know that her religious life was far more many-sided than I had been prepared to admit — and that there was a personal, *spiritual* life in her that was by no means to be equated with her *religious* life.

It is this evolving distinction I most recall today; its emergence constituted a critical place in my work with Connie and also in the recent research that preceded the writing of this book. I can still hear and see my child analyst supervisor, Dr. Abraham Fineman, going over my notes with me, trying to figure out this bright, troublesome girl who could one minute delight her teachers, the next drive them to distraction. As Dr. Fineman and I went back and forth, commenting on Connie's "ego strengths," noting her "acting out," we tried to hold on to our mission at the hospital — to "treat" a child who could get moody and sullen enough to worry the adults who had referred her to us. Once I was attempting a fairly ambitious psychoanalytic formulation — a discussion of Connie's "narcissism" that omitted mention of the narcissism evident in my very elaborate and self-important presentation. When I had finished, Dr. Fineman asked me what

I thought was the most irrelevant question imaginable: "Do you think she has her own religious ideas?"

I had no idea. I sat there silent. Dr. Fineman went on: Here is a bright child who is intensely involved in Catholicism. She is also having enough psychological trouble — truculence at school and in the neighborhood — to warrant psychiatric treatment (no small step for a working-class, culturally conservative, Irish Catholic family in the late 1950s, I now realize). Now, you are trying to get her to speak our language, to use the psychological words and images we find useful, congenial. She resists you, brings you lots of religious stories, themes, metaphors. You resist her, but she hasn't budged, and here we are trying to calculate how to work with her, how to make inroads on a neurosis, how to win her over, really, to a commitment toward therapy. Why not shift tactics, why not become seriously involved in her religious discussions? Why not let *her* educate *us* about her Church, and also about her? No doubt she would offer us some trite remarks, some memorized clichés — but who doesn't? Psychology can generate them as well as religion. She seems to have her own slant on things, and this defiant individualism seems to influence her religious life — making it *hers,* rather than a mere rote replication of Church truisms. Then Dr. Fineman posed this thought: "She's an *un*conventionally religious child. There's a spirituality at work in her, and we might explore her spiritual psychology."

What in the world did he mean? He saw that question on my face, and he seemed to be asking it of himself. He laughed — a welcome break in our seriousness — and tried to explain to me what was crossing his mind, the essence of which went like this: Look, we're not getting very far with this girl and her family, and perhaps we need a change of tack. He was not arguing for a therapeutic compromise or a surrender. Very important, he was not being condescending to Connie and her family, was not expressing a resigned willingness to put up with *them* and *their* cultural foibles for a while, coupled with a determination somehow to prevail with *our* way of seeing things. Dr. Fineman's attitude was quite different — a truly humble one, I began to realize, and one displayed at a moment in history when such modesty was not exactly common among specialists of our kind.

Decades later I find myself hearing gratefully his exhortation — that "we try to learn from this girl," that "we let her teach us her spiritual psychology." But I still had no idea what he meant by his use of that phrase, and I told him so with a polite question — only to hear that he was as perplexed and uncertain as I was, though obviously far more sure of himself than I, and hence ready for a gamble.

At wits' end, I also gambled — changed direction in my work with this young patient. For the first time in my short-lived, inevitably anxious and striving career as a hospital resident, I told a patient that I wanted some "advice." Today, so many years later, I recall my use of that word. "Connie, it would be a great help to me if you'd let me know how *you* see your life going, and what *you* think we here at the hospital can do to be of help. I really do need your advice — and I've discussed this with a wise, older doctor who has worked with children for many years, and he agrees. He, too, thinks I need your guidance as to how our meetings might be best designed to be of better use to you in whatever difficulties you're now experiencing." I gulp on those words now, as I write them, even as, back then, I'd begun to notice their ingratiating smoothness, their faint air of the patronizing, as I got to use them so often with boys and girls who were far less sure than their parents or teachers that they belonged in a room with the likes of me, and who might easily have responded with a "Huh?" to my overworked declarations of concern.

This young girl listened carefully. She was not impressed, I later realized, with my clinical mannerisms, but she did take note of my reference to my psychoanalytic supervisor. "Oh, you've got someone watching over you, too," she said. I scarcely knew what to do with that comment. I managed a self-conscious smile. As she saw it, and explained it to me, she had her God, and I had my supervisor. I fell silent. She said more — pointed out to me, in a reassuring way, how satisfying it can be to have "someone looking over you." Even now I can feel her words getting to me — and getting at a psychological truth.

Eventually Connie began telling me a lot about her religious life. She also began to share with me some of her private moments of awe and wonder and alarm and apprehension as she sat in church or at Sunday school listening to an imposing nun warn, lecture, promise salvation, threaten the scourges of eternal hell. Within a month or two we were having rather intense conversations, and I was indeed learning a kind of spiritual psychology, as Dr. Fineman had predicted might happen. I learned how a girl felt as she contemplated heaven and how she felt about the possibility of going to hell. I learned about a child's "talks with Jesus," her great devotion to Him, yes, but her anxiety: "I worry that I'm asking for too much of His time." How did *He* feel toward her? Did He have His favorites? If she slipped, made mistakes, did He not only become disappointed but fall into a rage? (Hadn't the nun described Jesus as "very angry" when He threw the money-changers out of the temple?)

What was heaven really like? The nun said, "You spend all your time with Jesus." Doing what? What was the devil like? The nun said, "He gets you and he'll never let go of you" — and the child, in the privacy of her thoughts, felt terror (but also a thrill) at the thought of such lasting possessiveness. Once she asked me, memorably: "How can He have so many people in His grip and never let go even once? I wonder."

These were not concerns easily shared, I realized, and they indicated a trust that had been slow in coming. But those concerns also told me a good deal about not only Connie's spiritual life but her ordinary, everyday one — family troubles that worked their way into her sense of who Jesus was and what she might expect or fear of Him. I stayed on the spiritual side of things, as Connie seemed to wish, but I discussed psychological matters, too. Yes, Jesus could be angry, though He was also forgiving. No, I hadn't the slightest idea how Jesus and the devil ran things in their respective territories, but I doubted that they acted like human beings — doubted that they literally spoke to people or grasped them in some physical way. She listened carefully, and I knew we were at those moments skirting her personal life, her strong bond with her father, her dread of his tantrums. She had turned her father, I knew, into a larger-than-life figure. When she contemplated spiritual questions and larger-than-life spiritual figures, she had difficulties not unlike those she faced at home and at school, as she herself began to recognize — and that recognition, I gradually realized, was therapeutic pay dirt. Her rebelliousness was the result of a fierce attachment to a parent. Her worry that Jesus might overlook her attested to a similar sense of jeopardy.

None of these psychological difficulties are all that unusual and surprising in a child, but I'd never have been able to work with Connie on their nature and consquences had I not learned of them as she talked about her personal way of being a devout Catholic. That way was to be musing, speculative; she dared to wonder, as theologians and philosophers have, about what such words as "heaven" and "hell," "grace" and "damnation," mean in human, practical terms. Of course, those words may not mean anything in such terms. But for Connie it went like this: "Heaven is right here, and so is hell — because we're choosing when we smile or we have that bad look on our face."

At first I tended to be dismissive and cynical. So that's what it all comes to — a big smile or a surly glare! But Dr. Fineman was more interested in the first part of Connie's statement — the earthiness of it, her insistence that the mysterious and speculative be tethered to this concrete life. Moreover, he pointed out, a girl not even a decade old had given herself a demanding daily responsibility — to choose with each move or gesture where she was going. No wonder she could be so sensitive, so quick on the draw emotionally.

In the long run I would learn to be more respectful of Connie's struggles — see her symptoms as evidence not only of conflict but of high aspirations and yearnings sustained by a faithful vision of what might be won, what a loss would mean. We two doctors kept focusing on this child's vigilant, even overbearing conscience as a source of trouble for her. Yet she had tethered this "agency" of the mind (the superego) to an enormous task: "I try to see whether it's God's eyes that are looking at me or that devil's [eyes]." For Dr. Fineman all of this was psychopathology, yes, but also something else — a child's psychological resourcefulness. "Look," he once told me, "she's trying very hard to control that tyrannical judge inside her, and she's enlisted not only parts of her own mind but a religion, and her version of a religion — fairly ingenious. I'm not sure the priests and nuns in her neighborhood would agree with the way she talks about heaven and hell, but she's breathed life into those ideas, her own daily life."

I realize that Dr. Fineman and I, for our own limited purposes, were attempting some second thoughts — much like the case Dr. Rizzuto would make in her book — on Freud's *Future of an Illusion* and, by implication, on an aspect of twentieth-century ideological orthodoxy. Instead of seeing Connie's religious and spiritual life as evidence of a disturbed mind, we tried to let that life be our guide and teacher; and, too, we began to understand how her spiritual life had kept the child together psychologically. "I see Jesus smiling when everyone else is looking real mean, even me," this girl had told me. Dr. Fineman, long a Boston colleague of Dr. Rizzuto's, had anticipated her sense of things when he wrote this in a supervisor's summary: "This girl has begun to settle down in treatment. Her use of her Catholic faith has been both a stumbling block and an opportunity for her doctor and me. We have stopped trying to take on her faith clinically! She has built her own version of that faith, and we have let her tell us all about it, and learned more about her. For her God is quite alive; He's a big part of her life. We're hoping He'll be of further help to her — and us, too."

I have always cherished those words. They gave a young doctor some encouragement, permission, sanction. A few years later, when I was in the South, talking with black children going through mobs to enter newly desegregated schools, I'd think of Connie and Dr. Fineman as I heard girls and boys even younger than Connie talk of God, talk to God, talk as if God were speaking to them, or indeed through them to others. At times I would still shy away from spiritual matters, try to keep those children conversing about familial or school tensions, about this or that city's progress or seeming demise, the result of serious racial turmoil. But at other moments I would listen (with increasing patience and finally respect) to these elementary school children as they let their minds soar to heaven, descend to hell, meet with saints and sinners. "I was all alone, and those [segregationist] people were screaming, and suddenly I saw God smiling, and I smiled," one North Carolina girl of eight told me in 1962. Then she continued, with these astonishing words: "A woman was standing there [near the school door], and she shouted at me,

'Hey, you little nigger, what you smiling at?' I looked right at her face, and I said, 'At God.' Then she looked up at the sky, and then she looked at me, and she didn't call me any more names."

Such a moment reminds all of us, whether our emphasis is sociological or psychological or theological, that even the most private of "illusions" can become part of a decidedly public event, and that barriers of race and class can rapidly yield to certain shared human experiences. The girl who told me of that event was convinced that God had suddenly intervened in the world's reality — even as I wondered out loud about the psychology that was at work in her.

Freud, correctly, found a good deal of the history of religion to have been mean-spirited, hate-filled, and all too ignorantly superstitious. Moreover, he was speaking as a brilliantly argumentative essayist rather than as a clinician when he wrote *The Future of an Illusion* — hence his tendency in that work to favor provocative and unqualified generalizations, in contrast with his use, in much of his clinical writing, of *instances,* his own dreams or those of his patients or anecdotes earned as part of a life's ups and downs. I have wondered what he would have made of Connie; or that black child, Laurie, from Greenville, North Carolina; or, for that matter, the white heckler who was stopped in her tracks by a child who knew exactly how and when to invoke God. Might a girl's devotion to God amidst the socially and politically sanctioned hate of the world around her have moved the great Viennese doctor not to the doors of faith but to a more nuanced sense of what some of us, of whatever age, can manage to do with our convictions?

At his most sardonic and combatively cynical, Freud saw organized religion as the institutionalization of wish-fulfilling fantasy — as a social lie based on the need individuals have for self-deception. Here a great moralist became sweepingly moralistic. Dr. Rizzuto's central argument reminds us that the mind's search for meaning and purpose through fantasy and storytelling, through a faith in received legends, handed down in homes and places of worship, in songs and poems and prayers, is not to be construed necessarily or arbitrarily as a lie or as a form of self-delusion. The issue, as always, is that of context and intention. Novelists spin stories aimed at the penetration (by writer and reader alike) of the many layers of truth, whereas liars spin stories meant to deceive, mislead, trouble, harm. Freud constructed his own story, a story of the human mind, its battles, its protagonists and antagonists, its victories and defeats. When he talked of a "metapsychology" he admitted as much.

Both Drs. Fineman and Rizzuto would declare such an approach as mine with Connie to be still psychoanalytic, and I would agree — it was a psychoanalytic approach toward religious and spiritual thinking (and daydreaming and night dreaming and reveries) rather than a psychoanalytic cross-examination. It is the intent that matters. A psychoanalytic "approach," then, can forsake ideological targets, conceptual ambitions, in favor of a phenomenological acceptance of the immediate, the everyday, the objectively visible and audible — all worthy of respectful attention for their own sake as well as for what they tell about a past subjectivity, one only surmised, one indirectly relayed through dreams and memories remembered. In Connie's words, still part of this listener's active neurochemistry: "The whole big world out there, it's God's worry, and it's mine, I guess, because I belong to Him." What a possessiveness! A possessiveness that joins together Maker and searcher, the divine and external "object" of religious faith with the investigator in each of us who puts in so brief an earthly appearance.

* * *

2

Method

HOW DOES ONE LEARN from children what they think about God and the devil, heaven and hell; learn about their faith and their skepticism with respect to faith? To repeat, I am a clinician, a physician trained in pediatrics and a psychoanalytically informed child psychiatry. I have never formulated or handed out a questionnaire. I have no "survey research" to offer, nor am I interested in making general psychological statements without reference to idiosyncrasies and exceptions. I do, though, rely upon certain assumptions about children — that we as human beings possess awareness or consciousness, and that, through language, we try to understand the world around us and to convey what we have learned to others. I have also assumed that if I talked to enough people who were willing to share thoughts and feelings, express ideas, then I would feel a bit more informed. I stop well short of large-scale generalizations about what does or does not happen to children with respect to their religious and spiritual life. When I tried to learn about the nature of children's moral life and of their political life, I heard the wide range of variation, the astonishing inconsistencies or contradictions in story after story — yet even so, I, the listening physician, anxious to order things, grabbed for conclusions and interpretations, rushed to begin classifying.[1]

There will be time, later, for some inferences and deductions, for a few of those "findings." These days, psychological and sociological statements or "data" are too often offered to us with no warnings about the limits of their usefulness, with no description of how they were obtained, with no context given for what is being handed down as a truth. Often, for instance, we are told, on the basis of questions given to children in a school or a social scientist's office, that young people can or cannot understand one or another line of reasoning. No doubt those claims are true — but what a child may not show comprehension of in a formal, academic setting, in choosing among multiple-choice alternatives, that child may well think about and talk about in his or her own manner and time. We are correctly told about "stages" of "moral development" — children's growing capacity to analyze complex moral issues, sort them out, think about them with resort to various ethical or philosophical points of view. We are told that children show "faith development" as well.[2] Surely, as boys and girls get older, they may well puzzle over religious or spiritual matters in progressively more subtle ways — call upon ideas or information unavailable to them earlier, not usable at eight but quite accessible at eighteen.

Nevertheless, so often our notions of what a child is able to understand are based on the capacity the child has displayed in a structured situation. If the child fails to respond to a researcher's predetermined line of questioning, the researcher is likely to comment on a "developmental" inadequacy. If an older child does respond well, he or she is considered developmentally advanced. The limitations of such an assessment are clear to me when I think of Hopi children who are illiterate, never learned how to take a test (there is such a thing as "test development," too!), and clam up tightly even if approached by an investigator who, anxious to get around "cultural barriers," has a few relaxed, personal meetings with the children before putting them through any tests. Indeed, a well-trained child psychoanalyst, certainly no stranger to the difficulties children have in sharing their ideas as well as their feelings, might find that after weeks or even months a Hopi child still seems relatively mute and impassive.

When I started working with Hopi children, I met them and talked with them in a school, thanks to the friendly willingness of a principal and a teacher to help my work along. After six months, a fairly substantial stretch of time in anyone's research,

I was preparing to forsake the entire project. The children were taciturn. They answered questions — just barely. They obliged my requests that they make pictures, but did not put their hearts into what they drew or painted. This invited in me a (retaliatory?) response: to define, to formulate, to categorize. I noted their distrust, their shyness, their cultural and social isolation, their lack of adequate education.

A Hopi mother, a volunteer at the school, was the one who tersely began to educate me. "The longer you stay here," she said, "the worse it will get." I was surprised, confused; before I could even ask her for an explanation, I felt a surge of anger in me, followed by a response that I suspect was neither original nor rare. I turned on her in my mind, heard myself begin to take her apart psychologically, even morally: she was officious, more than slightly self-important, a chronic busybody. I was all too well equipped by virtue of my life's education to keep my attention focused on the seeming gratuitousness of her hostile comment. Summoning a cool in myself that I didn't really feel, displaying a familiar mask of calm curiosity that belied other feelings, I threw out the predictable: "What do you mean?" Within moments I was hearing about the importance home has for Hopi children. "You see, they won't ever want to talk with you about the private events of their lives in this building. They learn how to read and write here; they learn their arithmetic here, but that is that. You are asking them about thoughts they put aside when they enter this building. The longer you stay here and put them in a position that forces them to appear silent and sullen and stupid, the less they'll be inclined even to answer you. Maybe they think: 'This guy isn't catching on!' "

Another occupational hazard of such work: *noblesse oblige*, if not outright self-delusion. I had been waiting for those (literally) poor children to "catch on," to begin to accommodate themselves to my interests. On a generous day I would use the word "trust." On a day when I felt I was getting nowhere — and badly needed someone, something, to blame — I'd remind myself how "resistant" to "Western values" the Hopis are known to be, how "withdrawn" they are, how "cut off" with respect to our nation's "mainstream values." Hadn't an official at a Bureau of Indian Affairs office used exactly that phrase?

When I went to Hopi homes there was no sudden miracle. But without question the work I did with those children really began only during those home visits. Indeed, within a month or two the children did seem altogether different. They smiled; they initiated conversations; they pointed out to me places that mattered to them; they introduced me to friends and neighbors; and, very important, in their casual and discursive moments — after months of acquaintance, and on home turf, and when I wasn't asking them anything in particular, just standing around idly, sipping Cokes, munching candy bars — they gave me some memorable thoughts that crossed their minds, so memorable that now I recall those children when I find myself saying that I began then to have some fairly solid notions about the spiritual life of children.

Here, for example, is what I eventually heard (in 1975) from a ten-year-old Hopi girl I'd known for almost two years: "The sky watches us and listens to us. It talks to us, and it hopes we are ready to talk back. The sky is where the God of the Anglos lives, a teacher told us. She asked where our God lives. I said, 'I don't know.' I was telling the truth! Our God is the sky, and lives wherever the sky is. Our God is the sun and the moon, too; and our God is our [the Hopi] people, if we remember to stay here [on the consecrated land]. This is where we're supposed to be, and if we leave, we lose God."

Did she explain the above to the teacher?

"No."

"Why?"

"Because — she thinks God is a person. If I'd told her, she'd give us that smile."

"What smile?"

"The smile that says to us, 'You kids are cute, but you're dumb; you're different — and you're all wrong!' "

"Perhaps you could have explained to her what you've just tried to explain to me."

"We tried that a long time ago; our people spoke to the Anglos and told them what we think, but they don't listen to hear *us*; they listen to hear themselves, my dad says, and he hears them all day. [He was a truck driver.] My grandmother says they live to conquer the sky, and we live to pray to it, and you can't explain yourself to people who conquer — just pray for them, too. So we smile and say yes to them all the time, and we pray for them." Her head turned skyward, and suddenly I realized she was beseeching the heavens, so to speak, on behalf of the Anglos of the United States, myself included. Here was a child's intense spirituality on open, unselfconscious display. When her eyes were again ready to meet mine, I was speechless. She had nothing more to say, either. Then she looked upward again and saw an approaching thundercloud. She looked at it attentively and for what struck me as a long time. Few if any Anglo children I knew would stare so protractedly at such a cloud, for all its ominously dramatic qualities. I awaited the end of her fixed gaze, the return earthward of her eyes. When they came back, she took the initiative, lifted her right arm, pointed to the cloud and especially to its thunderhead part — the swollen part on the top, "the home of the noise," she told me. I'd not before thought of noise as having a home. I decided to respond in that way, comment on her way of putting things. She smiled and said, "Noise has a home in us, too." I was waiting for more because, really, I hadn't given her credit for being able to be cryptically sardonic. She had seemed a quiet, aloof girl who never had much to offer during our discussions at school, and now we were standing on the side of a gentle hill near her home, and she was taking "nature" quite seriously and letting me know that we are also part of that "nature," not as outside it as perhaps I thought.

Children's responses to an outside observer will vary not only with the observer's "methodology" but with his or her own shifting work habits, his or her fluctuating moods, and, very important, his or her often changing sense of how to do the work, where to do it, for how long, and with which particular children. Rather obviously, some children are never going to say much, no matter how much time I spend with them and no matter how solicitous of their background and assumptions I learn to be. Other children are not only talkers but storytellers — and animated, voluble ones at that. I don't ask for them; rather, I wait to meet them by chance.

Of course, talk limited to those voluble boys and girls can have its own bias: an absence of just the kind of distilled and concentrated wisdom one quiet Hopi child managed to convey in her self-effacing, almost epigrammatic manner. That same girl,

months after the conversation about the thundercloud, talked
of a Hopi struggle with the Navahos which was then taking place,
a contest for land: "They [the Navahos] want the land, and we
believe it has been here for us, and it would miss us."

I asked how the land could "miss" a group of people.

"Oh," she replied, "the land can feel the difference."

I asked her, "How?"

"The Navahos want to dig and they want to build. The land
will be cut up."

I felt I need go no further in that direction with questions:
she'd made her point. But just as I abandoned our joint train
of thought, she advanced it, this way: "When it is quiet, really
quiet here, we'll all be with God — the Navahos and us, and the
Anglos. The land will be with God, and not with us." Did she
have any idea when that time would come? No, she most certainly
did not. But she was "pretty sure" of this: "Our people are here
to wait until the time comes that no one hurts the land; then we
will be told we've done our job, and we can leave." Again an
upward tilt of her head, as I tried to make sense of the complex
theology that had taken root in a girl barely a decade old, not
especially well educated, and within her school not known by
her teachers as "bright," as someone "good" for me to get to
know — and yet, I would gratefully realize over a couple of years'
time, a girl whose heart beat to Hopi rhythms and whose soul
lay open to an entire landscape.

Prolonged encounters with children are the essence of the
clinical work I learned to do in hospitals and of the work I do
in the homes and schools I visit. Each child becomes an authority,
and all the meetings become occasions for a teacher — the
child — to offer, gradually, a lesson. My job is to listen, of course,
and to record, to look (at the pictures done), and to try to make
sense of what I have heard and seen. My job, also, is to put in
enough time to enable a child like the Hopi girl to have her
say — to reveal a side of herself not easily tapped even by good
schoolteachers. The point, moreover, is that I let the children
know as clearly as possible, and as often as necessary, what it is
I am trying to learn, how they can help me.

Let me offer an only slightly edited version of what I said to a
group of seven boys and girls in a Sunday school class of an

Episcopal church in a Boston suburb, at a time when I was beginning the work that would ultimately make up the heart of this book. After some initial pleasantries, on a gray mid-November Sunday, I began my exposition: "I'd like to ask for your help. I've spent a lot of time — most of my life since I became a doctor — trying to understand what children like you think about a lot of things they go through. I'm interested in what they believe, in what they think is right and what they think is wrong, in how they want to live when they grow up, and where. Lately, I've been interested in what they learn in Sunday schools like this one — what the big lessons are, the important lessons. I've been interested in their thoughts about God, about the Bible, about going to church — for instance, how going to church affects your lives, and what difference, if any, Sunday school makes in your lives."

Suddenly a boy of ten or so raised his hand. I had yet to meet the children individually; I had been given a list of their names and knew their approximate ages (nine to eleven). I still had some sentences to deliver — I was just winding up, really — but nodded to the boy with the right hand waving. "Are you trying to find out if it means anything, going to church?" he asked.

"Yes," I replied, "that's part of what I'm trying to find out."

"Well, it does," he said, "because when you go home you think of Jesus — not all the time, but sometimes. That's the difference."

I didn't know whether to pursue the conversation or stick to my mental sketch of introductory remarks and my plan for a drawing and painting session: each child representing for me his or her notion of what Jesus looked like when He was here on earth. I hadn't even had a chance to mention the particular kind of art class I had hoped to get going. I had just decided to try to get back "on track" when another boy's hand went up: "But what if you *do* remember Jesus when you leave church — is that what you're supposed to do?"

I wasn't sure to whom the question was addressed, but almost immediately I realized that the matter was moot. About to resume my remarks, I heard a girl answer his question, which for her was clearly a challenge as well as a query: "You're supposed to follow Jesus, the way Matthew did, and Mark, and Luke. He's

not here the way He was, but He's here. I mean, when you go
to church, He's there — here — and when you go home, afterwards, He's with you, sort of. Isn't that true?"

The boy who had spoken first now again spoke up: "That's
what I said — you go home after church and you think of Jesus,
and so He's right here now, with you."

"Yes," said the second boy to speak, "but there should be more
to it than thinking of Jesus. My dad says, if you don't try to be
like Him, it's all a joke. That's what he says."

A girl who, I thought, had seemed a bit bored by all of us (she
had been flipping the pages of her Sunday school reader as I
spoke, and she had continued doing so as the others began
sharing their questions and ideas) now spoke up with no effort
to ask for permission first: "That's wrong, to call it a joke, going
to church."

She seemed to want to say more, but the boy whom she had
corrected was now up in arms: "My dad didn't say going to
church is a joke. That's not what I said, either. 'If you're a
Christian, you live like a Christian,' that's what my dad tells us.
When we come home from church — that's when he says that.
He wants us to remember Jesus and remember what we heard
in church, so we'll be better. If you go to church, and then you
come home, and you're just as selfish as you were before you
started out, then that's when it's a joke, like my dad says."

The girl still appeared rather bored. She was now flipping her
book's pages more noisily. She hadn't looked at the rest of us
for more than a second or two. When she had spoken she stared
down at her desk, and her eyes were still fixed on it. There was
a silence. I was about to finish my opening remarks and start
handing out paper, crayons, and paintboxes when the pages
stopped flipping and the girl looked up, first at me, then at the
others, including the boy who had by now become her antagonist.
When she spoke, however, she was looking directly at me, and
she didn't avert her eyes until she'd finished unburdening herself: "It's not fair; it's not fair when people start pointing fingers!
He's saying what his father tells him — so I could say what my
father tells me. He says if you go to church, then God knows,
and that's why you go, so He'll know you're thinking of Him,
and that's what He's asked you to do. So it's not a joke, even

if" — she paused and nodded her head toward the boy but kept her vision directed at me — "even if someone says it is."

With that final phrase she turned her eyes toward the son of that "someone"; he received their riveting attention and returned the favor. We were all stunned, and I was wondering, still, what to say, to do, when the boy replied: "You see, it's just like in the world. My father is a lawyer, and he says people fight over anything! They fight over their religion, too, he says. They say you're right and you're wrong, and they bring Jesus into it. That's not right."

"You're the one who started this," the girl instantly responded. "You're the one who said it's a joke, the way we go to church. You should speak for yourself and not us — not my family. My mother loves church, and so does my dad."

"I was not saying anything against your mother and dad, or you. All I said was what the minister says, that you can't just go to church and think it's the end of it, all you have to do. You have to follow Jesus. Isn't that what He said? Isn't that what the [Sunday school] teacher told us last week? I wasn't trying to be unfriendly. I was just expressing my opinion."

Another boy, hitherto wordless but listening and watching closely, intervened: "You're both right. We all have our opinions. You have yours" — he turned to the boy — "and you have yours" — he turned to the girl. "I have my opinion, too."

He stopped there, and no one seemed to have anything to say. I wondered what his "opinion" was, and was ready to ask — the question would be a way of signaling that we should go ahead full steam, never mind anything else I might have had to say — when the girl toward whom he'd just bent his head said, "Well, what's yours?" Her adversary joined in: "Yes, Carl, tell us."

It occurred to me that one of the children finally had a name in my mind. For a second, no more, I sat and watched Carl. He didn't want to ignore the challenge, I could see by his awakened face, the forward tilt of his head; and he didn't end up being at a loss for words: "It's like with everything else, there are lots of people and lots of opinions. A lot of time, I don't like church. I wish I was with my friends, playing. Some of them don't have to go to church. One of them told me he didn't think Jesus would like going to church."

Carl stopped only for breath, but he had given us great provocation. Three of the children, almost in unison, asked: "How do you know?"

Carl quickly corrected them: "I didn't say 'I know.' I said what a friend of mine thinks. There's a difference. That's the trouble. You guys" — he looked around at everyone in the room — "are more interested in fighting each other. My mother says the Bible is full of fights, and now we're having one, right here, and we're in church; we haven't left yet to go home, and we're disagreeing. You see why I'd rather go playing with my friends — a lot of times, I have — on Sundays?"

We sat and took that in. I found myself remembering my mother telling a much younger me, "We don't always do what we want to do in life. We do what is right, even if it's not always enjoyable." I never did dare ask her that big blockbuster of a word: why? Occasionally Dad would come guardedly to our defense: "I don't know whether going to church should be such a big deal, now, for the boys." We, my brother and I, were then off the hook: my parents would go at it, politely but with rising emotion, at which time we squirmed, because we knew the inevitable outcome — a car ride to church.

My reverie was interrupted. "I feel the same way lots of Sundays," said the girl again. "Last year I told my mom and dad that I get sleepy in church, and I wasn't feeling too good that morning. So, could I stay home? They said yes. I didn't expect them to say yes, but they did. They took my brother and went, and I sat in the kitchen and I wished I'd gone, and I was glad when they came back."

The boy with whom she'd been arguing now made his confessional gesture: "Me too — I still don't like coming all the time, even though this year I've been going. My dad and mother told us they'd never force us to go to church, but they do, sort of. They say we should go and pray, and then we'll come home, and they'll say we should pray on our own, and if we're good, then God will be happy, and that's what we should do."

A child who had yet to utter a sound, a girl with long blond hair, wide brown eyes, and an expressive face, now joined us with a big surprise of a question: "How do you know if God is happy?"

No one said anything. The children started looking at one another, telling through their faces that they were stymied. The stillness persisted long enough for me to become anxious to end it. The question had really intrigued me, and I wanted these voluble, argumentative young people to seize it. Silence, though. Finally I was ready to speak — but not entirely sure what I'd say — when I noticed the concentration on their faces. These children weren't withholding comment out of shyness, apprehension, suspicion, animosity; they were really at work thinking about how to answer that question. And then Carl made a comment (asked a question, really) that had everyone nodding or smiling in agreement: "How *can* you know if God is happy, or if He isn't happy, if He's sad?"

In an instant we all became one. The rifts and schisms, the arguments, gave way to a shared agreement. Carl had been rhetorical in his inquiry, and we all knew why. One by one we said why. One by one we declared our recognition of God's ultimate inscrutability. Carl listened, said "Yup" and "Right" and "Uh huh." When we'd each found our own words, Carl decided to make a summary of what we had concluded: "God knows us, but we don't know Him. Maybe we'll know Him when we die and meet Him; but that's only maybe."

Silence seemed to be an expression of unanimous consent. But suddenly the girl who had got us all going down this road, with her question about how one knows of God's happiness, turned to Carl: "Do you think we will really meet God sometime?"

A substantial pause. I thought to myself: we're about to turn onto a new road. Carl lowered his head and then, rather charmingly, looked up toward the ceiling. I thought right away that he was struggling mightily with a big question indeed. But the children, collectively, had another idea, expressed by the girl who had asked the question. She laughed, as did the others, and said, speaking to no one and to everyone, "See, Carl is asking God for the answer!" A big laugh, and I, the straggler who has finally caught up, joined in.

Carl smiled at this humorous distraction, but did not let his mind stop working on an answer. He took a deep breath and said, "I hope so. It would be great. People *did* meet Him, when He came to the world a long time ago. Maybe He'll come again.

When my dad sees a real bad news program on TV, he says, 'Gee whiz, the only one who can fix this mess is God, and He came here once, and He probably doesn't want to come back!' We are supposed to go meet Him, though — aren't we?"

The girl who had asked the question wasn't satisfied with an answer that was really a version of her question. She asked Carl, "But where would we meet Him? Do you think it'll happen — I mean, do you think you'll meet Him?" She stopped, but her mouth was slightly open and she was leaning forward in her chair, and we could almost feel the tension in her vocal cords until she uttered the concluding question, spoken softly, almost as if an afterthought: "I mean, what would you say — to Him?" Carl shrugged his shoulders but said nothing. No one else spoke. Then the girl hit upon an idea: "What do you think you'd say, doctor?" She had looked right at me, and just in case I had any doubts, she had thrown in that last word.

I didn't know what to say, didn't know what I thought. Uncomfortable that I had ended up in this impasse (who was trying to learn what from whom?), I sat there, looked at the children, and at last heard myself say, "I guess I'd start by saying hello."

The children laughed, and I figured I'd stalled successfully. I wanted to throw the matter right back at them: had I not made my stab? But Carl was too smart for me; politely but firmly he asked: "Then, what would you say?"

I told the truth: I said I hadn't ever given thought to such a moment and I didn't know what I'd say — and then I added, a bit desperately, "Maybe God would say something, and then we'd get going with a friendly talk."

Whatever the introspective thoughts that raced through my mind, the children quickly took over with an outpouring of imaginative constructions of such a conversation, at least their side of it. One of the boys announced that he'd confess all his wrongdoings and hope for forgiveness. One of the girls insisted that God already knows the mistakes we make, the bad moments in our lives, so there would be no point wasting His time with recitations in that vein. Another boy pointed out that God in the form of Jesus liked company, such as His disciples — liked to eat and drink with them, so perhaps the encounter would be over a table and over food. Another girl mused about the menu, at which point there was a mild general uproar, the gist of which was described by Carl (still the only one whose name I knew, an hour or so into this important phase of my research project): "We're getting silly, no?" But he had a quick afterthought: "I wonder whether God needs to eat or drink. I once asked my mom some question like that, and she sure looked at me funny. 'Now what made you think of that?' That's what she said. I said: 'I dunno.' She never answered my question! She put on her car radio."

There were more flights of fancy. Here were children who could conjure up in their own way the mystery of God's relationship to us, His creatures. But here, also, were children who felt constrained by the awesome responsibility of putting themselves in, so to speak, the Lord's shoes. One of the girls, the least talkative, spoke for the others: "No one has said anything about what God would think of us, say to us. We're all trying to tell Him something, but what would we hear from Him? I wonder what His voice would sound like. No one knows, I guess. Do you think He knows all the languages, so He can understand everyone and talk with everyone? He must!"

Immediately the children argued about that. A boy said it was ridiculous of us to try to second-guess God by putting words (or language) in His mouth. Another boy took issue and pointed out that God had spoken to Moses and that Jesus certainly talked to His fellow Jews "a long time ago" and so knew at least one language, a version of Hebrew. Hadn't they discussed precisely that in Sunday school a few weeks earlier? Yes, but "it wasn't Hebrew," a girl insisted; it was "some other language." No one could remember the word Aramaic, but the room was utterly still as they searched for it and also, I began to realize, imagined Jesus speaking it.

"I wouldn't be able to talk," Carl commented. He explained: "I'd be dizzy, maybe. I'd feel stupid — that anything I could say would be plain dumb."

"No," said a girl who had disagreed with him several times already. "He doesn't want us to feel stupid because of Him, so you wouldn't."

"Yes, I would," Carl reiterated, and then he added, "Hey, He'd be pretty surprised at us if we were just some 'cool cats' who weren't knocked over flat by Him being here — there — with us! Don't you think?"

"What do you mean by 'here' or 'there'?" the same girl asked Carl.

He answered in a bored, cryptic manner: "Beats me."

I was especially intrigued at that moment, about the looming conjecture regarding the geography of God's presence in our spiritual lives. But the children showed no evident interest in pursuing the question any further, and though I might have stirred things up with a question or comment, I did not. Parents had begun to accumulate outside the door, and the church bell fifteen minutes earlier had struck the hour that was to mark an end to our meeting. Soon we were standing, saying goodbye.

I present this early effort to understand spirituality in children because back then, preparing for the meeting, I did not know whether it would ever get off the ground. I was exploring something called a "research project." I was trying to figure out what social scientists (and foundation officers!) often called a "methodology." Long before, I'd learned from my wife that a good way to initiate such research is to sit down with children, tell them what you want to learn, and then hope that they will become colleagues, instructors, guides. When I left the meeting I had my tapes, with their "data," I had my notes, but most of all I had a sharp memory of a vivid experience, and a sense, now, that this idea had started having a life during the time we had spent in that room. I knew there would be more meetings, both with those children and with others in various settings around the world. One of the departing children had initiated an important exchange: "You didn't ask us to draw pictures."

"I know. I'm sorry . . . we got so caught up in our talk, didn't we!"

"Yes!"

"Would you want to do some drawing or painting next time?"

"Sure."

"I'll remember to bring the crayons and the paintboxes."

"Okay."

The heart of the research — the heart of this book — consists of such conversations, dozens and dozens of them, held in this country and in other countries, with Christian children, Islamic children, Jewish children, and children less interested in religion as such than in the kind of spiritual rumination many of us have had, regardless of our agnostic or even atheistic inclinations. The heart of the research, of this book, is tape-recorded meetings with individual children and with groups of children, worked into the various narratives that make up chapters; and children's drawings and paintings, done at my suggestion or at their own initiative, in an effort to portray God, Biblical figures, or a child's visual sense of the sacred or the profane.[3]

The children have been old enough to be in elementary school and young enough not to have entered high school (I speak here in the American vernacular). Most of the boys and girls have ranged in age from eight to twelve; a few have been as young as six or as old as thirteen. I have traveled far and wide, trying to learn from Protestant and Catholic children in North and South America and in Europe; from Jewish children in North America, Europe, and the Middle East; from Islamic children in Europe, Africa, and the Middle East. All in all, those who have worked with me and I myself have interviewed over five hundred children, some only once or twice, most at least five times, and many (more than a hundred) well over twenty-five times. It is the children who belong to that last group who have been the most patient and encouraging of our teachers.

After working with a child for a year or two, one knows enough to see the connections between a religious or spiritual life and other aspects of his or her day-to-day existence. "God is here and lives in all we do," Dorothy Day said, in one of her more hopeful assertions. An eight-year-old Jewish girl who lives just outside Boston told me, when I was trying to get my bearings in this research effort, that she could "feel Him nearby a lot of times," and that she hoped He'd stay near until "He's so close I can hear Him," at which point, she indicated, she'd no longer be here, alive. To learn of such a child's sense of spiritual connectedness and continuity, one has to put in, rather often, months or years of time.

As previously, I have talked with parents and teachers, too — but much less so than in the past, because more than ever before I have wanted to learn from young people that exquisitely private sense of things that nurtures their spirituality. "My thoughts, you mean, when they suddenly come to me, about God and the world and what it's all about — my really strange ones [thoughts], they are, lots of times," a Protestant boy in Westford, Massachusetts, told me a couple of hours after Sunday school was out. With those words — uttered only after seven months of weekly visits — I was reminded that so-called longitudinal research, for all its slowness, has its own rewards. "Stay with your patients long enough, through thick and thin, and you'll learn a hell of a lot more than you ever expected," Dr. William Carlos Williams said to me.[4] As that remark suggests, he could regard those patients as teachers, too.

I have tried to follow Dr. Williams's lead — tried to "stay with" a number of children long enough to earn their trust, and then tried to learn from them. The longer I have been at this research, the more I realize how much there is to recover from our Sunday school and Hebrew school past, from our nine-year-old or ten-year-old life, when the mysteries of the Bible or the Koran lived hard by the mysteries of childhood itself. The questions Tolstoy asked, and Gauguin in, say, his great Tahiti triptych, completed just before he died ("Where Do We Come From? What Are We? Where Are We Going?"), are the eternal questions children ask more intensely, unremittingly, and subtly than we sometimes imagine.

I have attempted to hear out children of various national, religious, and cultural backgrounds so that they might give us some idea of what the universal questions have meant to them, in all their diversity, as they begin their second decade on this earth. I thank the many teachers, priests, ministers, rabbis, Islamic parents, the world over, who enabled me and my wife, my sons, and my young colleagues to talk with so many boys and girls. Yet the week-to-week talks with children who live in my own comfortable hometown of Concord and those who live in the nearby city of Lawrence, where poor and working-class families predominate, were a foundation of this research.

I repeat: I am not interested in regarding the religious and spiritual reflections of children as collective evidence of childhood psychopathology. To be sure, children who are in psychological distress can use religion in ways that serve the purposes of a neurosis or a psychosis. I particularly remember a young patient of mine, schizophrenic at ten, who was convinced, beyond all persuasion to the contrary, that Jesus had sent him on a special errand to his hometown of Sudbury, Massachusetts. The boy's protestations uncannily echoed those of certain Christian saints and martyrs: "Jesus lives in me," he'd tell the nurses. This boy's intense and increasingly morbid preoccupation with Christ's voice qualified him for a prolonged stay in a mental hospital ward reserved for suicidal young people. I winced sometimes when the boy called me "an atheist who only pretends to be a believer."

That boy, a fragile patient, is not to be confused with children who are quite solid and sound psychologically, but who can become so immersed in religious or spiritual matters that a remark taken out of the context of their lives would sound very much like his. "I'm trying to let Jesus be my master, my complete master," another boy, also ten, told me a year into my research. By then, I knew him well, and knew how sincere, untroubled, and stable he was. He was as caught up in some of his regular school subjects as he was in his Sunday school lessons. "I think of Lincoln a lot," he once told me, with a moral passion that I found appealing. So it was, too, with his mention of Jesus. Without question both Jesus and Lincoln were called in as reinforcements because the boy, approaching the years of adolescent skepticism, was unwittingly having some second thoughts about his father and mother.

Even as this is not an exercise in psychiatric diagnosis or attribution, it is not, again, an attempt to impose a linear theory of cumulative cognitive awareness on the children interviewed, to examine their "faith development," an offshoot in recent years of what gets called "moral development." I have struggled to explain in *The Moral Life of Children* the limits of this kind of work, and what I said there surely applies here: a clinician's conversations with particular children are not to be confused with research done through questionnaires or by asking children to respond to a structured series of statements. I have no doubt that psychiatric interpretations of much that children say about religious and spiritual matters can, in a sensitive doctor's hands, be of great interest; and I have no doubt that a cognitively based analysis of the manner in which the moral and religious and spiritual thinking of children changes over time can also be of great interest. Do I risk pomposity when I describe this work as phenomenological and existential rather than geared toward psychopathology, or toward the abstractions that go with "stage theory," with "levels" of "development"?

To be sure, as a psychiatrist I have tried to explore the range of both feeling and thinking in the children I have met. I have watched for the bizarre, the "crazy," the psychologically worrisome or morbid. I have also watched for certain themes and trends, taken into account the variables that developmental theorists emphasize: age, social background, sex, race, nationality. But the major thrust of this book is narrative rather than abstract and analytic, consisting of the telling of religious and spiritual experiences in all their "blooming buzzing confusion," to quote William James. I do indeed try to make sense of such experience by examining the children's remarks, my response to their remarks, their pictures, my response to those drawings and paintings. But I don't move massively to the kind of formulations, the theoretical emphasis, that many social scientists and psychiatrists find so welcome.

As I remember times spent with children who have made clear what they hold dear about a given religion, or what they hold dear and sacred about life as they have come to know it, I think of novelists, of James Agee and his earlier self in *A Death in the Family,* of Charles Dickens's young Pip in *Great Expectations* or of *David Copperfield,* of Henry James's child in "What Maisie Knew" — children who, as they struggle to figure out the world, show the complex, ironic, inconsistent, contradictory nature of human character, and, too, of faith and doubt. Obviously, this book is one person's representation of what many young people have tried to convey — my story of the stories they kindly gave me. Others, too, might enjoy walking this road, one that has been somewhat neglected, even shunned, by any number of us who are significantly secularistic and scientific in our education. From such others we would, surely, learn more of what it means to be a human being, possessed of language and consciousness. And from the religious we might well learn what a great Teacher said of the spiritual life: "Suffer little children to come unto me, and forbid them not; for of such is the kingdom of God."

3

The Face of God

"I'LL DRAW HIS FACE" — that is a refrain I've heard spoken in many languages by children of Christian denominations and by those who deny any religious persuasion. In contrast, of course, Jewish and Islamic youngsters have been quick to remind me that the Jehovah summoned by the Hebrew prophets is not to be pictured, nor is Allah or his prophet, Mohammed. For certain Jewish children, in Israel and in the United States, this distinction has been an occasion for extensive further discussion. "Of course Christians will draw a picture of God; they see His picture all the time in their churches," a Jewish boy of ten told me.[1] "Our God hasn't come here. He has spoken to us, but He's not appeared." So his father had told him.

If I may be statistical: I have accumulated 293 pictures of God; all but 38 are pictures of His face, with maybe a neck, some shoulders, but no torso, arms, or legs. These are pictures made in response to my request for "a picture of God." When I ask for more, encourage children to go beyond the face, most of them oblige, though I have 53 drawings done by children who had no interest in going beyond His face despite my suggestion.

In Lawrence, Massachusetts, a nine-year-old fourth-grader had taken great care to draw "God's face" (not, she emphasized, "the face of Jesus"). I was sitting nearby in a classroom and looking at some pictures done earlier by sixth-graders. "Would you want to go beyond the face?" I asked her. There was a pause, and no response, so I spelled out the question: "Would you want to draw the body?" "No." Another pause, and then: "I don't think of God, except for His face; I mean, when I picture Him, it's His face." Even children who have pictured Jesus as a man and have seen Him pictured — walking, talking, eating with His friends and followers — are often reluctant to go beyond the representation of God's face.

In that same classroom another girl explained her considerable hesitation: "When God came here, He looked like a man; He was Jesus. But then He went back to being God, and I don't know what He looks like now, but you have to have a face!" She proceeded to give Him one: a big circle first, then much flowing wavy hair, then a neck — at which point she abruptly stopped. I noticed that she was scratching her own neck. When she stopped, she smoothed down her slightly disheveled light brown hair, at one point running her right hand through it. She put the hand on her desk. She kept her left hand on the drawing paper. She had put the orange crayon down after finishing the neck, and now her right hand moved toward the crayon and picked it up. Her eyes, though, were focused intently on the paper with its orange circle, the beginning of a face, and the brown lines that were meant to signify hair. Suddenly, out loud, she offered these ruminations to me, seated at a desk across the aisle: "It's a guess. I don't know if I'm on the right track. I'm not sure I should finish." Her eyes left the paper to gaze at me. I was silent for a few seconds. Thoughts crossed my mind: This has happened before and will happen again. Some children get right down to business and in no time render a portrait of God, of Jesus. Others are far less forthcoming — as if awe, even fear, descends upon them for a moment. This girl, Betsy, belongs to the second group. And then I spoke, to help move things along: "It *is* a guess. There's no correct answer — only you and me with our paper and crayons." Her head turned, her eyes took in my desk, my work, not easily visible because I was sitting at a steep angle to the rear. She resumed right away, perhaps grateful for another would-be artist's shared tentativeness. "I'll just do what I do," she said softly, almost to herself, well after she had begun doing exactly that. Soon she was giving the face eyes, a mouth, a nose. Next, she made ears, then supplied eyebrows. They seemed to prompt her to add a substantial beard.

For a while, the beard completed, Betsy sat and looked at the picture she had done, then at the crayons spread before her on the old desk, weathered by age and inscribed with scratches, ink spots, an initial or two. Once or twice she looked out the window, not toward the street but straight across a park toward a distant horizon of trees and buildings. She also looked upward and commented on what she saw: "The clouds are coming. It may rain before school is out."

"Yes, I heard the weatherman predict rain this morning."

"So did I." Silence for five seconds or so, then this question: "Do you think God gets rained on?"

"I don't know."

"What do you think, though?"

I shifted position in my chair before I said anything. I heard myself telling her that a boy had asked me the same question a couple of months earlier.

"What did you tell him?"

A tone of self-righteousness informed my rejoinder: "That I didn't know."

She was not as deterred as I had hoped she might be. She looked me right in the eye and asked me, "But you can guess, can't you?"

I noted that once again I'd shifted my weight in the chair. "Yes." In my head I heard a voice saying: Why not share your speculations with her, give her an answer, whatever comes to mind? But I honestly didn't know how to answer the question. "It beats me, Betsy, how to answer the question. I just don't know what to say. What do you think?"

The girl responded immediately. "I think He gets rained on a lot. Just because it's heaven doesn't mean there's no rain. Now, what do you think?"

"I know that when Jesus lived here He went through rainy days. I'm not able to imagine what the weather is like in heaven."

She seemed satisfied that I had in some way joined her in a speculative conversation — had not, as has sometimes been the case, held myself resolutely aloof through a relentless one-sided inquiry calculated to fathom her thoughts and hunches, her daydreams, her memories of a Catholic Sunday school education. She then turned a bit didactic. "God is with us, like He was with Jesus, and so He knows if it's raining or not, and He must feel the rain, or He couldn't know everything that's happening, and He does." A second's silence, an intake of breath: "If you don't think He's with us, then you're not sure about Him. That's when you should pray." At that point she decided, much to my relief, to resume her drawing. She seemed to know that I really didn't want her to say more. Out of kindness to me, perhaps, she shifted both of us to more concrete considerations: "I think I'll give Him a smile. He seems too serious."

Foolishly (greedily) I couldn't resist asking, "Do you think He has different moods?"

She flashed me a look of initial surprise, followed by impatience, conveyed in her tone of voice: "Well, if we do, He must, too."

"I don't follow you, Betsy."

She was quick to expand on her line of reasoning. She was, again, both forthcoming and instructive. "If God knows you, He knows of your good days and your bad days. Granny says she has both, and she's sure God watches her all the time. It may be tiring, a little, but He's God."

I could not resist blurting out, "Does God get tired?"

Betsy responded quickly and with animation. "Maybe He does; or maybe He doesn't — because He's God, so He can't get tired."

"What if God wanted to get tired?" I had by then decided that Betsy could take care of herself as well as me and my perplexed mind. Why, though, was I pushing our discussion without apparent let-up?

But there was no more time for such an arraignment. Betsy smiled and with a cheerful voice explained, "Well, if He wanted to [get tired], I'm sure He could." Then, after a second of reflection: "But why would He want to get tired?"

I was feeling a bit weary myself at this point. I smiled and remained silent, and she got the point. She returned to her drawing, decided to color the eyes, made them partially blue and partially brown — and as if to head off any question, she remarked, "I have blue eyes, but my sister has brown eyes, and God should have eyes like everyone." My mind traveled to a school on the outskirts of Stockholm, where a boy of ten had announced that when he tried to represent either Jesus or His father, he wouldn't use any of the crayons or paints offered to him: "The Lord is everyone's, so He's not white and He's not brown or black. He's all the skin colors and the eye colors. It's hard to imagine Him; that's why I'll just use a pencil." Betsy had some second thoughts of her own; she began adding some yellow and black to the brown beard she had done: "Probably He has all the colors of hair, just like with the eyes."

Often children give God their own hair color; indeed, a blond Lord, a blond Jesus, give way to darker divinities as one moves from Sweden to Hungary and Italy, thence across the Mediterranean to Israel, where a few Christian children live. The same thing happens with the eyes — a preponderance of blue eyes in the drawings of Swedish children yields southward to brown and dark eyes. In North and South America a similar pattern holds. Moreover, children themselves may be quick to notice such color-based distinctions and mention their significance. Several weeks after Betsy and I had the meeting just described, she and three others sat with me and looked at, one by one, a stack of drawings and paintings, each of them a rendering of God's face or the face of Jesus. Early on, Betsy remarked on the variations in hair and eye color, and pointedly said to Hal, a ten-year-old boy who had brown hair and blue eyes, that he was giving his own features to the drawings he did.

Hal was not reluctant to admit his action. "No one has ever seen God, not before you die. So how can you know? He probably looks different a lot of the time — I mean, you see Him your way, and maybe the next person sees Him some other way. My mum says He's a shadow — He looks like that, a shadow."

"But if He's a shadow," Betsy replied, "that means he's gray, and so how can He have blond hair, and His eyes be blue — He can't."

"Well, He *can*," Hal insisted, adding tersely, "He can do what He wants."

"You mean," Betsy asked, "He can change the way He looks?"

"Sure thing He can," Hal replied confidently. To expand upon his assertion, he pointed to a stack of drawings on the table in the small, comfortably furnished teachers' room where we were sitting. "There's no correct answer — they're all right. You [Betsy] see God, and I see Him, and He's how He looks to you and how He looks to me, He's both. I asked the priest, and he said so."

"But is the priest sure?" Betsy asked, half out of genuine interest, half rhetorically.

"He can't be sure, not a hundred percent," another boy, Larry, pointed out. No one disagreed. Dark-haired, with wide brown eyes, of Spanish-speaking background, Larry was eleven and tended to be taciturn, though not that morning. A Catholic, he was the most outspoken critic in that room of his own Church: "The priests here [in Lawrence] treat us [Spanish-speaking immigrants from Puerto Rico and various other Caribbean islands] like we're not as good as they are, their people. To them, Jesus must be Irish! They'd tell you — they'd draw Him as if He has the same color hair they have, the same eyes. The priests just guess, the same as we do! My father says the priests can make big mistakes. How God looks — it's up to me to draw, and everyone can do it, and the priest shouldn't be the teacher and give you the grade. He should just pray for you."

This youth, I knew, was bringing to our conversation the spirit of a neighborhood's racial struggles. Newcomers felt grievously ignored or scorned by those running the city (school officials, business leaders). A certain populism took aim at the Roman Catholic Church as an object of social and political criticism. Larry had not forgotten what his father, especially, had said on numerous occasions: "The priest will bend his ears to the sound of coins."

"If I drew a priest's face," Larry offered, driving his point closer to our topic of conversation during the school period immediately preceding lunch, "I'd have his ears plenty big."

"But God's ears must be big, too," Hal insisted. "He hears everything we say."

It was at this point that nine-year-old Maria, like Larry of Spanish-speaking background, entered the discourse with a cautionary note: "His ears could be powerful, even if they didn't seem any bigger [than anyone else's ears]. Maybe He doesn't even have ears — or eyes, or anything. Maybe He doesn't look like us. Maybe He looks way different."

(A week or so earlier, Maria had been quite willing to sketch, in pencil, a picture of Moses and the two tablets he received with their Commandments; and she had drawn a rather stylized picture of Jesus, also with a pencil rather than the available crayons or paints. But God was a different matter altogether: "Jesus visited the earth, and people saw Him. He was here. God, no one has ever got even a peek of Him! The nun told us to think of Him as a voice, not a person with a body. My mom, she says He talks, definitely, but you can't think He has arms and legs, and He doesn't eat and drink; He's different, so that's why I can't draw Him.")

"Even so, even if He's different," Betsy promptly insisted, "you can guess. That's what you do, you guess. We don't know what Jesus looked like, either. They didn't have television then, and there were no movies, and you had no cameras, either, so we guess when we think of Him — what He looked like. You close your eyes, and pray you'll see right. The teacher [in Sunday school] told us that's what to do. She said, if you have faith, you'll 'receive' Him. She said He'll just come to you with His words, and what He wants you to do, and you'll see Him, you can, sometimes. I mean, you won't actually see Him, but you'll try to, and if you're really sincere, then He'll be there for you, and whatever way you see Him, it'll be Him, it will be."

She had put a lot of herself in that statement. Most children who draw God's face more than once, or that of Jesus, repeat more or less the same thing again and again — the same proportion to the features, the same use of colors, the same overall shape. Not Betsy. She once colored God's face brown and told me that if she were black, as some of her classmates are, she'd want to draw God's face that way "all the time." But a second thought took this expressive form: "I'd want to make Him white some of the time, because He's white as well as black. Don't you think?" To that question I answered yes.

Betsy was prepared to let the God she was beginning to know be elusive, changeable, multicolored. In her religious drawings she could be imaginative and playful, but she avoided sentiment or self-indulgence. In truth, she was responding to her family's religious life: "Daddy said each person can have a visit from God. He'll be smiling, or He'll be sad — it's up to you, because it's you He's visiting." Hence in a series of faces she showed God smiling, frowning, light-skinned, dark-skinned, though mostly

He did respond to her genes, her background, a natural consequence, she reminded me several times, of *His* nature: an
accommodation, of sorts, to each person.

In the same city of Lawrence, the same (Henry K. Oliver)
school, a black girl of twelve, Martha, was concerned about more
than racial significance as she drew and talked about her notion
of God: "I'll try to picture His face, and I hope I get it right.
He might be black; He might be white. I don't care. All I know
is He must be disgusted with the bad people He let come down
here. He must have wanted to get rid of a lot of trash. I heard
on the TV about 'the environment,' all the trouble; well, there's
folks here who are trash, never mind what they'll be doing with
their garbage. When I think of what God looks like, He'll be
shouting and cursing His head off, or He'll be crying, because
of all these no-good folks."

That said, she put some tears on the long, brown-faced God
she had drawn. Then she ran a black crayon over them, leaving
the face defaced, as it were. The ears were quite small, the nose
mere dots, the mouth wide open, baring teeth. But the eyes ruled
the portrait, big and black, their visibility accentuated by the
thick brows placed over them. This was a God who missed nothing and was not at all pleased with what was taking place on this
planet. Interestingly, as an artist who had definite opinions about
what to emphasize in the divine face, Martha was not without
her moments of doubt, even skepticism; "I was going to give
Him some hair, but maybe He doesn't have any. Who says He
has to look like us? Maybe He doesn't look like us at all! Maybe
there's no face to Him! Maybe He's all eyes! He must keep track
of us, and how could He do it but through looking? Beats me!
Maybe He doesn't care, until He decides on that [judgment] day.
My uncle will stand up [in church] and say we're all going to get
it, get it bad, when we go before Him, but some are worse than
others. Some are pretty good folks. God must know what He'll
do!"

She wrote a message under her picture: "Watch Out, He'll
Spot You!" Retaining her faith in the visual side of the Lord's
judgmental procedure, she was connecting her drawing to her
uncle's fiercely admonishing participation in a neighborhood
evangelical church attended by poor black families. She had

several times told me about what happened during those long, heated Sunday services, about her fearfulness when older men and women (among them her uncle and her grandmother) seemed on the verge of losing control as they shouted warnings, appeals, lamentations, denunciations. She tried not to hear, but she remembered all too well certain phrases, and much to her alarm, they worked their way into her dreams. She woke up in a cold sweat, her legs "shaking," her head hurting, her stomach in pain. "After one [dream] I thought I was dying," she explained, "and I was scared for a little while, but all of a sudden I stopped being scared." She explained why quietly, briefly: "I remembered God."

She herself had brought up a subject that interested me a great deal, as Martha and the others in her sixth-grade class knew. After an awkward silence (I was trying to figure out what to say and was intent on not being intrusive, even though I wanted to hear more about Martha's dream), she spoke about the God that was remembered: "I think I saw Him, but maybe I just felt Him. When I woke up, I thought of a face with a smile, but I don't know whose face it was. I couldn't draw it. [I had asked.] With God nearby, I stopped being so scared. My gramma used to tell me that when you need God, He'll show up; He'll come and touch you, and you'll be all right afterwards. I'd ask her what He'd look like, and she'd say He doesn't look like anyone; He's a spirit. But they have pictures of Him in church, I knew that. She'd say: 'Child, those are pictures of Jesus, when He visited here with us. But when He left, He stopped being like that; He became a spirit, too.' I guess I was remembering my gramma and what she said while I was having that dream, and maybe that's why I felt better, or maybe, like she said, God looked down on me and He touched me, and I was OK after that. Even if He's a spirit, you can see Him, I think. When I woke up and was scared — I pictured His face: the big eyes and a smile. *He* wasn't scared, so I decided I shouldn't be either."

The phrase "I pictured His face" is one I have heard in schools and in homes all over the world. It is a phrase associated not only with an emotional rescue of sorts, as happened to Martha early one morning, but with a range of other psychological experiences — with times of accomplishment as well as those of jeopardy or alarm. A twelve-year-old, Mark, the son of devout Seventh-Day Adventists living near Chattanooga, Tennessee, talked with my son and me about his already impressive athletic career — he had a formidable record as a runner in local competitions. He looked ahead to further achievements both in school and on the track. He also made sure that we understood his notion of the sources of his energy: "I want to do the best I can, but I won't be able to unless God is with me all the way."

My son Bob, a medical student, gently emphasized Mark's great powers of concentration, his determination, his obvious good health, the physical strength he had achieved through relentless, carefully planned and executed exercise. Mark quickly indicated that the emphasis on what his mind and body had managed to do was not quite enough. Yes, he had indeed worked hard to excel, but in so doing he had been, he told us, "a servant." We were both struck by the intensity and sincerity of Mark's casual conclusion: "I've been lucky that God has picked me. It's His smile." A moment's hesitation, then an elaboration — perhaps offered because he knew it was needed at that moment in that company: "When I'm running and I see His smile, I feel my body change — it's like shifting into high gear, my daddy says. My legs want to go so fast, I'm afraid they'll leave me behind! I've even heard myself saying to them, 'Please, not *too* fast, or you'll get there before I do!' It's like — they've been taken over. Once, when I ran my fastest race, I knew at the start that I was going to fly, just plain fly: I saw the biggest smile I'd ever seen on His face, just as I was waiting for the bell to ring. I had my eyes closed, and I wasn't trying to see Him, or ask for any special help from Him. No, sir, I didn't even say a prayer. Sometimes [before a race starts] I do, but not then. I said my prayers in the morning, and I asked God, please, to let me do the best I could. I didn't ask Him to make me the winner, no, sir. I used to want to win the races, but my daddy and our minister said it's not the winning, it's the running with God's blessing, that's what counts. Just because you think of God, and you pray — He's not the One who will take sides and push you so you can beat out others."

At that point he stopped. He was sitting across from us, his head a bit bowed, each of his hands folded into the other, and both of them placed a bit awkwardly over his flat, trim lower abdomen. His father often sat in that position — guarding, however, a substantial belly, a memorial to the enduring power of fried chicken. ("Daddy always cooks me lots of fried chicken the night before a race. He says it's good for the muscles, and it makes you stronger all around.") My son, who had come to know Mark and others in this small community well, got right into the thick of the boy's way of thinking. "It's true, as you said, God won't take sides and push you — but do you think He knows there will be a winner, and if He does, do you think He's had some say in who the winner is?"

Silence held us, to the point that I became aware of my watch. I began thinking of some words to speak, some nondescript comment, perhaps, that would carry us along further. A complex theology was under discussion here. My son came to the rescue: "Well, anyway, Mark, you seem to keep on winning."

That observation — the simplicity of a truth recalled — stirred the boy mightily, to our surprise. "You can't say God wants you to win. I don't believe He wants any of us to win, not any one. He wants our faith in Him, and then we try our best, and if you've given Him that [your faith], then you've done the most important thing. The night before, I'll pray, and I can see His face; it's a large face, and He's smiling, because He loves us and He wants us to love Him. God's face is the face of love, our teacher said [a fifth-grade history class in the spring of 1988], and I think of him saying that, I hear him saying it, and then there's God, coming to me with a smile, and I thank Him. I'll be asleep soon, and when I wake up, I'll see Him again, and I pray, and I say, 'I'll do my best by You,' and that's all. When I start the race I might have one more prayer to say, and I keep my eyes shut tight, and I don't want Him to come and be on my side so I can win. No sir, I don't always see His face — only sometimes. I just say my prayer fast ('Please, God, let me be your servant'), and then right away my eyes are open and I'm going to run as fast as I can, and get to the end, and I'm looking at the end, and it's the end that's on my mind, and nothing else. I might see His face when I'm running; I might. But lots of times — no. When I'm running, it's as if my legs are trying hard, *so* hard, and I can't keep up with them; and there have been moments when I think they're not my legs anymore, they belong to someone else."

That last remembered feeling of Mark's begged for an inquiry. Yet I also felt ashamed: "Who might the 'someone else' be?" I gulped, trying to swallow the words before they became audible.

A bright, intuitive boy with a mind that also did some racing, Mark turned out to be a lap ahead of this self-conscious doctor: "Your legs are your own, but your strength is given you. When you pray, it's for strength you're praying. I guess we belong to God, unless we fight Him. That's where the devil comes in — he'll chain those who are ready to let him. I've wondered why some folks give in to the devil, and others don't. It's up to the person, to me, I believe. I have a friend, he's gotten into trouble in some races. He says the devil gets into his [running] shoes. It's not right, to think like that. You have to stand up in your shoes and say they're yours, and you aren't letting them belong to anyone else, not the devil, that's for sure."

He had helped clarify his remark that sometimes he felt as if his legs belonged to someone else — but he had still not put to rest my speculation that at times he felt the Lord had in some ineffable manner taken possession of his legs, made them a victorious instrument of His. I posed this question to him directly: "Do you feel every once in a while, Mark, that your legs are going so fast, doing such a great job, that God Himself is the One who is guiding them — that He's the 'someone else' you were referring to, when you said your legs 'belong to someone else'?"

"No, I didn't mean it that way. No, I meant that my legs were going so fast, they just seemed out of my control — and so [they were] someone else's. But I didn't mean that they were in God's power. That wouldn't be right, for me to think such a thing. I mean, He's the One who looks over us, but we have to be on our own, and that's how we get judged. It's up to us. He looks, and He smiles, or He gets upset, but we're the ones doing what we do — that's how I believe it goes." He went back, finally, to the face of God as he reminded us that he heard a lot about God at home and in the Seventh-Day Adventist school he was attending and, of course, in church; and that he had tried hard to make sense of what he had heard; and that his own achievements prompted him even more to think about who he is and how his performance has turned out so well. "I look up to God, and I think of Him looking down on me," he told us. We needed ask for no elaboration; he offered it to us immediately and un-self-consciously. "I was named after [the disciple] Mark, and I wonder what he looked like. I once asked our minister why God chose the disciples He did, and he said he didn't know, but he was sure everyone is special in God's eyes. It's *His* eyes that are real special, I'm sure. I mean, *He's* as special as you can be, but it's the eyes that He uses, to see all of us down here! Sometimes I'll do what my mom and dad have told me; I'll pray to God and I'll think of Him, and then I'll see Him, His face, His eyes. That's all I see, His eyes, mainly, and His forehead, I guess, and His hair, not much else. He's looking down, and I pray He'll smile on us. That's what I'll see sometimes, too — His smile; He'll be smiling."

Mark's pictures, done over a year's time, have often featured that face, those eyes, that smile. The eyes have varied in size; the smile in its fullness, its breadth — signified by cheek lines, by the mouth opened wide or not so wide, or, on a grim day, the mouth closed. Here (pulled together from a number of separate talks) are some of his notions of what would bring a dour or melancholy look to God's face: "If you ignore Him, that's the worst thing you can do. He'll be sad, and you'd see it on His face. He doesn't want us to praise Him just to be nice, though. He wants us to praise Him because we've realized who He is — He's the creator of all the people.

"There was a terrible accident on the [interstate] highway, not three or four miles away. A man was driving a truck, probably headed for North Carolina, and the police think he fell asleep. He crashed into a car and there were five people in it, and not one of them was alive when people came to help out. My daddy was going in the opposite direction and he saw the wreck, and he crossed over the grass [median strip] and wanted to be helpful, because he's taken a lot of Red Cross courses, and he can give first aid real good. But they all were dead — a father and a mother and three kids, and one was my age, I believe. Daddy got right down on his knees and he prayed for the family, that God should take them into His house, and be real extra nice to them, considering. It's times like that He must be in tears Himself. Probably those folks were crying on the way to meet Him, and He must have been crying awaiting them. He wept when

He was here, I think, and there's lots of trouble, still, since He left long ago.

"I picture Him, mostly, trying to smile on us, but with all the troubles, the wars and the murders — drugs, you know, and all that — He must bow His head a lot and shake His head a lot, and like my mom says, you'd see all the pain of the whole world in His eyes if you saw the eyes. When I think of Him, He's smiling, and that's because we've been lucky, our family. Why, we could have been wiped out, all of us, just like the folks in that car on the big road. In a second, when you least expect it, the end can come. That's what our minister preached to us on the Sunday after: when the end comes. He said we should live each day like there won't be any more of them coming, and be ready every morning to meet our God, and every night, too. I'll say my prayers, and sometimes He's listening right to me, and other times I know there's a lot He has to do besides give me a pat on the back! But I'll see Him, looking down here, and that's what will happen when I die — I'll go meet Him, and He'll look me over and make up His mind! You're here to do the best you can so when you see Him and He sees you, it'll be a good meeting. I'll admit, yes, that I wonder some days how He keeps track of all of us, but the answer is He's God, and when He looks, it's different than it is with us, with a person down here.

"On some days, I'm sure He's cross — He'll close His eyes and not want to look at any of us! There was a day — a year ago — I was set for a race, and I woke up: I was feeling lousy. I had aches in my legs, and I had a headache. No way I was going to run. I had no appetite. My mom had hot cereal for me; it's my favorite: oatmeal. My dad offered to make pancakes; he's great [at] making them. I wanted a glass of water and nothing else. 'Pray to God,' they both said, 'He'll heal you.' I did, I closed my eyes, and I tried to picture Him smiling; but He wasn't. He didn't even want to look at me. He had His face turned. I tried to keep praying. All of a sudden I saw His face, right before me, and He sure didn't seem friendly. I told my folks that I was praying, and the Lord was sort of telling me this wasn't my day. My dad wanted to know what I meant: 'Where do you get the idea that it "sort of" isn't your day, according to God?' He asked me that. I said: 'From my prayers, the way he looked at me.' Daddy got a little upset; he said I was jumping to conclusions, and I shouldn't. We all sat and said our prayers, and God was nicer — He looked friendlier. It was the smile, yes [I had asked], and it was His eyes, too. You can see in the eyes if a person is with you or he's not a friend and doesn't like you. It's not that God is like a guy in the playground, on your side or on the other side! No, sir, He's different; but He has to pick and choose with us, here; the Bible says that, and it's up to each person to try to meet Him, and open up to Him, and then you can appeal to Him, and He'll listen and He'll pay attention. Why? Well, if you know someone, then he knows you; and if you don't it's hard. The same with God."

He stopped cold then. He appeared to be looking inward: he stared into space, his face turned decidedly away from us. After five seconds or so — a longer time than one might think in a conversation that had had practically no lapses — Mark surprised me by turning the tables: "What do you think?"

I wanted to make sure that I was answering the question he had in mind, so I replied, "About what, Mark, about what we were just discussing?" I hoped he'd spell out the nature of our conversation. I had been so busy trying to listen, to fathom *his* ideas, as they were being presented, I had lost any sense of my own thoughts on the matter.

But Mark wasn't going to state his position again. Rather, he said, "Yes" — the shortest reply, obviously, to my question.

I took a breath, and then I replied, "I don't picture God keeping tabs on each of us in such a way that He sorts out on the basis of who prays a lot to Him, and who doesn't, and who has come to feel familiar with Him and who hasn't — who sees His face a lot, as you do, and who doesn't. That's my opinion. I'm not at all sure what is the right thing to say — but that's my thought on how God works with us, among us."

Mark listened closely, I could see. He frowned a bit a few seconds after I had finished, as if he had all of a sudden had a thought that was rather distressing to him, and then he shared it with me: "But you pray so God will know you, and He'll answer your prayers. If you don't pray, He won't know you."

I wanted, immediately, to blurt out my impression that God knew all of us, whether we appeal to Him or not; yet I did not want to argue with Mark. He had been kind enough to share his spiritual life with me, and my reason to be there, in that town just outside Chattanooga, was to learn from him. I handled such thoughts by saying nothing about them. Instead, I offered a feeble "Yes, I see what you mean."

My son Bob's face registered annoyance, and he intervened, addressing Mark directly: "There are some people, Mark, who don't pray to God as you do. Maybe they think of Him, or maybe they hope that their lives, the way they live, are their way of praying to Him. I mean, they try to be good people, and so all they do is *that* — try hard to be good — and they hope He'll notice and approve."

Mark was not at all put off. He smiled. He said that he surely didn't want to lord it over others: "My daddy always says we're here to practice our own religion, and we don't want to tell others what to do, and they shouldn't want to tell us what to do: you should be fair, and you should hope the next person is as fair to you as you are to him."

Mark's further reflections on prayer have been assembled from an hour and a half of subsequent talk that day and, two days later, another two hours: "There's no right and wrong way to pray. I agree. My momma once told us that, too; she said it's up to you to find your way of getting to know God. You shouldn't be praying so you'll be God's favorite. In church we'll hear that, and my momma will make sure I hear because she's always telling us you can use prayer like anything else — get into trouble. 'Don't *brag* about your praying,' she says every once in a while, and I sure get the shakes afterward, when I'm praying. I pray that I'm not bragging! I try not to [brag], I try to be 'open and aboveboard,' like Daddy says I should. My mom says, 'Give your heart to God.' My daddy says, 'Be open and aboveboard with God.' Maybe God smiles at people, some of them, and they don't know it. He could do that, I'll bet! I'd miss praying to Him. It wouldn't be the same. Yes, I know some people don't think of God, don't even believe in Him. In school our teacher said we should pray for them, so God must know them, too. He probably thinks: that's OK, that's OK, even if they don't think of Him much.

"I tried not to brag with anyone when I won the big race last month. I prayed to God, and I thanked Him, but I didn't say for what! I just thanked Him! I said my prayers, and I pictured Him listening; He was looking interested in my prayers and it seemed like He looked me right in the eye, but He didn't smile, and I was grateful. I didn't want to see Him smiling — like He was saying, 'Mark, you did a good job.' That's what my parents were saying, and my grandparents, and lots of friends. I thanked them, but I didn't feel I'd done anything special, and I was trying to tell God that — tell Him thanks, but I'm not being a fellow who's becoming stuck on himself. If God sees any of us becoming like that — you get to thinking you're the cat's meow — then He'll let you know. How? [I had asked.] He'll just turn away from you."

At that point I asked Mark how he would know such a response of God's, such a cold shoulder. "I don't know where I heard that the Lord will turn away from you sometimes, if you do something He doesn't take to, but I've been pretty sure it [such a turning away] can happen — and it does. It seems natural that if you're the Lord, and a person hasn't been good, then you'll be unhappy, and it'll show on you, and you just might turn in another direction. My granddaddy, he'll get pale and he looks like he might just pass out, if people talk and he doesn't like the words they use, and maybe with God that happens: *He* gets pale, too!"

A particular child may well build his or her very own imaginative construction of God's face; in this instance, Mark saw paleness. Ears vary in their prominence, vary perhaps according to the child's inclination to see or be seen, the child's relative preoccupation with hearing what is going on, with listening as a means of being part of the world, joining in its activities. The mouth also differs from picture to picture, depending on a child's concern with eating, with smiling, and, too, on the sense of vulnerability a child may have — hence a notion of God as angry, even devouring. One child's God of smiles gives way to another's alarmed deity, ready to chew up and swallow, or spit out with disdain, the world's sinners. A friend of Martha's in Lawrence, Massachusetts, talked of God's "disgust" — His willingness, she was sure, to denounce "drug dealers and gang people," and, beyond words, His interest in "blowing them away with a hurricane" or "using his teeth to make mincemeat of them." Such vivid ways of summoning God and evoking His actions remind a listener that the emotional volatility of children can find, in God, an ally. "Someone has to come here and clean up our block," Martha's friend insisted one hot summer day, and God was her first choice to do the job. A great devotee of Saturday television cartoons, she had every inspiration to harness their magical power to the task of doing what seemed to be the impossible — clean a city of many serious injustices. No wonder her God's face had teeth that were pointed and raggedly sharp; they were instruments of the indignant God she visualized. She gave Him concrete expression in a series of five portraits, each distinctive. His look in those portraits surely expressed hers, as the one who has to walk every day past the scene she would have God mercifully grind up.

Children living in more privileged circumstances may present to the viewer divine faces of an altogether different sort — full, well formed, wide-eyed, smiling. Yet, these faces, too, can be remarkably idiosyncratic — as if, in heaven at least, questions of class and race and nationality carry diminished effect. A girl of eleven, in New Orleans, let me know how she imagined God's appearance, His "looks," as she put it: "I don't think of Him as handsome, not the kind of man I picture myself wanting to meet when I grow up. God is different. He looks different. He's the only one who looks like He does — I mean, no one looks like Him. That's why I don't know how to draw Him, because He's so special." Still, she had many times seen pictures of Jesus and pictures of God, too, with his long, gray-white beard, much white hair, and deep-set, penetrating eyes. She was quite willing to attempt her own reproduction of such images, but she took pains to let me know that she would "just be copying" — putting on paper the notions given to her by the Sunday school books. Moreover, she made an interesting point to me one day as she readied herself for a drawing session: "They tell us [in Sunday school] that Jesus is God, but He's the son of God, too — so they must look different, Jesus and His father." Then she, as have others, wondered out loud how anyone really knew what Jesus looked like: "My daddy says there weren't any cameras then, so there's no picture of Him, and that means you can't look at one and copy it. I know that in the black churches they'll tell you

Jesus is black; he's colored. Our maid told us that's how He looks in her church — the pictures of Him — so there's the difference. I asked my grandma who's right, and she said Jesus was not a colored man; He was a white man, but all people want Him to look the way they do, and that's 'natural.' I asked her if I drew a picture of Jesus, or God, and His skin was brown, and not white, would that be wrong. She said, 'Honey, I don't think it makes any difference up there — skin color.' "

These remarks prefaced a drawing by a fifth-grade private school student of considerable independence of mind. She featured God's face provocatively, and with an arresting use of color: she gave Him a triangular face, with triangular eyes and a triangular nose; a sliver of a mouth; ears that looked like isosceles triangles that had lost their bases; a short haircut, a vertical crew cut; and a green-blue complexion. The face was placed on an orange curve — a line that might, in another picture, have been a bowl, or maybe a sliver of a moon in a sky. I was surprised and perplexed by the picture, though I quickly reminded myself that this girl, Sara, was a precocious, artistically talented child. Indeed, her mother is an artist, and one who generally favors an abstract impressionist style. Nevertheless, here was a child who dared experiment rather boldly with God's face.

When I questioned Sara about her drawing, I discovered that she had found for herself an ideological justification for her unusual rendering. "You can't know what God looks like, because He may not even look like us. I don't think He looks like anything else, no. [I had asked.] I think He might be some force, like the winds — a tornado, a hurricane! — or He might be the stars, maybe some invisible rope that holds all the stars together. How can we ever know until we die? My grandma will say to me, 'Sara, one less day before I meet my maker,' and so I asked her what she thought He'd be like — and look like — and she said you have to wait and see. So I told her I was drawing the pictures for you, and she said, 'Anyone's guess is OK,' and so that [the picture she had just drawn] is my guess, and it could be right and it could be wrong."

Sophia, twelve, the daughter of a maid who lived a few miles away in another part of New Orleans, followed her mother's advice, drew Jesus as black, and told me He is God, He is black, and she is sure "white folks" will discover a similar truth one day, though it may not come until He comes back here, and then "everyone will see." I asked Sophia the source of her information, her certitude. She was immediately responsive: "Our minister knows." I wanted to hear more but I said nothing for a few seconds, though I was convinced by Sophia's direct gaze at me, and the thinnest of smiles on her face, that she fully appreciated my state of mind. Finally, I asked whether she had given thought to *how* the minister knew. Now her face broke into a full smile and her eyes lit up, a prelude to the animation her voice displayed as she spoke: "On some day the Lord will come down here. We'll see Him, and He'll speak to people. He was a poor man, like us, and He'll talk with us folks. He spoke to Martin Luther King, and our minister knew him. My momma and my daddy — before they were grown up — got to see Martin Luther King; they can remember him talking. Our minister was there. God was there, too, visiting us. He'll pay some people attention on Sundays, if they really work in their prayers to hear Him. He'll speak through you, and you can see Him if you just let your eyes be free to wait and look until He comes."

Sophia had told me of the long hours she put into churchgoing on Sundays; each week she was there, in the same pew, amid her large, extended family. She herself, when she was little, had glimpsed Him: "I wasn't yet in school, I don't think. I was there [in church] with my folks, and with their folks, and my cousins, and then my momma cried, and said she'd just seen Him, the Lord, and so did I. He had a big black robe, and all I could see was His face, and He had a big face, and He was saying something; it was important, but I couldn't make out what it was. He had big eyes, the biggest I'd ever seen, and He had a big, big forehead, with lots of wrinkles, and then the hair, some white and some regular, not white. He was talking, so His mouth was open, and I don't remember anything else about Him, except that He wasn't looking at us; He was staring, but not at us. God doesn't look at people, I don't think. He looks right through you, but not in your face, I don't think. Maybe He's looking over us all, and not into anyone's eyes."

I had heard Sophia's parents talk about God, and I knew that some of their ideas and speculations had come to inform their daughter's images. Her God's fiercely attentive yet austere and distant posture helped her — as it did her parents — comprehend the life of poor blacks in New Orleans. "God is up there looking down on us every single second," she told me one morning, and then she commented, "He adds things up later. For every line on his forehead, He'll do something later." I had been told, finally, the reason for the prominent and creased forehead given by Sophia to her dark-skinned Lord.

In a working-class white neighborhood of Boston, a nine-year-old boy, Tommy, a bright fourth-grader, told me that he had no idea what God looked like, or how to draw Him, "unless He looks like you see Him in the windows in church." A certain hesitation? I encouraged the boy to draw God in whatever way he wanted, but he persisted: "Do you want me to copy the pictures of Him in the church?" I reminded the boy that those pictures weren't nearby. He nodded but said he could close his eyes and come close to remembering what he had noticed in church. I told him that I'd be delighted to look at what he could recapture in that manner, and I'd also be delighted to see any picture of God he might want to construct on his own. He wanted to pursue this discussion further, unlike many children, who were content either to draw a picture of God similar to others they had seen, or to improvise and draw their own personal version of Him. I was asked this: "Isn't it a big secret, what He looks like?"

I answered, "Yes, I think so."

"Do you think He looks like us?"

"I don't know."

I was about to toss the question back when he announced his considered opinion: "I don't think He does. He might look real different."

"Like what?"

"Oh," said Tommy, "like something that doesn't even exist here."

I wanted to know whether this lively, energetic boy had long been prone to such a conjecture. He told me, "In Sunday school a nun showed us a picture of Jesus and asked us to copy it. She told us to be very, very careful, because it's God we're copying.

My friend asked if God and Jesus look the same. The nun told us they *are* the same! I wanted to ask some more questions, but I could see she wasn't liking us asking any. She told us to 'get down to business,' and we sure did, right away! She carried this [blackboard] pointer around with her, and if she didn't like what you said or the way you questioned her, she'd slam it down on your desk, and you knew what she was telling you: next time it'll be on your hide! My dad has told me: never fight with a nun! My mom says they're the toughest people on the whole face of the earth."

After he delivered himself of that statement he seemed lost in further thought, uninterested either in conversation or in picking up the box of crayons, which sat at the corner of his desk. I tried to think of something to say, but nothing came to mind. I found myself looking out the window. It was a rather unremarkable April day, not too cold or too warm, neither especially nice nor rainy and unpleasant. The American flag hung quietly in the front center of the room; a list of key vocabulary words was on the blackboard underneath. My mind suddenly went back to my own fourth-grade classroom — Miss Herlihy's. I saw her at her desk, "dictating" (as she put it) "words" to us. "These words will be your companions for life," she would tell us. I undid my spell and returned to the year 1988 just in time to hear Tommy say, "Maybe God looks like a star. Maybe He looks like this planet." A long pause. "Maybe *He's* the one who is the toughest on the face of the earth."

I was struck dumb. I tried to figure out what this boy meant and how he had gotten himself to that meaning. "I don't understand you, Tommy," I said.

He looked surprised, as if I hadn't remembered what he'd told me earlier, what his mother had said about nuns. He explained: "The nuns told us God rules the whole world, every place in it. He must be all over the place. Maybe He's not someone like us; maybe He's hiding, and He looks different. Maybe He's big, as big as the moon or our whole planet. I'm sure my mom would agree He's tougher than the nuns!"

No more words. Tommy now looked hard at the crayons, reached for them, decanted them on the desk, looked in the box to see if any remained, found three still there, took them out carefully — and as if, thereby, they had earned a special status, placed them slightly apart from the somewhat used twenty or so others, one of which rolled to the floor. Tommy picked it up and promptly sent it back to the box — for now an exiled status. He drove this point home by setting the box on the furthest corner of his desk. Ready at last, he picked off the top piece of paper from a stack I had placed on a neighboring desk, and right away he began his work with an orange crayon. He drew a large circle, and then, abruptly, put the crayon down, picked up a yellow one, with it drew another circle, smaller and above the first. Then he forsook the yellow crayon for the orange one and used it to make a face — round eyes, a thin line for a nose, another thin line for the mouth, two small half-circles for the ears. He put the orange crayon down, then decided to be more emphatic: he placed it in the box — the end of a tour of duty. Resuming with the yellow crayon, he imposed identical features on the upper circle he had earlier made. The yellow crayon, too, was then dispatched to its place of enclosure. Now Tommy picked up the black crayon, held it for a few seconds poised over the paper, directed it toward and then away from that piece of paper, and after two more such movements, back and forth, laid the crayon to rest on the desk, but still held between three of his right hand's fingers. Those fingers moved a bit on the crayon, ready to go; but the mind that makes decisions had not figured out what to do.

I wondered whether to say anything — and if so, what. I told myself to keep quiet; this was not the Tommy I had come to know, a quick-witted and fast-moving child. He looked out the window — up at the sky, I noticed. I found myself doing likewise. Then he returned to his drawing while my eyes stayed with a cloud; I observed its largeness, its heaviness, as it moved across my field of vision. The next thing I knew, the boy had begun to use his black crayon. He capped the orange face with black hair and then gave a similar head of hair to the yellow one. In a second or two the black crayon had also been dismissed to the company of the three confined ones while the artist looked first at what he had done and then at all the unused crayons. They prompted from him a regretful observation: "I wish I could have used more of the crayons, but there are so many of them." He prepared to stash them away, too; he did so, methodically and more thoughtfully than I had realized. When three or four were still left on his desk, he let me know his reasoning: "I decided to save these, so I can draw a rainbow; it can be seen all over — the whole universe!" I was surprised and impressed. The boy's smile was large and lingering, a rainbow in itself. He was obviously delighted with this idea and savored it for a few seconds before implementing it. Tommy picked up, in succession, a green, a purple, a red, and a yellow-green crayon and made his large rainbow in such a way that it bracketed and sheltered both faces; it had an enormous, dominating presence on the rather large piece of paper he had chosen.

When he had finished this project — enacted an inspiration, really — he methodically put away the last of the crayons, always harder to do than to fit the first crayons into an empty box. He closed the box. He could now turn his full attention to the drawing. He moved the paper so that it was in center stage on the desk. He looked at it intently. Ten or so seconds elapsed. I watched him while he was looking at what he had accomplished. Eventually he picked up the paper, and I thought he was going to hand it to me, as he had done in the past. But no, he held the drawing up for my inspection. I looked at it, and I was intrigued: an unusual rendering of God's face, I decided, and a suggestive one. I wanted to ask Tommy some questions, ask him to explain what he had intended to say, but I wasn't sure how to. Tommy rescued me with a confident analysis, delivered in a brief, eager, vigorously balanced expository manner: "I thought I'd give us God the father and God the son! The sun is the father, and the earth is the son! You see?"

I most certainly did. I smiled and said an enthusiastic "Yes." He was pleased. He was quickly anxious to proceed, and did so: "The rainbow is the Holy Ghost, maybe!" I must have looked quite interested and surprised. "Well, you see, God has a face, and so did Jesus. The nun will tell you they are the same, but the priest told my mother that's not true; they are different. I'm with the priest! Then there's the Holy Ghost, and I never figured It had a face. Maybe a ghost *does*, like in [television] programs, or movies — ghosts run around and have faces and they talk. But I don't think the Holy Ghost is that kind of ghost! No, sir!

I'm sure the Holy Ghost must look different, but I don't know how different — what it would be like to see the Holy Ghost. It's only when we go to meet the Lord, then we'll see the Holy Ghost too, I think."

Tommy was trying with all his might to visualize the complex, tripartite deity he was learning about in his classes: Father, Son, Holy Ghost — who are, he pointed out to me several times, "all together, but they are separate also." His drawing was, for me, revelatory in its originality, in its dense symbolism, all tendered to the viewer with a disarming simplicity. His vision — the sun as the face of God, the earth (where Christ arrived, the incarnation) as the face of the son of God, and a rainbow (which is what we see on earth, and owes its existence to the sun) as the Holy Ghost — was a thing of great and overarching beauty. I told Tommy that he'd given me something unique and valuable: God in His possible or various forms. He paid close heed to my language and asked me if his "faces" were what I meant by the "forms" I had mentioned. "Yes, it is those faces I'm talking about," I reassured Tommy. He answered with this bold leap: "The rainbow is one face the Holy Ghost might have. There could be others, maybe there could. I asked my [great-]uncle (a priest) how the Holy Ghost 'comes down' — because he would tell us that It does. He said it's one of 'God's mysteries' and we'll never know until we go to meet Him. Maybe some birds carry the Ghost down to us. Once I saw some birds sitting on a telephone wire outside our house, and one of the birds flew near us and then flew off. It might have had a message for someone, my [great-]uncle said. He told me never to forget that God has His own way of reminding us of Him — that He's around!"

For many Christian children, drawing God's face does just that — gives Him to them concretely, brings Him "around." I have never asked a Jewish or Islamic child to draw a picture of God, nor have I asked children who assert their indifference to formal religion to represent what, after all, they doubt or deny as believable. On occasion I have, however, heard both confessions and fantasies. In Jerusalem, a Jewish boy of twelve, almost thirteen, told me, after drawing a picture of Moses holding the tablets of law, of his sometime transgression: "I think of Moses a lot; he is our greatest teacher. My brother [only five] asked me what God looks like and what Moses saw when he went up the mountain. 'Did he see God?' I said, 'No, of course not: you cannot see God.' 'How can that be, if he gave Moses the tablets?' I was stymied. I said, 'These things happen.' I didn't convince him. He was all set — I could tell — to ask me a million more questions. I raised my voice and said, 'Don't ask me; ask Father, ask our rabbi.' I wanted no more questions!"

But he heard his own mind continue to work restlessly, and try as he would to stop the thoughts and visions, they kept arriving: "I saw Moses up there, the clouds under him; I saw someone who looked like Moses talking with him and giving him the tablets, the commandments. I closed my eyes, but that didn't work: I wasn't seeing through them anyway! I decided, then, that I knew what the word 'devil' means: it means breaking rules, and letting your mind try to become the boss, instead of being a loyal, good student. I remember having questions, like my brother's, but I stopped them; when he asked them [of me], though, they came back. My father tells us we must do what is right, but we will always make our mistakes, because no one is perfect. I think it's a big mistake to forget what you learn [as a young observant Jew]. In school the teachers tell us to use our minds any way we can — to be clever, to be 'inventive,' they will say. But you can go too far. With God, the rules are His, and we have to listen."

In London, a Pakistani girl, almost twelve, told my son, firmly, what he had heard from other Islamic children: no pictures of people, of living creatures — "only patterns." Yet, after drawing many intricate patterns, and after many discussions centered on her everyday hopes, her aspirations, she broke a particular chain of thought one afternoon in London to tell her American visitor about her prayers that "in a future time" she would "meet Allah" and "meet Mohammed," that she would "see both of them, their faces." She hastened to say that she would be "in another life" when such a meeting took place. On another visit her mother asked my son about his work with children who were not Islamic. The matter of drawings came up — not for the first time! — and the mother confided this: "My children, when they are quite young, want to *see* Allah, and Mohammed as well. If I had pictures of them — their faces — the children would be *so* happy! I tell them that not everything appears on the tube [television]. I tell them we must close our eyes sometimes, not always try to see more and more: movies, videocassettes, the stations you get by pressing the buttons or turning the dial! Well, what does He [Allah] look like, they ask? Shut your eyes when you have such questions, I tell them! If they keep on asking, I will answer, I have answered, 'Try to see Him, His face, and you'll be blind — no more sight!' I cover my eyes to show them what blindness is — only the dark [is seen]."

In quite different neighborhoods, other children also learn to stifle interest — as I learned in a rather fine elementary school which for decades has catered to the intelligentsia of a Boston suburb. A boy of eleven, interested in what God looked like — his friend was of a devoutly Catholic family — asked another friend for the answer, only to be told, "God looks like nothing, because He doesn't exist; He's not real." The boy turned later to his Catholic friend: did he "really" believe in God? Yes! The Catholic boy eventually showed his inquiring classmate and neighbor a book with pictures of Jesus. The friend looked, looked away, thought to himself, said nothing. But several weeks later he told me he had tried "to picture what God looked like, if He exists," only to decide the exercise was futile: "You can't see Him, if he's not there, and Dad says it's all a superstition, religion — but for a second I saw someone when I was trying!" His decided skittishness as he told me of that "second" persuaded me to let the matter drop there. In his own way, he had stepped into forbidden territory (a strange land, ruled out-of-bounds at home). Some religions say no to visual representation of God, whereas others for centuries have celebrated Him by showing Him in paintings, in stained glass, on ceilings, in the pictures children see in the books they read while growing up.

Working with children over the years has taught me that they are quick to connect themselves, in all sorts of ways, to whatever it is they do. Picturing God's face turns out to be no exception. A child's race, class, sex, family experience, and idiosyncratic personal experience may work their way into the drawings he or she does, though such influences contend with religious and cultural conventions that have exerted their own hold on the

child. Many Christian children have been eager to present me
with a fairly conventional face of God — one witnessed in a book
or in church, and now turned into their own drawing. Many
others let their minds meet mystery with surmise, or maybe a
flash of drawn guesswork that embodies, also, a few private
dreams, worries, anticipations. The prominence of the face, and
often a single part of the face, has been for me a constant source
of interest and wonder — God as glaring eyes, as ears picking
up human static, as a mouth that smiles constantly or seems
angrily ready to devour any number of devilish enemies in the
universe; and God as someone whose wisdom and experience
are signfied by lined features, gray and white hair, a full or
partial beard. Though some children do give God a full body,
as we shall see, the many who don't have made clear their reasons, and the child Tommy's are quite representative: "God
doesn't have to worry about eating and drinking, I don't think.
My [great-]uncle said He's 'sprung' — He got outside the skin
and can go where He wants." That notion, of a Lord liberated,
as it were, "sprung" from the flesh, lingers in the thoughts of
many children and is conveyed quietly, sometimes compellingly,
by the use of crayons and paintbrushes: faces full of so much
authority, or grandeur, or power, or love, or mystery, or judgmental passion, or insight, or alarm, or worries, or vulnerability
(God as the one who suffers for humankind) — but also, faces
suspended bodiless, it seems, in the infinity of space, the eternity
of time.

Sometimes, as I sit and watch a child struggle to do just the
right job of representing God's face, His features, the shape of
His head, the cast of His countenance, I think back to my days
of working in Dorothy Day's Catholic Worker soup kitchen.[2] One
afternoon, after several of us had struggled with a "wino," a
"Bowery bum," an angry, cursing, truculent man of fifty or so,
with long gray hair, a full, scraggly beard, a huge scar on his
right cheek, a mouth with virtually no teeth, and bloodshot eyes,
one of which had a terrible tic, she told us, "For all we know he
might be God Himself come here to test us, so let us treat him
as an honored guest and look at his face as if it is the most
beautiful one we can imagine." At the time I had a great deal
of trouble seeing God in that face, even as the faces of God some

children have presented to me seem improbable candidates for such an honor — "and yet," as Dorothy Day would sometimes say, never finishing her sentence, thereby leaving open any number of possibilities. God's face is *His* to reveal — so she and any number of children seem to have known. In Tommy's words, uttered after he glanced yet again at his Holy Ghost drawing, at his rainbow that had become so much more: "You have to trust in God when you try to imagine Him." To be sure, he had been given some advice along those lines at home — but then, in the fresh presence of his picture, had shown a boy's independent spiritual life to be sturdy, affecting, and persuasive.

4

The Voice of God

"I AM SURE you will understand," the boy said politely. He waited for a second or two before going on — time enough for me to notice his concern that I might not grasp an essential aspect of his religious and spiritual life. When he resumed he said: "I talk with Allah, and He listens. I pray to Him and Mohammed, and they speak to me." The boy was named Haroon; he was eleven, of Pakistani ancestry and now a Londoner. I tried to explain that I had talked with a lot of children of various backgrounds, that I had heard them speak of the prayers they offered to God and of the responses they received. Perhaps Haroon was intending to let me know that a Westerner would inevitably have trouble understanding him?

With time I learned the various meanings of the phrase Haroon often used, "I am sure you will understand." One time it might represent a gesture of reassurance: you are clearly on target. Another time he was reminding me, ever so courteously, that I seemed confused, maybe even wrong-headed. Often the remark was something else, a child's assumption of a teacher's job: let me help you figure things out, so you "*will* understand." Once in a while I heard in that phrase a note of decided impatience or annoyance: like so many others in this city of London, this island of England, you seem so convinced — how mistakenly — that your sense of things is sound.

Still, Haroon was tolerant, forbearing, forgiving. He wanted to educate me. His father and mother, deeply religious, had enjoined him to try to bring me "closer to Allah, and to His prophet, Mohammed." The more visits I had with this bright and talkative boy, the more I heard not only his everyday words, but special messages he felt privileged to have, messages he pointedly directed my way: "I am sure you will understand that Allah has a lot to tell us, and that is why we are here, to receive His words. If we pray to Him, He listens, and then we must listen." I did some attentive listening, and that morning I found myself impatient with Haroon's didactic, if not patronizing, tone. He was trying to share his spiritual life with me, and his manner of doing so — I would only slowly learn — was quite similar to that of his parents.

One day, as we talked, I asked Haroon about his exchanges with Allah. "Is it His voice you hear?"

"He does speak to me. He hears my prayers and He answers them."

"How does He do that?"

"With words for me to remember."

I wanted to ask him *whose* words they were, his or His, but I didn't dare introduce a skeptical note into the conversation. Instead, I settled for "What words?"

"Oh, many." He paused, and I wasn't sure whether to press for examples or let things drop, in hopes that we would get at this matter another time. Haroon had by then got my number, as I confirmed when I later reviewed his reply. When I failed to respond to his "Oh, many," he asked me if I'd ever heard anyone address me who wasn't there in body.

"Oh, yes," I replied.

"Then you do understand," he said. In fact, he was telling me that *he* understood what I was trying to understand about him.

Two weeks later we got down to some specifics — the lessons Haroon was learning as a consequence of daily prayers: "I ask Allah to give me strength, and He says I already have strength. All that day I heard Him: 'You already have strength.' When I was at school I looked the bully [another boy in his class] in the eye, and was ready to take him on. Maybe he would have won if we'd fought, but I was ready to test him, and with that, he lost interest in me! It was Allah who had given me strength."

I decided now to become cranky, dubious. We had become

friends, Haroon and I, so we could respect each other's points of view, I thought. Indeed, I was almost ready to preface my remarks with "I am sure you will understand." Instead, I heard my voice lowering, my words coming out only hesitantly, but I reminded my young friend that the bully might well say his prayers, too. The observation hit Haroon in the face, I could see. I was appalled with myself. Why did I say that? What distrustful core of twentieth-century psychology prompted me to respond in that way to this boy's heartfelt story?

In a second my mind had jumped back decades to recall the fifteen- or sixteen-year-old boy who bullied me in our neighborhood when I was about eight years old. My father used those confrontations to share with me his beliefs — a sense that it was a tough world, and that one had to learn, in some way, how to survive. "Stay out of his way," Dad suggested. "He's almost twice your age, and there's little else you can do." But I didn't quite manage to follow my dad's advice. I tried my own version of Haroon's strategy. When the bully (Richie was his name: one never forgets such details) got aggressive with me, I tried to glare at him, and when he came close and shoved me, I asked him what I had heard my mother ask, rhetorically, at the dinner table: why did he pick on me — why me instead of someone else he *really* wanted to hit? I can still see his face reddening and feel the pain of his punches. The next day (it was the only time in my life such a thing happened), Dad came out of the house when Richie walked by, grabbed his arm, and gave him the lecture of his life: if Richie could assault me, Dad could assault him — that was "the rule of hoodlums," a phrase I can still hear in my father's voice. Thereafter I felt safe, of course — yet strangely weakened and fearful. Dad let me know that what I had experienced was merely the beginning of the bitterness and violence I'd see as I grew older. (Hitler was approaching the height of his power then, 1939, and Stalin had already murdered legions of onetime idealists, and the two dictators had just diplomatically embraced.) Nor did my mother's point of view provide much satisfaction to me or to my father. She urged on me what Haroon had availed himself of — prayer: "Bobby, we have to feel sorry for those so weak they must strike others; we have to pray for them." I had already learned that this mixture of psychology and Christian piety did not work with Richie, and my father let my mother and me know how effective such an attitude would be in 1939 Europe. Hobbes's famous dictum ("Life is solitary, poor, nasty, brutish, and short") seemed to be the rule, regardless of prayer. Worse, all sorts of ministers and priests had signed up willingly, even eagerly, with Hitler and his henchmen. While my mother, in later years, would hold on to Bonhoeffer's example for dear life, my father would shake his head.

In clinical work, a child psychiatrist has a private childhood to live with — the by now well-known "counter-transference" that has us responding to patients in ways that echo our own early experiences within a particular family. When I talked with Haroon and he told me of the efficacy of prayer in a concrete moment of his unfolding life, my own past instantly awakened and became as fresh and persuasive as it had ever been. My surly rejoinder to this decent, introspective, and well-behaved child signaled that his story had touched my raw nerve. As for the boy's reaction to what I'd said, his silence unnerved me. I waited for words, anything, even the ever-recurring "I am sure you will understand." I yearned for a bit of Haroon's occasional con-descension as a sign that he had not been unduly cut down by my sharp-tongued logic. Instead, the boy seemed rather hurt and offended. I was about to apologize when he spoke up: "Yes, I am sure he [the bully] does say his prayers." I felt a bit relieved. But after another long silence, Haroon gave me this to ponder: "But I'm sure Allah listens carefully to all the prayers He hears."

The academic part of me was ready to continue this duel. My mind wondered about the prayers that must have been sent to God from Auschwitz and Buchenwald, from the Gulag, from the terrible slums of Calcutta, from Haroon's relatives, so poor and ill, he had told me, in Pakistan. Fine, God listens, I thought, yet millions get trampled daily by crooks, liars, murderers, let alone the relatively minor bullies with whom Haroon and I as children have contended. I noticed my legs cross and uncross, and I heard a gurgle or two in my stomach — for me always a sure sign of rising anxiety. It was my turn to talk, but nothing came to mind, so I looked at my watch and told my young friend that we were long past our allotted hour. Haroon thanked me, as always, for the visit. He asked after my sons, whom he had met. He did me the great favor of showing me some books he was reading in school — enabling us, really, to resume our friendliness with one another. As I took my leave Haroon said, "I will pray to Allah that you and I find the right answers!" I was speechless just long enough to feel self-conscious as I thanked him.

A few days later both of us had given thought to our last meeting, and Haroon told me that he was ready to talk once more "about prayer." I cringed a bit. Haroon didn't wait for my explicit approval. He told me that he had asked Allah for guidance, several times, and that Allah had sent no definitive solutions: "I prayed, but I kept hearing nothing, only my own words, or I heard Father and Mother saying you must believe [in God, in Allah, in Mohammed as His messenger], even if you're in bad trouble."

I told Haroon that I had reached my own kind of impasse — that I believed, finally, that the world is full of trouble and evil, and that it would always be so, prayers or no prayers. Haroon listened carefully, looking directly at me. He nodded. In response to me he had only this question: "Isn't that what we are told — that only when Allah comes to save the world will it be saved?" I didn't know he had been given such a message as a young Islamic worshipper. Haroon had something else, though, to put forward. That very morning had found him at prayer, and he had heard a voice — Allah's, he hoped but would not dare assume: "Pray to be worried all your life as you are now. Pray that you don't put away your worries in some closet." This voice had made him nervous and confused. He had been hoping for a release from the dilemmas we'd been examining, and now he was told that at all costs he should treasure their perplexing, plaguing presence. He had asked his father for an explanation. (Father and son were close confidants; they had an impressively strong bond.)

Haroon had to wait a day or two for a reply, and when he received it he passed it along to me at our next meeting: "My father told me that when you pray you should wait and listen. Allah speaks to you. I told him I'd been waiting, and I *had* heard Allah, and He told me I *should* be worried — because there's so much trouble. My father asked what still had me so upset, then. I told him that I was now worried about what *you'd* say!"

At that I smiled. I did more: I laughed vigorously. I told

Haroon that I thought he and I were together sitting on a riddle familiar to many devout people, and also to many who worship no God but worry honestly and deeply about the world's many wrongs. I told him how moved I had been by his recent story — the strength he felt as a result of his concerted prayers to Allah, the real self-confidence that had accrued to him. I told him of my own childhood experience with a bully and of the lessons my father taught me. To all that Haroon listened with great care and attention, his head nodding or occasionally somewhat averted so that he could gaze reflectively into space. When I had had my say, he thanked me. He also let me know quickly that he thought we stood close together in important ways, though our postures were not identical: "We're both worried. Allah said we should be. I hope all the bullies in England begin to worry — but they may not. I guess we need to pray that Allah has time to worry about them."

A child here was touching upon the vastness of this universe, the mystery of God's time, His capacity for attention, for responding to the billions of requests He hears day after day. In the face of such mind-boggling matters, Haroon was clearly ready to throw up his hands, beg assistance where he could find it, at home and in the mosque. He was not fatuous about prayer, about the world's prospects. He expected a life of more bullies down the line. But he hoped (maybe against hope) for his own self-respect and dignity. One thing he *could* do, he told me that day as we ended our meeting, was pray for his own moral survival: "I hope Allah will remember me. I hope He will speak to me. I hope He will call me when I am near the edge, so I won't fall down too badly. I hope He will keep me from becoming a bully. I would not like to join the ranks [of the world's bullies]." I think as he looked at my face he saw the high regard I then felt for him: I saw him as a boy who had already staked out a tough but eminently worthwhile challenge for himself, and who had, maybe, shed a few illusions, accepted some aspects of secular "reality," yet held dear his faith in what Allah had to say to him.

To listen to God's voice[1] is no less essential to children of other religious faiths than Islam. Haroon's attentiveness to Allah's *voice* often reminded me of a Jewish boy of Haroon's age who lives in Brookline, a suburb of Boston. I first met Avram when he was nine, and I kept in touch with him through his early adolescent years and attended his bar mitzvah. His parents, Conservative Jews, are devoted to their religious faith yet also successful in America's secular life — the father is a lawyer, the mother is active in a number of community projects. She was once a librarian but abandoned her career for marriage and her three children's care, and now, after their departure for school, has become, by her own description, "a full-time professional volunteer." Avram, a bright, sensitive, voluble boy with a delightful sense of humor, is the oldest child and only son. He has done a lot to educate me about the important principles of Conservative Judaism, taking pains, at times, to let me know how he and his fellow Conservative Jews differ from Orthodox or Reform Jews. He has attended Hebrew school for many years, and has also been very close to his father, who was the son of a rabbi. (Avram's grandfather died before he was born, and Avram is named after him.)

"Our God worries about us down here," Avram told me a month or so after I'd returned from England and the discussion with Haroon. The word "worries" caught my ear right away — Haroon having been told by Allah that he ought to keep worrying, and now Avram attributing worry to God. Immediately I wanted to know more from Avram, and he was not loath to oblige: "We [Jews] are always trying to understand God, and He is always interested in us — we're His children. He's been worried about us for a long time. He sees all the trouble [down] here, and He must be sad. When I pray, I ask God to help me. I think I'm trying to find out what is the 'best,' by asking Him.

"I hear Him; I hear Him saying that we should obey the Commandments and live good lives. I hear Him saying that one day He will bring all of us [Jews] back together. He made a pact with us, and He will help us — but we have to show Him we are deserving, we are ready [for His help]. God's voice is in you when you are making choices — it turns you towards the right direction. It's not only our decisions that count; it's His decision — to teach us the right way to be. If it was only your voice and mine, and everyone else's [down] here, we'd all be canceling each other out — fighting, saying I'm right and you're wrong, and [hearing] others saying the same, and my dad says we'd all be like you see those people in the commodities market, shouting at each other, so you can't really even hear your own voice. That's why God has to speak — so we'll stop and get the right direction to go."

As I listened to Avram, I wondered: Exactly whose voice does he hear when he tells me it is God's "voice" that addresses him during his time of praying? I became increasingly precise in my questions: "Avram, is it your dad's voice you hear, or the rabbi's, or your own? I mean, do you actually hear God's voice?" I thought I knew what he meant when he talked of God's "voice," but I had enough confidence in our friendship, its give-and-take, to go through this kind of close analysis, and I thought it was necessary for me to do so — because it is important, as Avram himself has told me, that we separate our own ideas (and wishes and concerns) from God's.

Avram could be good at clarifying. Here are some of his efforts in that direction, which I garnered from several talks: "When I pray to God, it's not like I'm talking with my friends. No, it's not the same as being with my dad or mom. They have told me to talk 'special' when I speak to Him, God, and I try to do that. I bow my head; I lower my voice; I close my eyes. I say my prayers [in Hebrew]. I wait a while; then I ask Him for His help. I mention some people who are sick. I mention some people I've seen on the TV who need help; I try to give him a report — [something] like that.

"I hear Him saying that I should work hard, and do my share. I guess He'll do His [share] if we do ours. It's my voice; it's Dad's and Mom's; but we don't talk to each other like that. It's His voice, I guess — because it's different. Just like I don't talk any other time like I do when I pray, no one talks to me the way God does — He gets me thinking, and then I hear Him. It's not His voice — I mean, He doesn't speak to us when we pray; we speak to ourselves. But it's Him telling us what to say — to tell ourselves. Do you see what I mean?"

I nodded. I remembered a prayer I once heard Dr. Martin Luther King make in Alabama — one in which he asked God to speak to him at a time of great danger, so that he would in turn have some idea of what to say to others, who were paying him the closest of heed and who were also scared and in clear danger. "Speak to us, dear God," Dr. King implored repeatedly, "so that we can hear You, and thereby ourselves." I have those words on tape. I played them once for Avram. He smiled.

A year later Avram was busy preparing for his bar mitzvah and experiencing from day to day the rigors (and occasional obscenities) of junior high school and of adolescence itself. An inward-looking youth, he was also a first-rate athlete. Idealistic, he nonetheless wanted to enjoy the pleasures of a comfortable, upper-middle-class life. Devoutly connected to his religion and the cultural life associated with it, he was a well-born American who knew his country's history exceptionally well and took a strong interest in its politics. Avram was a self-described "juggler," or, as I thought of him, an adroit, sturdy tightrope walker who had no trouble walking the wire, even if we onlookers, watching, felt a thump or two in our chests. I began to realize how earnestly he conversed with God. The verb "converse" was his, used to indicate what transpired in his home every day, early in the morning and late at night, when a boy (he was not yet the "man" an observant Jew becomes at thirteen) tried to "hash things out" (another expression of his) with his Creator.

"Last night I really looked forward to a conversation with God," he told me one afternoon with no evident shyness or embarrassment, nor with any trace I could detect of self-importance or melodrama. He had been studying hard for two tests, one in math, one in history. He was both tired and wide awake: "All those numbers and equations were circling around and around in my head, and the dates and names of [Civil War] generals and the battles they fought. My arms and legs wanted 'out,' my head had 'the study fever' — that's what my cousin [in college] calls it. Around eleven or so I'd had enough, but I knew I needed to wind down, or I'd toss and turn and never go to sleep. I'd been eyeing the Bible off and on all evening, and I thought I'd read it. I like Isaiah — it's Dad's favorite. I started reading it from the beginning: 'The vision of Isaiah . . . Hear, O heavens, and give ear, O earth: for the Lord hath spoken . . .'" I've read that so many times, and I still can get excited reading it again. 'The Lord hath spoken'! I sat there; I lowered my head, and I asked the Lord to speak to me. I mean, I prayed to Him.

The Lord has other things to do than speak to me! I know that! But our rabbi says that God has nothing more important to do than to speak to us, to anyone who really and truly wants to speak to Him. He's there, watching and hoping for us."

At his use of the word "hoping," my face — unbeknownst to me — reacted, as Avram noticed: "Did I say something that bothered you?"

"No," I quickly replied, but by then the word "hoping" had moved directly into my consciousness, and I found myself grasping a bit frantically for words. As usual, I bought time with a question: "What do you mean when you say that God is 'hoping for us'?"

Avram paused not a second before starting to talk: "Oh, I mean that he really takes an interest in us, and He really hopes for the best — that our lives will work out well. He's not a magician. He gave us our freedom. It's up to us! But He didn't walk away after He let us be on our own. He's *hoping* — He's hoping we'll remember His Commandments and try to live up to them.

"This evening, when I was cramming, and I sat there, and crossed my damn feet and uncrossed them, and took off my loafers and put them on, and wondered what was on TV and tried to forget the damn thing was ever invented — and suddenly (it was nine o'clock; I counted the church bells) I thought of the prophet Isaiah, and of Moses, over and over: 'And the Lord spoke to Moses . . . ' I'm sure not Moses! But our rabbi tells us: 'We're all part of what Moses was, and *is*,' that's the way he [the rabbi] says it, and he always emphasizes '*is*.' We'd say: Moses lives! Someone will put that on a T-shirt, and I guess a lot of folks won't know *which* Moses. To me he *does* live! I guess last night I sat there thinking of him and Isaiah — the two of them talking with God."

He stopped. We were distracted by a low-flying plane. He looked up, then back in my direction. He resumed. "I said my prayers, and I tried to tell God afterwards what my life is like. I said I feel I don't have the right values some of the time — there I was praying to Him only after I was through stuffing history dates into my head. The people of Israel (the Jews of centuries ago) ate dates and prayed to God; we *memorize* dates.

The way it is now, lots of us don't give Him a second thought. My father says: 'For a lot of Jews God means nothing, but it's nice to go to a temple on the high holidays and be seen there!' The same with Christians, I'm sure. It's a real pity! And there I was, doing the same thing: math and history all night — and five minutes for a conversation with God. He might have been hoping for more."

He heard himself use the word "hoping"; and remembering my earlier inquiry, he became, in the best Talmudic tradition, acutely aware of the subtleties of human communication: "We think of ourselves — that we're the ones who need God, and are supposed to pray to Him. Right, we sure need Him — but doesn't He want to be in touch with us? That's the other half of the equation. (I've been studying math too much this week!) He's out there and we're here, and it goes back and forth, or it should."

I broke in briefly to ask about "it," because I wanted very much to hear him talk about the "conversations" he has with God. I was not disappointed: "Well, 'it' means messages, I think, sending them back and forth. After I pray, I listen, and I hear God letting me know what's important and what doesn't matter half as much as I might have thought five minutes earlier. It's not God's voice — I mean, I'm not a religious freak. It's my voice, but it's not my usual voice: it's different, it says different things, and it even sounds different! My voice is beginning to change — it cracks every once in a while, and boy, can it be embarrassing. But you know what: my voice changed years ago, going back to when I was eight or nine, and I first started thinking of God and what *He* wants, not only about me and what I want."

He stopped and seemed unlikely to continue on this course. I asked him, as forthrightly as possible, "Avram, can you tell me exactly what God said to you last night?"

"Yes. It wasn't much; but it was enough to give me plenty to think about. He told me enough was enough, and I should be myself, and not just someone trying to get two A's tomorrow morning. I mean, He told me I should keep my mind on where I was going, not just on these tests. 'Avram,' He said, 'remember Moses and Isaiah — especially tonight, when you're filling your head with algebra and the battle of Antietam.' 'Avram,' He said, 'there will be other days, not just math quiz days and history quiz days. Live for them, too, those days!' That's about all. 'Tomorrow will be a "math quiz day," ' our math teacher told us. 'Tomorrow will be a "history quiz day," ' our history teacher told us. Good enough! I'm glad I can turn to God and hear Him mention other kinds of days!"

I decided to question him. We were, after all, virtually within hailing distance of the Children's Hospital, where I'd trained in pediatrics and child psychiatry. I could hear the voices of my old child psychoanalyst supervisors, wondering about the 'parental superego,' as one of them often put it upon hearing one of my case presentations. I spoke to Avram as quietly and casually as possible, lest he feel I was intruding on him. I said, "Avram, do your mother and father, your parents, talk like that to you sometimes, as God did?"

He didn't rush to answer. When he did respond, he did so wordlessly, with a shake of his head. Then he offered his explanation: "My mom is nice to me, but she wants me to do well. Her idea of what I should do at nine or ten or later is this: 'Avram, when you think you've learned all you can, go to bed and get a good night's sleep; then you'll be rested and do better in the morning.' My dad would say something else, like: 'Avram, keep working until you've got it all down cold. Sleep is important — but you can always catch up on it later! The best way is to prepare in advance, but if you can't, you can't, or if you didn't, you didn't — but hell, get through with it and do a good job!' "

He smiled at the way in which he had captured both the content and the delivery of each parent: the mother's affectionate concern, the father's not so subtle encouragement to go out there and win, win. Like many other children, Avram had managed to combine aspects of both his parents and fashion his own quite distinct personality, and to construct with their help his own moral viewpoint: one does the best one can, one works hard, but one keeps one's overall perspective — three themes I've heard him bring up repeatedly. Avram asked me to remember what he'd told me a moment before, God's words to him. "You see, the God of Israel isn't pushing me in the same direction my parents are. When I hear God talking, I realize He's different, lots different. I don't hear people talk like Him. I've asked my folks about that. My mom says, 'Of course He's different; He's God, not you or me.' My dad says the same, but he'll say, 'God understands if we can't be perfect, the way He wants us to be. He understands it takes time to know how to honor Him in the right way.' Dad can be pretty caught up in his business, even on weekends. It kills him to have to work on the Sabbath, but sometimes he'll just have to. Dad says God puts everything in the right perspective, but I'm not sure God's perspective is my dad's or mine. Our rabbi talks a lot about that — how we try to make God a partner in our businesses, and it's wrong, and how we think of God when we need Him, and we forget Him otherwise, and that's the worst, because it's taking Him for granted, and He should be on our minds as much as possible, and not just when it's convenient for us. When I pray and God's words come to me, I feel I've at least remembered what the rabbi said, and I'm at least trying."

I began to realize that this boy had most certainly found for himself an uncommon voice, perhaps a preternatural one — that was about as far as the skeptical listener in me dared go. For Avram it was a supernatural voice, one from the Lord himself, mediating his language, his family life, his situation as a twentieth-century American living in a well-to-do, well-educated, mostly Jewish, East Coast neighborhood. At no time did Avram claim to be addressed by God as Moses and Isaiah were. To be sure, He *is* that very same God who spoke to the Jews of centuries ago. He is the God of Time as well as Place. Nor did Avram want to fit God conveniently into the requirements of a contemporary life. This was a young *Conservative* Jew, but he was studying at Brookline High School, not in a yeshiva.

A year later, after his bar mitzvah, he wondered what God's message would be to him had he gone to Israel, as a cousin had, and been educated in the Orthodox Jewish tradition. This prompted me to ask him whether he thought God's "voice" might then be a good deal different. He answered, "Yes, I'm sure," and we both reflected in silence for ten or fifteen seconds. Then Avram said, "If you are the Father of your people, you have to speak to them so they can understand you. It's each one of us He'll talk with, if we give Him a chance. I talk with my friends differently, depending which one I'm with; that's what you do.

God must speak every language there is. I guess He does." He was groping a bit. He didn't want to turn God into a relativist or an opportunist, but he very much wanted to regard Him as marvelously, miraculously able to hear those individual souls who over the centuries had called to Him, who had prayed with all their energy and hope that He would hear. It was at such moments that Avram and I fell into a silence that lasted long enough for us to know that we had exhausted the subject.

For an eleven-year-old Catholic girl, Anne, who lived not so many miles from Avram — in West Roxbury, another suburb of Boston — nighttime prayers were also of great importance, though for her God's voice did not usually stir anguished self-scrutiny. "I get on my knees beside the bed," Anne told me once (I thought immediately of Avram standing at prayer near his window, head bowed), and then she briskly waved aside all further detail: "I say my prayers, and I hop into bed, and the next thing you know, it's morning, and I can tell by the smell of coffee that my mum is up and 'cooking with gas.' " Her mother was as energetic as that descriptive phrase implied — in fact, the family stove used electricity — and Anne tried constantly to act like her mother, even when praying: do what has to be done, and then get on with the next of life's assignments. She was a reasonably good sixth-grade student when I started getting to know her, and an excellent athlete. She thought at the time that it would be "fantastic" if she could be "an Olympic swimmer" someday, but more realistically she dreamt of being a nun, or maybe, if she got good science grades later on, a physician. Her mother had been "trained as an RN, but gave it all up for us." There were five of "us" — Anne was second oldest. Her father was a high school athletic coach and student counselor. His sister, also named Anne, became a nun, but left the order she had joined after almost a decade. A great-uncle was a priest who died in an automobile accident just after celebrating his twenty-fifth year in the Jesuit order.

"I say my prayers a lot," Anne informed me as I was learning about her life, including her religious habits. She went on: "I pray before I go to breakfast, and I pray before I go to sleep, that's twice a day. We all say a quick prayer before meals — 'not too long,' Mum always says to Daddy, because she wants us to 'eat up,' and then we're the ones who clean up, and she collapses in front of the TV. She's going all day until then!"

On the other hand, Anne had seen her mother, every once in a while, "stop everything" and sit down on a favorite living room chair in order to hold her rosary beads, say her prayers, or even "just sit there," itself a noticeable event for her children, all of whom commented on her vigorous, high-gear style of running a home, not to mention doing myriad volunteer jobs: "Mum raises her hand whenever someone calls for help, and she's there first and leaves last," said Anne with admiration and a touch of annoyance. The reason for the latter was revealed when she admitted that the price of her mother's generosity to others was high for Anne and her sister, a year older, who look after their three brothers and their father in certain ways: "We help with the cleaning of the house. You should see their [her brothers'] rooms!"

In this conservative, traditional home, Jesus, His life, His sayings, His stated ideals, His expressed admonitions, stimulated Anne occasionally to rebellion, to outspoken dissent. She had learned, I began to notice, that Christ's outspoken challenge to "the powers that be" worked well for her as she chafed at the everyday constraints of a well-run household: "I think of Jesus when I've got so much to do, too much. He said we should follow Him, even if it means we don't do a lot of things we're supposed to do. But we get lost in all there is to get done, and we're not much thinking of Him. It's not right. I told my mum we need more time just to stop and think in this house. She said, 'Well, Annie, what would you think about, once you stopped and had all that time put aside?' I told her, I said, 'I'd think of Jesus, and how He said you should concentrate on what's important.' My mum looked up, and she said I was 'dead right,' and I think then I could have taken the whole afternoon off, if I'd have said I was going to say my prayers in my room!"

She did have moments of more prolonged, genuine piety, times when (no matter what was happening at home, for the good or for the bad) she stopped and really gave herself over to her prayers. Her aunt was the one who had taught her to do so: "Aunt Anne told me she had a 'special obligation' to me, and she would teach me how to pray, and how to listen to Jesus. She said that when things get too much for her, she finds a quiet place, and she gets on her knees and prays for Jesus to come and talk with her, and He does. I don't ask Him as much as she does, I don't think — ask Him for advice. Maybe, when I get older —" She broke off abruptly.

I asked her about those times when she did follow her aunt's lead and prayed in a more sustained manner. She said: "I go into the sunroom [a small den at the back of the house's second floor, filled with plants, a couch, a small desk and chair] and I look out the window — up at the sky. If I stare long enough, sometimes, a funny thing happens: it almost looks like Jesus is up there — the clouds look like a man. He's not really there — in the clouds, I mean. He's in heaven. I don't know where that is, but I do wonder, yes. I don't get down and pray in the sunroom; I just sit and think of Jesus. It's quiet there. I do what my aunt said I should do: I just think of Him, and I talk to Him. It's not like my regular prayers. It's like — well, I'll say, 'Dear Jesus, I'm a little tired, and I can feel myself getting moody, and I'm not being "charitable," the way they tell you in Sunday school to be, like You were, and so, please, if You can, help me.' Sometimes I'll just get up and go back where I was, and that's that. Other times I'll close my eyes and I'll picture Him. He looks like He does in our Sunday school books, and He might speak. He might say, 'Anne, you've got to think of others, and not just yourself. Anne, even if your mother is pushing you a lot, you've got to help out.' But He'll be kind, and I get the feeling He's on my side; He understands what I'm going through!"

Whose voice was this? More precisely, whose voice did Anne believe she was hearing? I asked, "When you were just talking, you told me you were getting some helpful advice from Jesus. Was He the one talking to you when you were in the sunroom that afternoon?"

"He was," she answered, and then right away she added, "But He wasn't." She elaborated briefly: "He did speak to me, and I saw Him — pictured Him. But I don't know if it was Him, really. My aunt says He comes to you, visits you, so I guess that's what happens." I asked about His voice, His way of speaking. She hadn't thought about that. She looked down at the floor and thought — and thought and thought. I was ready to ask something else, just to break our silence. But at last Anne looked up, told me she'd been "eliminating" people, one after the other, and she couldn't come up with anyone, though maybe "there's a little of my aunt in the way He talks, but it's a man's voice, so it's not her all the way, no." Her mother, her dad, her grandparents? No, not them, for sure. A teacher? A priest? "Maybe a *little* like our priest, but He wasn't the priest mainly, no."

I asked her about the content of the remarks, their possible similarity to statements she had heard elsewhere. She drew a blank. She decided I needed a lecture. "Dr. Coles," she began. She looked down toward the floor again, and I braced myself. Her eyes lifted and her mouth opened and her voice started again. "Jesus answers our prayers, if we keep praying and we deserve it. I'm not boasting. Maybe He's not happy with me a lot of the time! But if I do pray and He does answer — then it's *Him*, He's the one I'm seeing, and He's the one I'm hearing. Don't you think?"

That last question puzzled me. Why had she asked it? She seemed a trifle irritated with me, as if I didn't really believe her, or rather as though I were denying her reality, rendering the experience merely "psychological." I felt slightly uneasy. Further, I found myself comparing her with Avram. Why was it that when I explored this same territory with him, I felt more relaxed, and things went so much better? Because Avram was a more subtle psychologist and theologian? How could I know? As of that moment I had spent much less time with Anne than with Avram. Perhaps I was failing to do justice to her (apparently) less self-examining spiritual life. Perhaps Anne had asked me what I thought as a way of telling me that, like all of us, she had her skeptical side. In a sense, her willingness to ask that question was itself a measure of the very subtlety I had been inclined to deny her.

Meanwhile, a child had asked for my opinion, having shared a personal religious event with me, and I began to realize that my mind's turning away from Anne at this moment had to do with my own difficulty. What *was* I to think of this "religious experience" — how should I, as a listening doctor, not to mention as a fellow human being, regard it? What was I to say with respect to her assertion "It's *Him*, He's the one I'm seeing, and He's the one I'm hearing"?

I hesitated. Anne had no intention, however, of letting me off the hook. She sat there and looked right at me. I said, "I don't know what to think, Anne," after which — such evasiveness! — I immediately contradicted myself: "Many children have told me stories like yours. They've seen God as they think about Him, and they've heard Him, too. He has come to them, and they are grateful."

I wasn't at all satisfied with what I'd said; it was too formal and detached, a research summary rather than a response to a confiding girl's request. As I heard myself, I began to realize why Anne had, in a way, provoked me. She had expressed a certain unselfconsciousness in her spiritual life, and then, for my benefit, perhaps, she had implicitly questioned that aspect of her experience; moreover, she had asked me to offer sanction, either to the religious unselfconsciousness or to the secular skepticism. Immersed in a psychological study, mindful of moments in my own life not unlike the ones she (and Haroon and Avram) had described, I felt torn, maybe cornered, and thus irritated. With Haroon I could act the somewhat aloof observer and listener; with Avram I became the intellectual who savored these somewhat mystical moments; but with Anne I felt, for some reason, on the spot.

A tactful, kind girl, she released me graciously from my impasse: "I'm sure grateful when I hear Jesus speaking. It's real helpful. I can remember what He's said later, when I need to remember. I can be calm then, and not goof up!" It sounded a bit sticky with sentimentality: were these merely rote satisfactions reminiscent of the evangelical testimonies on Sunday television? Or was the child trying hard to garner enough strength to get on with life as best she could?

She made plain her struggle weeks later as we continued our discussions. "The priest says we should get to know Jesus. I wanted to raise my hand, right there in church, and ask him how we're supposed to do that. But I was afraid to — I'd never have the nerve! I asked Mum and Daddy later; they said you pray, you keep praying. I asked my aunt; she said the same thing. It's true, you must pray; but Jesus hears prayers from

everyone, and I hope He answers all our prayers, but you'd have
to understand if He didn't! Some days I pray a lot, a whole lot,
but I don't know if Jesus has heard me. There must be others
who have worse troubles. Like Daddy says: we have a nice home,
and two cars, and all we want to eat, and the place we go to
during the summer [on Cape Cod]. So what's there to complain
of? I guess others should be the ones for God to visit."

Such generous self-effacement, coupled with a charming humility and an ever-present gratitude for life's favors, was, nevertheless, not sufficient to quell Anne's outbursts of loneliness,
moodiness, even fearfulness. "I hear the priest tell us to be better,
to try to be better, and I feel worse! I don't like my [homeroom]
teacher this year. She's got a bad temper. She likes the boys, not
us girls. She's not married — and she likes the boys! That's not
nice, to talk like that. My mother says we should sew up our
mouths. I try to, but things slip out! I look at the picture of Jesus
[in her room] and wonder how He could be so nice to everyone!
He's God, that's how. Lots of time I don't feel nice at all. I'm on
a 'hate tear,' my aunt says. Not really; I like most people — most
of the time. To tell the truth, [I like] everyone but that teacher.
I never like her!

"When I start praying, and when Jesus does answer, when He
tells me that I've got it good, and I should stop and take it easy
and try to put on a smile with people, and not turn my head
away from them — that's when I'm all better, and the day seems
sunny again. Rain has been pouring on my whole life — that's
how I feel — a real heavy rain, and I'm wet and shaking, but
then the clouds just go away, and it's warm and I can hear those
words the priest says, and the ones my aunt says, and I've learned
them: 'I am the light of the world; if you follow Me, you won't
walk in darkness, but you'll have the light of life.' I hear that,
when I hear Him, when I pray to Him as hard as I can, and I
need to hear Him, and I do."

I have included here remarks scattered over a month's time,
an abridgment of the girl's continuing attempt to convey the
meaning God had for her as she went from day to day. The
culminating thoughts were difficult for her to put into words,
and by then (I'd known her over a year) I found them strangely
affecting. I was still, of course, trying with Anne, as I had with

Haroon and Avram, to understand God's voice as she heard it, to gain some sense of its origin in her life. I had come to be a little less psychologically skeptical when I heard the affirmation, at once solemn and casual, that Anne made to me — the poignant quote she offered me from St. John. Her face lit up as she spoke those Gospel words about light that she'd been hearing.

As I look over my notes now and try to make sense of what I have heard, I worry that sometimes I deny the children I have met a capacity for gullibility or superstitiousness. Surely, Anne in particular has often gone through a sort of quick-fix routine — conjured up a spell of listening, supposedly, to Jesus, then returned to her busy life, as she herself has acknowledged: "I mustn't be in a hurry when I pray, really pray. There are the fast prayers, and I don't think they're very good. It's when I can go to my room and settle on my knees and stay there and *talk* with God, not just try to get something out of Him — it's then that I'm on the right track and not turning my prayers into a joke."

With such self-arraignments she spoke to satisfy an outsider's critical ear but also declared her membership in a confessional religious community that has extended over continents, centuries, and denominations — a community that includes children. Here is one final moment with Anne — her story about an encounter with Jesus when she had just turned thirteen: "I had a whole afternoon free. We were going to Brewster [on Cape Cod] later that evening, when Daddy came home. I had a terrible case of poison ivy. I was covered with it, head to toe. I felt so stupid: I know what it looks like, and I let myself forget. I tried to blame it on the dog, our poor old dog. I accused him of getting into the leaves, and I was sure I'd picked him up and caught it that way. But that's unfair. I take him for a walk, with a leash on all the time — and if it's not me, it's Mum, and she's even more careful than I am that he stay away from the poison ivy leaves. It was *me* who gave me poison ivy — and after a few days of scratching myself crazy, I remembered how I got it. It was at my friend's house, when she had the party. Too much was going on for me to bother about poison ivy!

"I went to my room that afternoon, and I was scratching, and I began crying. I felt so dumb and so lousy — and the summer was just beginning! I don't feel pretty anyway, and now this! I looked in my mirror, and I completely broke down. I just cried and cried, but I didn't want anyone to come and comfort me. I was crying, but I wasn't making any noise. I've cried other times, and the whole house has heard! That afternoon I wanted to be alone with myself — well, not completely. I wanted to talk with God. I wanted Him to listen to me. I know it was selfish of me to throw all my silly troubles at Him, but I wanted to.

"I asked God please to forgive me for being so selfish and conceited. I just stayed still, on my knees. I tried not to let a single muscle move. I could feel the poison ivy, the itch. I thought of getting up and putting on calamine [lotion], but I decided no, I will stay right here — maybe forever. For a minute I think I'd convinced myself that I'd at least stay there until that damned poison ivy went away. I bent over toward the bed, and I put my head on the mattress, the spread, and I think I must have fallen asleep. It was the strangest thing — I suddenly opened my eyes and I realized I'd had a short dream, it must have been: I was down [at] the Cape, and I was walking, but not near the ocean; maybe near this meadow I know. It was a nice day. The sun was out, but I saw a big cloud, and it began covering the sun, getting right between it and me! I looked down and there was a shadow, my shadow, and then as I was looking toward the ground, I saw poison ivy, lots and lots of it. I was ready to scream and run when I felt this hand on my shoulder, and I whirled around, and there wasn't anyone there, no one, but I heard a voice, I heard Him — I knew it was Him — saying: 'I am the light of the world,' saying my favorite words from the whole Bible. I felt so good, hearing those words. I was even ready to smile at the poison ivy instead of running away from it! That was when I came to. I was there in my bedroom, on my knees, my head on the bedcover. I just kept it there, and let my mind be still. I remembered the whole dream — it must have happened fast, but it seemed like I was there [in that Cape meadow] a good long time! I felt warm inside; I felt at peace with myself. I was waiting for the poison ivy to start up again, but I just didn't care. I smiled at the thought of it; I almost dared it to try getting the better of me. I guess God's words had taught me — for a while! — what's important and what isn't."

*

Occasionally, as Anne talked of such happenings in her life, I found my mind straying: returning to work done in Brazil by my sons and me during the early 1980s,[2] or to work done by my wife and me in the South during the early 1960s — when, again and again, children told us of God's words, delivered to them by day and by night. I have written about some of those children, and was able, back then, simply to accept the contact they felt they had with Jesus, with the Lord. With these three children — Haroon, Avram, and Anne — I seem to have become a bit more anxious. Perhaps, when I was far away from the scene of my psychiatric training and mainly interested in other aspects of children's lives — such as the poverty those Brazilian or Southern children experienced, or their political thinking — I would hear them out without yielding to psychiatric insistence about the "voices" they heard. Now that I was formally engaged in a *study* of the religious and spiritual side of childhood, I felt obliged to be observant first and thereafter as analytical as possible — especially with children like Avram and Anne, who live in the middle-class New England world that was and is my home. Yet Anne did, indeed, prompt my mind to turn backward to earlier work; most often she nudged me toward Rio de Janeiro's *favelas*, and in particular to one girl, who was ten, a year Anne's junior, when I was living in Brazil. After a while I went back to look at my Brazilian notes and listen to my Brazilian tapes rather than to keep worrying about the question of Anne's "voices" and the reasons, personal and professional, for my response to those voices.

Here, then, is young Margarita, whose life is contained by a *favela* and its terrible suffering and humiliations; who regards the Catholic Church, as she has known it — a small chapel stands at the base of the *favela* where she lives — with no affection at all, quite the contrary. These assertions by an uneducated but outspoken and often unforgettably eloquent girl are gathered from many talks: "When I look at Jesus up there [the well-known statue of Him, arms extended, that stands on a hill and overlooks Rio] I wonder what He is thinking. He can see all of us, and He must have an opinion [about us]. I try to talk with Him. When I am most upset, He is all that I have. My mother is sick. She still works in Copacabana [as a maid in a hotel], even though she coughs, and she bleeds. [She had tuberculosis and died soon thereafter.] She is all we have — and Him. [She points to the statue.] A lot of time I ask Him why He does things like this. [She moves her right hand across an arc, encompassing the *favela* where her family lives.] He must see what we see, Copacabana and Ipanema [wealthy parts of the city] — and then this place. Mother used to tell us we'll go to heaven, because we're poor. I used to believe her. I don't think she really believes herself. She just says that — it's a way of shutting us all up when we're hungry! Now, when I hear her say it, I look up at Him, and I ask Him: What do *You* say, Jesus? Do You believe her? Do You believe the priest who says the same thing? Do You notice that big car he drives, and do You notice that big house he has? This is a priest who spends most of his time with the rich, and they give him some extra *cruzeiros* to go pray for us once a week. What do You think of him — and of his rich friends? Don't forget them, dear Jesus, when you're looking us over and making Your decisions [as to who gets into heaven]!

"I shouldn't blame Jesus! I do, though, sometimes. He's right there — that statue keeps reminding me of Him — and the next thing I know, I'm talking with Him, and I'm either upset with Him or I'm praying for Him to tell me why the world is like it is."

Margarita wasn't anxious to stick to the subject. She preferred talking about her mother's health (a doctor friend of mine eventually got her admitted to a hospital, but too late); or to talk about her hopes for the future — to get a job as a salesclerk in a Copacabana store. But in the midst of those talks she did come back often enough to the statue of Jesus, so that I once tried to explore the matter carefully. She did, finally, tell me in detail of her dialogue with God, and I well remember how her face lit up, how wide-eyed she seemed, as she talked of it: "When I'm at my lowest, and I look into the future and see us all [her four younger sisters and two older brothers] alone, with Mother gone, I want to scream. I get angry at Him. I go and tell Him off: 'Why are you going to take her? What has she done to deserve death? Don't tell me — as the priest does — that she'll go to heaven! All of us here can't eat off our mother's life in heaven! Have you asked her what *she* wants? You know how to do that,

if You want to! You can talk with us when You decide You have
something to say! They keep telling us [in church] about all the
miracles: You've shown up all over, so You can show up here.
Or are we not good enough! That's what a lot of Your priests
and nuns think, the people in Your church: they suck up to the
rich, all the time. And they live like the rich — in big homes,
with big cars parked outside. We know! We see! My aunt works
for an Ipanema family; she sees pictures of our bishop having
a love-time with that family. You know who that man is [the head
of the family where her aunt works], You know what he does —
and You let your biggest bishop here hold hands with him!
Shame!"

For the first time, my doctor friend, a pediatric surgeon, who
was translating, intervened; he was worried by the girl's anger,
and a bit shocked, too, I began to realize, as he told me how
"surprised" he was by her vehemence. We had a long discussion
about it in English. He, a devout Catholic, expressed his alarm
for the girl's spiritual life while I slipped into the child psychiatrist's mode of analysis: listen, this girl is terribly frightened
and sad; her mother may soon die; her father is long gone; the
family is desperately at risk, and so her rage is not only under-
standable but much better expressed than pushed aside — covered, for example, by gestures of piety. But there was a limit,
the Brazilian doctor told me, and besides, the girl wasn't really
angry at Jesus. I agreed and made the usual psychiatric avowal:
in time, let us hope — with more talk — we will "help" her to
realize the scapegoating, the "displacement" at work in these
religious tirades.

Margarita and I resumed our talk. Her anger persisted for a
few minutes, and she spoke in a way (and with words) I knew I
would never be able to repeat in articles or books. I was getting
ready to try to distance her and me and the translator from that
anger when she happened to notice something above us in the
darkening midafternoon sky: "See! It's already raining, over
there." She turned fully around, her back now to the ocean, and
surveyed the heavens: "See, lightning! Listen!"

We heard the thunder. Margarita's gaze was fixed on the sky:
more lightning, more thunder, a roll of it, as if the whole city
of Rio de Janeiro were its object. We were high on a hill — as

with many other *favelas*, the one Margarita lived in offered a commanding view of the entire metropolitan area — and while we watched and listened she pointed: more coming. Now and then she paid attention to the city itself, the shadows over this part, the dramatic light that suddenly descended. But her eyes kept returning to the origin of the storm: "You see, there is action up there. He doesn't only sit and suffer; He walks and He talks — He lets us know what He can do when He wants to! He must laugh at that statue sometimes." She turned toward the statue and started scorning it, in language occasionally blasphemous. I didn't need my doctor friend to translate; by then I could tell, more or less, what she was saying as her face expressed, in turn, wry amusement, fierce scornfulness, heated indignation.

At a certain moment, unwittingly, I shut off the tape recorder. She immediately turned toward me, toward it: "Why did you do that?" I told her — a half truth — that I didn't have all that many blank tapes, and I was here to talk about *her*, not Jesus, not the Catholic Church, not the winter storm, beautiful as it was. She then argued with me, and, because I realized she was right, I turned the machine back on: "You two should be knocking on the door of the priest's house and asking him why he eats so well [he is a bit overweight] when my little sister [she is a year old] is always crying, because she doesn't get enough food! I hope Jesus sees everything that goes on here. I hope He doesn't just stare into the ocean, like that statue! If you want to know about us in this place, ask Him. Maybe He'll answer you."

She stopped abruptly: more lightning and thunder. She was excited by it and, I noticed, silenced. Thunder and lightning now became our common ground: a fireworks display that enforced silence and elicited full attention. Only when the skies began to quiet down did the alert, sometimes truculent girl turn her face back toward us: "When I talk with Him, I ask Him why He doesn't knock down that statue. Why should He be locked up in it, like someone in jail? I suppose it's nice for a lot of people; they've got Jesus just where they want Him, in the concrete up that hill! I'd rather have Him way up there, way above the clouds, standing on the moon, or a star, maybe, throwing lightning and pounding His table with His hands — thunder in case we don't see what He's done! I'd rather have Him send a flood of rain down the slopes of our *favela* so that the priest's car won't start. Then he'll have to walk, as my mother does, or take the bus, as she does. Then that 'cooler' in his car won't work anymore. At least Jesus is up there, under the sun all the time. No 'cooler' for Him! It must be plenty hot for Him in the summer, around Mardi Gras [in February]. I've asked Him about the weather, but He won't say anything, not on that score!"

By now I was ready to pick up on what I realized, in retrospect, had been a repeated invitation to discuss her religious and spiritual life. "What *does* He speak about?" I asked her — a question I might have posed weeks earlier.

She was ready with an answer. "He'll say something to me at odd times. When I leave [the shack where she lived] to go on a walk and tell Him what's on my mind, He doesn't give me the time of day. If I shout, He shuts up. If I tell Him how much I love Him, He won't blink — no sounds. But if I'm really in low spirits and not thinking of Him — thinking of myself, and worrying what will happen to us, what will happen *next* to us — it's then that He takes me by surprise, completely. I hear Him and He'll say: 'Margarita, you are looking too far ahead. First, try to get to the evening, the sunset; then try to get to the morning, the sunrise.' When I hear Him, I feel calmer. Oh, I'm not totally persuaded. Listen, who knows what can happen between the time the sun goes down and the moon comes up — never mind the time between the sun setting and the sun rising! But hearing Him gives me everything to hold on to. I think I go walking to try to find some strength, and just when I give up, He's there. He tells me to remember His own life — it was full of trouble. I try to remember what He said, and I try to remember what His life was like: we used to hear about it in church, when mother took us. She stopped [going] a year or two ago. When I hear Jesus talking to me, I wish I knew more of Him. I'm ready to go back to church — once or twice. The priest doesn't seem so bad then. He used to tell us all we should be patient, we should be patient! Over and over! God has a better way of addressing us!"

This monologue did not come flooding out. There were interruptions, distractions, silent moments, questions from me, and more weather troubles, a strong wind that put the fragile shacks on the hills in jeopardy. But by the evening I had heard a sentence here, a phrase there, that touched and stirred me. Her speech was blunt, slangy, quite powerful in its down-to-earth canniness. (Translation is always a problem in such encounters, of course.) Her interest in God, I realized much later, was far more important than I allowed myself to notice at the time. The listening she did to God turned out to be the mainstay of her life. His voice uplifted her spirits when nothing else could. To her, His voice was *sui generis* — not that of anyone she knew, certainly not the priest's; and yet I gradually discovered a certain resemblance between the thrust of his comments, his homilies, and what she heard God say in His moments of expressed concern for her.

She did not take the priest's words and put them in her imagined Christ's mouth. Nor did she hear the priest's voice as that of Jesus. On the contrary, she tried hard — and ultimately in vain — to set the two against each other: Jesus as an outsider, and as an opponent of the rich and powerful; the priest as a hopelessly flawed supplicant of money and privilege. Still, she knew that this might not be the whole story. There he was, bringing food and clean drinking water and medicine to some of her fellow *favelados*, even though he also spent time in Copacabana and Ipanema and drove in a comfortable (but not extravagant) car, a Brazilian-made Ford. As Margarita once said angrily, he was not Jesus. She didn't expect him to be Jesus, but she wanted Jesus badly in her life, knowing, I suspect, that only a miracle of the Lord would have a chance of reversing her fate and that of her family.

When the priest's humanity gradually revealed itself to her — she who was growing up and learning day by day just how complicated and unyielding life can be — she found it tempting to go after him with vehemence. After she did, however, I noticed that she made amends: she would recall one of his kind gestures; she would grant him a pleasant smile, a friendly manner; and, very important, she would find some charity in her heart for him, say out loud what she surely knew within, that the corrupt wealth her mother as a hotel maid had seen in Copacabana was not the priest's doing, for sure, and not his preference, either.

He begged from "them," she once admitted, to give to her and those like her. When she raged, she had contempt for him; when she was calmed by God's voice, she pitied him, even respected him for his efforts, and at times of meditative perspective and deep feeling, she held him up as one of the few decent people she ever had met.

I knew this priest, Father Ricardo, and had heard him often talk of the *favela* where Margarita lived. He knew of the girl's outbursts against him; her aunt, a faithful parishioner, had reported them to him. Not interested in or conversant with contemporary psychodynamic psychiatry, he still knew how useful those rages were to Margarita and others; he saw the importance of having an outlet for all that resentment and frustration. But he also knew that for this girl, and others, he had come to mean something positive, too: "She is so polite to me; I can see her struggling to smile, even though she has no reason in life to be happy now. Her lower lip will tremble just a bit: the holy anger of Christ in the temple is ready to pour forth! But she holds the tide back until she can be away from me — and later I hear of the tirade!"

Once, as we talked of the girl's love of Jesus, her daily search for His vocal presence, fleeting though it was, I could not resist playing the didactic psychiatrist. I assured the priest that Margarita was troubled and troubling, but, after a fashion, quite solid and sound, not to mention unusually bright and perceptive. He responded initially by lamenting the tragedy — such a smart and forceful person, headed nowhere fast. If only, if only . . . his voice trailed off while his right hand reached for the crucifix worn around his neck. But he did not continue with that refrain and recite how many he knew like Margarita; rather, he took me up on my psychological assessment: "Oh, yes, I know she has her wits about her, I'm sure of that. She'd be in much worse shape if she didn't stick her finger in my face every once in a while, and tell our Church how far it has to go to be worthy of Him — and of her!"

I found that statement, especially those last three words, almost unbearably poignant. I sat there, glad to have a Coca-Cola to lift and put down, lift and put down. He seemed caught in a reverie, and I had nothing more to say. Soon his housekeeper, who lived in the *favela* near Margarita's family, was ready for us to have a meal, and we moved to the dining table and did our eating amid more talk about various *favelado* children I'd been meeting, including, again, Margarita. At one point, as we talked about her interest in the statue of Christ, about her conversations with Jesus, I once again commented on the strangeness to me of such an interior experience on the part of a child. "Jesus doesn't talk to the children you treat in Boston?" he asked. "No, father, not really," I replied. "Too bad," he said. Now I summoned my medical concerns and threw in a few philosophical and theological ones: what *were* we to make of all this, if Margarita (and some others) kept hearing those voices of God as they got older? Hysteria? Auditory hallucinations? A scandal to the Church and its institutional life? Primitive, uneducated thinking? Superstition? I didn't spell all that out, but in a glance he let me know he knew the litany that was occurring to me; it was written on my face. He chose to break our silence with this: "Oh, I think God does His work in many ways. All things come from Him, we are told in seminary, so with a child like Margarita I'm sure He wants a way to reach her — and I guess He has found one." Now, nearly a decade later, all the research done and examined, I'm not much further along than I was that suppertime with Father Ricardo in his home at the foot of a Brazilian *favela*.

❊ ❊ ❊

5

Young Spirituality:
Psychological Themes

IN HER LATE SEVENTIES, looking back at more than half a
century of work with children, Anna Freud[1] was remarkably
candid about the limits of psychoanalytic inquiry: "We have our
own interests to pursue. Yes, we let the children set the agenda,
as we do with adults when we ask them to tell us what comes to
mind. But our patients come to us because something has gone
wrong, something isn't working well, and we have learned how
to figure out why things don't work. I remember a boy who at
ten knew more about computers than I would ever know. He
was brilliant and very talkative. He wanted to spend our time
together talking about science — computers and their ability to
sort out information. I tried to follow him; I noted that he
wanted — he needed — a conversational friendship with me.
(His parents were scholarly and had little time for him and, I'd
learned, little time for each other.) At one point he and I had
quite a time because I had to tell him that psychoanalysis is not
meant to be an exploration of the intellect! Well, he asked right
away: How about the soul? Not the soul either, I had to tell him.
If I'd asked him what he meant by the soul — as I might have,
if I had been working with a different child — he'd have been
all too happy to engage me in a discussion of that subject for
many weeks! I was trying to tell that boy what I've had to explain
to some of my adult analysands — that we [psychoanalysts] do
know something about the emotions, and we are interested in
'normality' as well as 'pathology,' but we are not to be confused

with intellectual companions or discussants, or with philosophers who are trying to discover 'answers to life.' "

She had a wry tone in her voice as she spoke that last sentence, and her face showed a thin, momentary smile. Lurking in the background of her narrative was the issue of "resistance" — the manner in which anyone in analysis explores various ways not to deal with certain subjects. We try to distract both ourselves and our doctors, because the closer we get to our rock-bottom troubles, the more anxious and fearful we are likely to get — a truism, by now, of how an analytical patient finds himself or herself attracted to "rather too inviting digressions," as Miss Freud put it. Not that she disclaimed an interest in some of those "digressions." She had read widely, and was especially interested in poetry; she also had an idealistic side that could prompt an engagement with social and political problems. But she was wary and modest when she contemplated the application of psychoanalytic thinking to other intellectual activities.

On the other hand, she was both interested and encouraging to me so long as I planned to do research in the psychoanalytic tradition. "You won't be 'treating' those children; you'll be asking them to be your teachers, to help you learn. You will no doubt discover that they have many psychological matters to discuss, indirectly more often than directly. Biblical stories will have become their own stories — but which ones for which children, and why? At other moments you'll be further afield [from psychoanalytic child psychiatry]; you'll be having talks about philosophy and theology — and children can hold up rather well, sometimes, in those kinds of discussions, provided the adult doesn't assume too little of the child being interviewed."

Again, she evinced her shrewd, tactful way of being encouraging yet guarded. She knew how daunting it can be to sit, with a particular line of questioning in mind, in a room before a child, only to find an utter lack of interest on the part of the boy or girl, whose politeness or charm conceals detachment from adults trying to press matters too urgently. She also knew that other children can be rather too obliging and forthcoming — ready in an instant, it seems, to grab at whatever direction is offered by a teacher, a doctor, someone who comes armed with questions, paper, pencils, crayons. She reminded me at great length that

day, drawing confessionally on her failures as well as her successes, how important it would be, in a study of young spirituality, to set aside my preconceptions and let the children "do
with the opportunity what they will." She was espousing once
more her well-known conviction that "direct observation" ought
to precede the theoretical classifications that characterize what
she called "a later stage" of research. I can still hear that marvelous phrase of hers, her confidence that boys and girls would
indeed "do with the opportunity what they will" — share what
sense (if any) they make out of life. "I often think," Miss Freud
went on, "that we must work harder conceptually with our research data when we are at our desks writing than we do when
we are sitting with the children and asking our questions of
them." She paused and then added a delightful explanation:
"Perhaps it is because then [when we are writing up our work]
they are not there to help us!" I loved hearing those words at
the time, loved seeing her smile, her eyes awake and lively; and
I have remembered them while writing this chapter.

Children try to understand not only what is happening to them,
but why; and in doing that, they call upon the religious life they
have experienced, the spiritual values they have received, as well
as other sources of potential explanation. My first awareness of
religious and spiritual reflection as an aspect of a child's development came early in my residency years when I worked as a
pediatrician with children who had contracted polio amid an
epidemic in Boston during the middle 1950s, just before the Salk
vaccine became available.[2] Suddenly, hitherto healthy children
found themselves paralyzed, unable to walk or to move their
arms or even to breathe. Those afflicted with that last kind of
polio, the so-called bulbar kind (a paralysis that affected the
breathing center in the brain stem), would have died were it not
for the massive "iron lung," a dinosaur of a respirator, that we
had available at the Children's Hospital and the Massachusetts
General Hospital. A child's whole body except the head and neck
was inside one of those machines, kept alive, as one child put it,
by an electric plug.

   The hospital staff worked around the clock to take care of
them. Dozens of children were suddenly faced with the prospect

of a crippled life, a life whose very breath often could not be taken for granted. Indeed, rather quickly the children learned the score with respect to their medical prognosis — they'd gradually improve, or they wouldn't much improve. They also learned about the rehabilitation efforts they'd be making once the acute (febrile) stage of the illness had passed. Another resident and I spent long hours listening to those children; eventually we reported what we'd heard to our colleagues, and wrote up what we'd heard for professional journals. We were more than tempted, of course, to emphasize the psychiatric significance of what the children told us. Yet, as Erich Lindemann, the psychoanalyst who was chief of the psychiatric service of Massachusetts General Hospital, kept reminding us: "These are young people who suddenly have become quite a bit older; they are facing possible death, or serious limitation of their lives; and they will naturally stop and think about life, rather than just live it from day to day. A lot of what they say will be reflective — and you might respond in kind. It would be a mistake, I think, to emphasize unduly a psychiatric point of view. If there is serious psychopathology, you will respond to it, of course; but if those children want to cry with you, and be disappointed with you, and wonder with you where their God is, then you can be there for them — and help all of us here in the hospital."

His advice may strike the reader as the purest of common sense, yet we eager young doctors were all too interested in medical and psychiatric pathology. Still, Dr. Lindemann, who had achieved a national reputation when a serious nightclub fire in Boston caused hundreds to die and others to suffer terrible burns, knew something we would only gradually discover: that when people suddenly lose a loved one or lie in a hospital in great pain, they may not so much become undone as become aroused psychologically — prompted to look with the utmost intensity at their past life, their present condition, and their future prospects, if any. Under such circumstances, psychological themes connect almost imperceptibly, but quite vividly at moments, with a spiritual inwardness.

In those days recording conversations was possible, but I cringe as I remember the large, awkward machines we lugged around. I was embarrassed one day as I asked a boy of eleven, an "iron-lung patient," as we called him, for permission to record our conversation. I was acutely aware of how slim his hold on life was. He surprised me: "Please record every word I speak. I may be dead tomorrow, and this would be a chance for my words to outlive me!"

Soon we were having daily conversations, beyond our medical exchanges. Tony was of Catholic background, the son of a Boston civil servant, a good athlete, and the oldest of four children. He had been waking up with nightmares. He would pull a cord, immediately summon the nurse, and tell her he was dying, he knew it. Each time, after a careful check of his vital signs, she found nothing amiss. Two nights in a row, however, she called me, as a necessary precaution. By the third night we had begun to write this phrase on his chart: "[needs] psychiatric consult." By the fifth night I *was* that "consult," and by the next afternoon we were having the first of what Tony would eventually term our "regular meetings."

He didn't easily let go of the significance of that tape recorder; he let me know that his anxieties, his nightmares, deserved from me a kind of comprehension he worried I might not summon. His speaking had a didactic thrust, I began to notice a bit uneasily; it seemed that this paralyzed schoolboy athlete, this able student, felt misunderstood by me and others who were working hard to be of help. One afternoon, with the sun shining on us out of a cloudless, brisk October sky, Tony took note of the weather, us doctors and nurses, and his short, now eventful life: "I could be there [in parochial school] playing football, basketball. I could be doing math, my favorite subject. Why me? How did this happen? What did I do? That's all I do, ask these questions. I figure, there must be someone to answer them! God is the one, my mom says, but can He hear each one of us? I wonder. I've got so much time — to think and think, and ask these questions. When I go to sleep, I have these scary dreams. I'm in a car — my cousin's — and he's driving, and we're going faster and faster, and I can see that we're going to crash, and I shout, 'Joey, Joey, put on the brakes,' but he doesn't, and I hold on to my rosary beads, and I figure: Jesus, here we come! Then I look, and there's no one in the driver's seat, and I don't know what to do. I can't drive! I try to, though — I move into Joey's seat and hold the wheel, and I reach down with my right foot for the brake, but my foot doesn't work, and the car keeps going, and I can see the edge, the edge of the hill, and below, there are all these cars, that have crashed, gone off, and that's when I wake up, and I'm wondering where I am. I mean, am I here in the hospital, or is it someplace where you meet God, and He decides what'll happen to you?

"The nurse keeps saying [each time he woke up, night after night, shouting] I'll be all right, and I shouldn't be scared. You say that, too. I wonder why I shouldn't be scared! I could just stop breathing — anytime. We had a blackout in the hospital yesterday. It was a lightning storm. All right — they had extra juice, emergency juice, for our machines; they told us not to worry. But what if the 'auxiliary power' went on the blink and these machines just pooped out? Then what? You folks ought to climb into one of these things, and see how it feels! Like a prison — only you can't walk up and down the cell, and you can't even breathe without the machine doing it for you! That's what I ask: OK, God, I must have done something to deserve this! Tell me!"

A long silence. For the first time I imagined myself lying on my back inside an iron lung. I already felt claustrophobic in that small ward room. I found myself wondering: Why are you doing this kind of work? Why are you taking these risks? What would you do if you got polio? What would you do if you knew you might die soon? We'd all volunteered to do extra rotations, and I had the absurd notion that if I kept willing it, I could stay well and keep up the pace I'd maintained already for three weeks. Tony, however, knew better about how life works, and interrupted my worried reverie: "When I heard there was a polio epidemic, I said, 'Too bad, someone will get sick.' It's never you! That's how you think: *someone else!* Now it's me; I'm the 'somebody else.' Everyone comes to see me. My mom would sleep right there [at the foot of the iron lung] if you folks would let her. My dad is so broken up by this, he comes here, and he's crying all the time he's here, so my mom has to take him home, and then she comes back alone; but I tell her to go back, because Dad can't cook, and my grandma is sick, and the kids [his younger sisters and brother] need her. She says *I* need her; but

I don't. I'm not kidding! I need God to save me! In that dream, that's what I decide: Tony, you can't save yourself, and there's no one here to save you — because Joey is gone — so you're in God's hands. He'll keep you alive, or you'll go visit Him — fast!"

Tony needed no help from me in interpreting that recurrent nightmare. It told of his lonely, recent travel through time and space to the very edge of things; it told of his brave, desperate struggle to gain control of what life he had, to master a machine which might well, he knew, be his last "home" before he died. His cousin, Jocy, seventeen, had always been his hero: "He's the kind of person I wanted to be. He's captain of the football team [in a Catholic high school], and he's a real good student. He wants to go to B.C. [Boston College] or Holy Cross. He comes to see me, and I can see he's scared, and I know he's trying not to show it, but it's natural. I'd be frightened to death if I came here to see *him!* Well, I'm not frightened to death now! I could be dead any day, and I know it. The priest came and he said he's praying for me, and everyone is, but I'm not sure it will help. I remember in Sunday school, we read of Job, the guy who got sick, and everyone around him got sick or died — I forget a lot of what happened — and he was fed up, real fed up. He didn't know what to make of it all, and I don't either. The priest told me I should have faith, and I hope I do, but you can have it and you'll still die, even if you're only a kid. I was praying last night, thinking of Jesus, and then I remembered — He was young when He died, and even being God, it didn't save Him from dying. I felt real low then." He had no more to say that day. His eyes filled up; I wiped them. I felt, for the first time, that Tony "might not make it," a phrase he'd been using that had prompted me to reach heights of vigorous reassurance: nonsense, he *would* make it!

I dreaded the next meeting; I'd heard beforehand that Tony had been cranky and sullen with others on the house and nursing staff. But he was thoughtful, calm, almost self-possessed, if quiet, when we talked, and he seemed to take some surprising pleasure, still, in the fact that his comments were being recorded: "They'll [his words] be around for a long time. I could be dead and people could listen to me! What if they had a machine like that in the old days — we could hear George Washington, we could hear Jesus! I guess I'm going soft in the head!"

We talked about future technology — the day when we'd be able to take "moving pictures," easily, of one another, so that we'd be able to see as well as hear people decades after they'd died. He was quite matter-of-fact during that discussion, but at the end of it, suddenly, unexpectedly, and quite softly, he said: "I pray I won't die. I'd like to live longer." He seemed so calm; but for some reason the simplicity and directness of his statement unnerved me, and I said nothing. Finally, anxious about the silence, I spoke: "You'll be fine, Tony." I had been saying words to that effect all the time during those tense, fearful weeks, but now they rang hollow. I was almost (stupidly) ready to apologize for my banal ways when Tony thanked me and allowed the first note of cautious optimism I'd heard in two weeks of knowing him: "I'm still here, so I guess maybe God has had a conference, and He's decided He might keep me 'on hold' for a while, and maybe let me hang around here, until I can die with my friends, when we all get older. I'd like to go to heaven right away, if I'd be admitted, but I've been thinking: I'd be alone there — my friends are here, and they'll stay here a long time, I hope." A quick stop for air and strength, a sip of ginger ale, and then he said, "If I stay here, if He lets me, I've told myself — well, I'll thank God every day, every single day, until I *do* die, every day!"

He slowly improved, and I well remember the day he could leave the iron lung. In a way, he was luckier than some of the other patients, whom he for a while had envied — the boys and girls who hadn't needed an iron lung but whose limbs were paralyzed, and who would remain impaired for the rest of their lives. Once he recovered fully, he was able to resume a normal life — though, of course, on that first day, when he was able to depart his captivity for only a few minutes (gradually we'd lengthen the stay "outside"), he had no sure knowledge he was on the way to a full recovery; neither did we. His remarks a week later deserve to be part of this description: "It's an illness, I know. But if I live, and be like everyone else, I'll think of it as something else. I'll think of it as God grabbing ahold of me and saying, 'Tony, you'd better watch out, and you'd better try and be as good as you can.' It's God testing me, it's been that, I guess. I hope I can get through this, and show Him I'm grateful, and I won't ever forget — forget Him."

I have no idea how Tony's life went after he left the Children's

Hospital late in November of that year, just after Thanksgiving. We had plenty of other children to keep us busy, and I had no great ambitions, more than thirty years ago, for "longitudinal research" — to stay with one's informants, one's teachers, for a long time. But this boy had gotten to me, as certain young patients do to those of us who become witnesses to their crises. He had become anxious and afraid. He had become moody and even felt bouts of panic. He had experienced terrifying nightmares. He had become — so the nurses reported — wordless and withdrawn one minute, overtalkative and full of pretended cheer the next, only to collapse in sadness when his mother tried to tell him he'd eventually survive his ordeal. Through all those psychiatric ups and downs, those medical trials, he underwent a concomitant religious trial, a spiritual challenge. He listened to his priest. He said his prayers. He held his own rosary and his mother's in his hand inside the iron lung, sometimes one in each hand. Then he stepped from religious routines to spiritual contemplation, and doubted his Catholic faith as he never had before. He identified with Job's suffering. He found himself, once, wondering quite explicitly whether the young man Jesus "really wanted to die, even if He was going to see God." He became, without question, religiously skeptical: "How can all of us here [on the ward] figure this out, according to the Church?" He went further — told the priest not to "bother" coming, told his mother he must somehow have been "excommunicated," or else why this illness that threatened to take his life?

At the same time, often minutes after he had embraced a religious ritual, or upheld — or abandoned — a religious tenet, he would ask himself and the world questions about meaning and purpose. A mysterious streak of "lousy luck," as he put it, had befallen him. To be sure, he was trying to keep on a relatively even psychological keel. Depression, however, threatened to claim him. Severe anxiety broke through, as his nightmare certainly showed. His strict conscience pushed him toward self-criticism, toward an avowal of all the small mistakes he had made in the course of a brief life. Desire taunted him: the strong legs, so used to exercise, confined to the iron box; his muscular arms, so accustomed to pushing a lawn mower, catching a football or a basketball, holding on to a bike, now stretched flat along the sides of his torso. His rational, intelligent self worked hard to keep control through stretches of humor, politeness, cooperative good cheer. His remarks often mingled psychological and religious introspection: "The priest says pray, but I don't feel like praying. My uncle [a high school athletic coach] says I should 'keep smiling,' and I'll get through it all. I try to — I get low, and then I talk myself out of it. But a lot of the time I'm thinking to myself — if you go, Tony, then where will you go to? I ask and ask. I know I'll never get the answer until I go, and I don't want to go, not until I'm as old as my grandpa! But I might, so I should be wondering, I guess. Better to wonder than just lie here and feel lousier and lousier."

A close textual reading of that child's casual account of his mental activity shows him seeking and abandoning religious practices; endeavoring to keep himself emotionally stable; and, not least, giving himself over to questions our philosophers and theologians and novelists have asked over the centuries and ordinary human beings have posed to themselves. His spirituality was, I think, evoked by the distinct possibility of death.

Months later, when I showed Dr. Lindemann my notes on what Tony had said, I tried to anticipate a psychoanalytically relentless response by embracing that approach myself. Was not this spiritual inclination, finally, a kind of psychological defensiveness? The boy himself had given us the clue in his remark that his spiritual questioning, his musing about what lay ahead, might well spare him the "lousier and lousier" time he was having emotionally. "Yes, you could say that," Dr. Lindemann said, and then, unforgettably, he added: "I suppose everything we try and do is 'defensive' in some way. So where are we? More important, how do we best understand this boy, Tony?" He went on to add the obvious — that a particular child of a particular religious background and psychological makeup had responded to a life-threatening moment in a particular intellectual and moral manner: the boy had asked searching questions about the nature of things and tried to comprehend the ineffable, the intangible, the mysterious. "Perhaps," said Dr. Lindemann, both seriously and mischievously, "we can refer to his 'defensive spirituality.' " I have thought of that phrase with the same mixture of seriousness and ironic amusement many times in recent years.

As I go over the interviews I've done with children, I find certain psychological themes recurring. I hear children (on tape) talking about their desires, their ambitions, their hopes, and also their worries, their fears, their moments of deep and terrible despair — all connected in idiosyncratic ways, sometimes, with Biblical stories, or with religiously sanctioned notions of right and wrong, or with rituals such as prayer or meditation. Indeed, the entire range of children's mental life can and does connect with their religious and spiritual thinking. Moral attitudes, including emotions such as shame and guilt, are a major psychological and sometimes psychiatric side of young spirituality. In this regard, the discourse of children rivals that of Christian saints, such as Augustine and Teresa of Avila and St. John of the Cross. Here, for instance, is Tony when he had been able to leave the iron lung and was on his way to a full recovery: "I hope I'm worth it — for God to smile and say I can stay here. I could have been a better person, I know that. I could have helped my folks out more. I've been lucky, but I'm not sure I deserve it. Maybe God just gives you a second chance. Maybe He says, 'They're young, those polio kids, and they can have another chance.'

"Why do some who get sick die, though? I know some bad things I've done. I ran away from home, and my dad, he came and got me. He told me I should be ashamed of myself — I was 'ungrateful.' When I was sick, real sick, I began to think God was saying the same thing to me — that I was 'ungrateful.' I've been 'slow to help' at home; my mom told me so a year ago, I remember. It hurt, hearing her be tough on me, but it was good, because I tried to do better. I'd pray to God: Please give me a boost, so I can be stronger.

"I sure hope I remember this iron lung for the rest of my life. I hope every time I don't do something I'm supposed to do I just stop and close my eyes and picture this lung, and me in it. Maybe then I'll pile up a better record with my folks and my friends. There are times when I get grouchy, and I don't appreciate how lucky I am to have the good friends I do [have], and my family! Jesus tells you to be kind, and think of others, not just yourself, and I wish I was better at that. When I was almost dying, I wondered what He'd think if *He* was sick and in a machine all day like I was. I guess Jesus wouldn't have been feeling sorry for himself. He'd have asked about others on the ward, not be squeezing the alarm to bring the nurses and doctors over, the way I kept doing. I wish I'd been a better patient! I feel a little ashamed now. I'll be saying my prayers, and I'll think: If Jesus didn't spot me, because He had others to help, then He won't be too disappointed with me. I pray to Him, that I'll be 'worthy,' like we do before we eat [at home]. I guess He knows everything, though. I guess you can't 'slip through His net'; my dad says that! I've done stupid things. I planted gum on a kid's seat, and he got into a fight with someone else, this guy he thought did it, and they both got into trouble with the teacher, and I didn't say anything. I did wrong. I told the priest. He didn't tell me to do anything. I think he figured it was water over the dam. But now that I'm here, and I've got all day and all night to think, I sure remember every mistake I've ever made!"

Accidents, illnesses, bad luck — such moments of danger and pain prompt reflection in children as well as adults. A boy's vulnerability becomes an occasion for prayer, for remembrance of past encounters with the clergy as well as parents, for a scrutiny of the mind and the soul. Religions are known, of course, for their insistence on upholding various moral principles and standards, for the reinforcement they offer to their adherents' consciences and to the culture of various nations. But less evident are the strategies boys and girls devise to accommodate a secular and familial morality, on the one hand, and the religious morality they hear espoused in churches, mosques, synagogues. The task for those boys and girls is to weave together a particular version of a morality both personal and yet tied to a religious tradition, and then (the essence of the spiritual life) ponder their moral successes and failures and, consequently, their prospects as human beings who will someday die.

For children, even those quite healthy and never before seriously sick, death has a powerful and continuing meaning. They hear what their elders hear in sermons and stories, in songs, in scriptural warnings. They also experience death personally when grandparents and other older people depart. I teach a fourth-grade art history course in a Cambridge public school. A picture titled *The Doctor*, by Sir Luke Fildes, a British painter (1844–1927), has each year stirred a great deal of conversation among the children. In it, a physician sits by the bed (a makeshift arrangement of chairs, actually) of an ailing child; the doctor's left hand is held to his beard-covered chin. On a table nearby, a cup and spoon are to be seen, and a bottle of medicine. The child (most likely a girl because of her longish hair) is sleeping, her left arm outstreched, her right arm on top of her chest, a blanket covering her. In the background the dim outline of a man, presumably the child's father, can be discerned. The children are unusually hushed once they see the slide of that sickbed scene, and they refrain from immediate comment. I have learned to ask nothing, to say nothing. Eventually the questions always come — inquries that, of course, make their own statements.

"That's a girl, right?" asked one talkative child. "And she's sick, right?"

"Yes."

"What's the matter with her?"

"I don't know."

"She looks very sick," that child observed, and then she asked a further question: "Do you think she'll make it?"

"The picture doesn't tell us, does it? I hope so."

"I'm not sure she will," a boy announced. "You know why?" He didn't wait for an answer. "She looks really sick, and you said that picture was made a long time ago, so the doctors weren't as smart then."

"Hey, that's not fair," another boy countered. "Just because it was the olden days, and there weren't the drugs they have now, penicillin, doesn't mean the doctor there, he was dumb. What do you think was the matter?"

They were utterly silent (a rare moment) and united as they awaited my answer: "I don't know, but she looks as though she's had a fever and has been wasted by it."

"Yes," several children agreed.

"Will she die from it?" asked a girl.

"I don't know."

The girl who asked me that last question now became a narrator, personal and expansive, rather than a child prompted to conventional curiosity by a picture. "My cousin was very sick. She almost died. She was only seven. They thought she had a bad blood disease for a while, but she didn't. She got high fevers, too, just like that girl. We all prayed and I guess God heard us."

"How do you know [He did]?" asked a boy sitting beside her, instantly.

She turned toward him, gave him a fast glance, turned abruptly away, and with her face gave him a piece of her mind — a sharp frown. She replied to his question with noticeable disdain: "If you don't believe in God, just say it."

"I didn't say anything about God not existing. I just asked you something, that's all," he said. She sat in cold, contemptuous silence, looking away from him. He looked right at her and asked her the same question again, now explained and phrased more gently: "If you pray, you want to know if you are reaching God, so that's what I'd like to know. Isn't that all right, to want to know?"

The girl who had spoken first now answered for her classmate, who clearly had no intention of deigning to have any more talk with her skeptical neighbor: "Don't you see, there's no way you can be sure, because God doesn't go around bragging that He did this, and He did something else! God does His stuff 'behind the scenes'; our priest told us that. I had a brother, and he died. He had a blood vessel that broke — in his head. Just like that [she snaps her fingers] it happened. My dad said there's no God if He lets that happen. My mom said you can't blame God; He just put us here. I didn't know what to think. The priest came and visited us, and Dad wouldn't come out. He stayed in the bedroom. He [the priest] told us we shouldn't get upset with Dad — because it's natural, when someone dies like Tim did, so young, that everyone will ask why God lets it happen. But He didn't, that's what you've got to remember. He tries to be helpful. He's always in there, pitching for us. It's 'behind the scenes,' that's how He works. So you pray to Him. But you can't expect Him to make everything perfect. Our priest said it would be heaven — we'd be in heaven — if that's what God could do down here."

Her long theological discussion and clarification held the children's attention throughout. When the girl had finished, her audience had no rejoinders, and a few nodded their agreement.

I began to wonder whether I should proceed to the proverbial "next slide." Suddenly, the first girl, the one who had told us she and her family had beseeched God's help and received it, began to speak: "You can tell that God is hearing you when you pray to Him. Sure, He can't do everything, not until you go to the next world — and He's the boss there. But He'll listen to you if you really want to talk with Him. He will."

"How do you know? I just want to know," said the boy again. "That's all I'm asking; I'm not against God. I just wish I knew how you pray and hear back; I mean, how He talks back — how you know He talks back. That's all. That's all."

His jumbled prose, his earnest, almost pleading manner, his obvious sincerity, his essentially amicable intent — we all responded with friendship: smiles on faces, heads tilted toward him, mouths open a bit, ready to speak. A chorus of "yeahs" arose — not applause for him, but an acknowledgment from others that they had felt as uncertain or puzzled as he. The girl who had assured us that the Lord does, for sure, listen was now nonplused. She looked at me and finally at her neighbor, the boy she had obviously regarded, so far, as a wicked presence, best ignored. Then, rather dramatically, she looked up at the ceiling, prompting more than one of us to think she might be testing, then and there, her faith in God's answerability. At last she spoke: "You can't prove it, because He's not someone you can see and touch! But he looks out for people, and if He saw that girl [in the picture], He'd feel sorry for her; and if she prayed to Him, He'd try to answer her prayers. I know."

Another boy, obviously unimpressed with that statement, creased his forehead, put his hand on his head, even pulled his hair a little, and got ready to talk, then paused. With no competing remarks and the stillness uncomfortably lengthening, he finally spoke up: "If you say God would try to help that girl, then you mean she lived, she got better. Right?"

He was looking directly at the girl who had spoken, but she refused to look at him or react to him. Again she looked up at the ceiling; then her eyes drifted down and settled into a stare directed through the window to the outside. Another girl intervened, somewhat on her behalf, but also in the spirit of the boy: "You can't expect us to know if that girl lived. Maybe she didn't even exist! She's in the painting, but did she actually live? Anyway, that was a long time ago. And besides, if God wanted to help someone, He wouldn't tell *us!* He'd do what He does — I don't know what He does! I'm not sure there *is* a God! *Is* there a God? My dad says no, and my mom says maybe!"

The room came alive then. "Yes, there is a God," said one boy; a murmur of approval followed. The boy who had just declared his doubts, and his parents' doubts as well, immediately asked, boldly: "How do you prove it?" A boy sitting in the front row who up to this moment had been not only quiet but apparently uninterested in the entire discussion — he had been looking at goldfish swimming in a bowl located on a table beside my desk — suddenly spoke: "What has all this got to do with the picture?"

"Well, when you get sick, you pray to God you'll get better," answered another student who had also kept out of the fray until that moment. Everyone agreed — there were nods, smiles, and expressions of relief that some common ground had been found. We all looked at the picture once more. The children asked interesting exploratory questions. Where was the mother? Why was the doctor thinking, rather than doing something? Where was his stethoscope? Did doctors use stethoscopes then? Was the girl "really" asleep, or was she "just exhausted"? Who owned the picture, and did it make the owner "sad" to look at such a scene "all the time"? (I found out, a few days later, that the picture is located in the Tate Gallery in London, and I told them that.)

But soon thereafter we were back to God, prayer, and spirituality. One of the quieter children, a boy who had murmured a yes or a no but had said nothing substantive, got us thinking with this speculation: "Maybe she's dreaming of God. He could be telling her she'll be all right, or even if she won't be all right, He'll be nice to her when she comes to Him. Don't forget: if you're a kid, you'll probably go to heaven — that's what our Sunday school teacher told us once, that God smiles on kids!"

No one spoke for a while. The children seemed quite lost in their own thoughts. An ambulance's siren broke our silence, ironically enough. One of the children, usually taciturn, wondered if there was a "grownup" in that ambulance, or if it was a "kid." The boy next to him, another observer rather than participant in our earlier discussion, wondered out loud what the rest of us were thinking — how sick the person was, and where the ambulance was headed. Then he asked: "Do you think God knows what's happened? Do you think the person did something wrong, and God knows, but He won't do anything to help?"

Lots of lively thoughts were exchanged at this point. I noted, yet once more, how often children (like adults) think of God as a judge, a critic, or a benefactor: one who rewards and punishes. The children also managed to give God a psychology, one not unlike their own. One child emphasized His moodiness, His overworked life — "all the people He has to keep up with." Another child stressed the wisdom of God, His ability to spot what is wrong or "dumb," His ability to find and concentrate on "the good side of things." A third child declared God to be "like the doctor." We all now looked at the picture, and the girl told us of her reasons: "That doctor is thinking about the girl; and so is God. I'll bet every minute God thinks of sick people, and He wonders what will happen [to them]. It must be hard to be like that — everyone is trying to get your help!" Others chimed in, worried about an occasional slip-up. That last concern, addressed to the class by a girl who was a bit shy and rather easily overlooked, gave us a new reason to stop and think: "Maybe God never knew she was sick. Maybe He was busy. Maybe the doctor wishes God would come and help, but He hasn't come, and the girl is getting sicker and sicker."

So we resumed with a theological vengeance — some children arguing, in essence, that God, by His very nature, misses nothing; others insisting that there is a distinct chance He does get overburdened or distracted. He is interested in how "honest" and "good" we are, I was told. He does not like "liars" at all, or "people who hurt other people." He also dislikes selfish people and, conversely, favors those who think of others, not only themselves. Under such circumstances, the children let me know, they had best try to be thoughtful, sensitive to others, and as law-abiding as possible. Yet, they quickly admitted that "no one can be perfect" — that they stumble along, often making mistakes, and that as a result they worry sometimes about God's opinion of them, worry that they may well be judged quite harshly by Him at that distant but, to them, real moment when He and they shall meet.

Some of those children had a different kind of worry. Reared in agnostic or only perfunctorily religious homes, they indicated a skepticism about God's existence, not to mention His purposes or values. Yet the sight of churches and synagogues, the words of faith uttered by adults or other children, have an impact on these doubters, making them "nervous," making them feel they might "get into trouble" down the line, when and if the Almighty should prove to be more than a collective fantasy. "I don't know if there's a God," a boy declared, "but I've wondered what would happen to me if He was real and He knew I wasn't on His side!"

Not all the members of this group turned God into a potentially vindictive or punitive figure. I was interested by the way several of them (three girls, two boys) really worked hard at linking him to the doctor in the painting. God for these latter children is pensive, even a bit perplexed — which is a measure, perhaps, of their own thoughtful, questioning attitude toward organized religion, and a measure, too, of their natural spiritual curiosity, something in them that is not yet firmly shaped, that is restless and subject to continual consideraton and reconsideration. "I'd rather have God [be] like that doctor," one boy said, "sitting and trying to be a friend, and maybe praying, than [be] waving His arms around and shouting, the way some ministers [on television] do." His image of God as not only devoted to a sick child but praying on her behalf prompted an explosion of comments, of imaginative leaps from those childen; it was a major moment for me in my research. I was glad that we were meeting in the afternoon, that our discussion could spill over, occupy a second "period," otherwise designated as "study time"; and as a consequence of our especially spirited talk about spirituality, I arranged to meet with a number of these children individually, both at school and at home. They became involved, that is, in the home-to-home study I was doing.

The question that got the children going, right after the boy suggested an image of God as a prayerful physician, was: "What do you mean, God 'praying'?" A girl in the back of the class asked it so quietly that I didn't quite hear it. I was going to request that she repeat herself, but right away a girl sitting beside her asked the same question, this time louder and with an obvious edge of derision. Before the boy could reply, the second girl revealed the conviction that had prompted her inquiry: "God is God, so why should *He* pray to Himself? We pray to Him, we should; then He listens, and He decides."

"How do you know what He does? Have you talked with Him? Why couldn't — why wouldn't He want to pray?"

The boy who spoke those words stunned us not only by saying them, but by how he said them. He stood up, his face flushed, and looked directly at the girl who had obviously provoked him. This sharp face-off got me thinking of the Supreme Court and its cautionary rulings about the relationship between religion and public education. Were we in danger of violating some law? In this "art history" class devoted to a painting, *The Doctor*, we were moving fast toward highly speculative theological reflection. What would the children's parents make of all this? But those parents had already set the stage, as became clear when the boy thus challenged added a bit of fuel to the fire: "Anyway, my dad says God isn't owned by ministers and priests and rabbis, those people. He's got His own ideas — and just because there's a church, and inside it they tell you they speak for Him, don't believe them!"

"Hey," a girl pointed out, "that's your father's idea, but it's not my dad's!"

"I agree with her," another girl said.

"I'm with her, too," a boy noted.

"Well, not me," another boy shouted. "On television you see these ministers, and they are crooks! Why should we be pushed around by them? They'll steal from you! That's no good! If I was God — if I was God, I'd like being a doctor, sitting beside that girl, and I'd sure pray for her, to get better!"

"Well, you're *not* God," his friend sitting beside him wryly and softly said.

That observation prompted a much stronger echo from another boy: "So don't get any big ideas!"

The conversation was clearly deteriorating until a boy asked, "Didn't Jesus go around being a doctor?"

We all fell silent. I was going to answer the question with yes, but realized the children all knew about Christ's healing — hence their quiet contemplation. Now they looked at that picture on the wall with fresh interest. A girl wondered out loud, "Do you think *he* could be Jesus?"

A boy said no, then explained: "He's a doctor; if He was Jesus, the picture would look different."

"What do you mean?"

"Well, He'd have that circle [halo] over His head, or He'd carry the big stick you see" — the Good Shepherd's crook, shown in Sunday school books.

"I don't know if you're right. He could just come here and try to be like us, like one of us. He could do that. He could if He wanted to."

"Who says so? You! Don't you think a priest would know better?"

"No!"

"I agree [with the one who said no]. God can decide [to do] whatever He wants, and it's up to no one but Him. That's true, isn't it?"

"Yes, it is. But what's the point of arguing! Let's get back to the picture! Let's say it could be God and it could be just a doctor! Isn't that a compromise?"

"Yes, it is. It's silly to try to say what God can do and what He can't do, and what He's like and what He isn't like. According to my mom, He's different for each person, because He can be like that."

"Well, now *you're* saying what He's like, right?"

"No, I wasn't! I was just saying He can be anything He wants to be, and so He could be like that doctor in the picture. He *could*. I didn't say He *is!*"

"OK."

Hands were still waving in the air. More children had more to say. But the school bell rang, and so that last "OK" put an end to our colloquy.

As we all prepared to leave, the boy who had proposed a radical versatility for God came up to me and wanted to pursue his idea further, and we eventually did, in talks both at school and at his home. During one of those discussions he enlarged on his point of view, an interesting one both psychologically and theologically, one I have also heard other children suggest. Here I combine comments made in the course of three interviews, eliminating my side of our exchanges: "When I think of God, I think of Jesus, and how He was a good friend to the disciples who followed Him. He wasn't trying to make people feel bad, like those priests do a lot of the time, and ministers. My dad says the churches fight over who owns Jesus! They try to steal Him [from each other]. He was a person as well as God, so He could be a doctor or something else, a teacher or a businessman, maybe. Why not? There's this man who has been giving money to kids to go to college, if they stay in school and study. He's a business-man, and he might be better than a lot of priests. Well, yes, even if he's Jewish [I had mentioned that fact], that man could be Jesus. I mean, Jesus was a Jew, wasn't He? So, if He comes back again, he could be a Jew again.

"When I don't feel good, and there's no one I want to talk to, it's then I'll think of Jesus — more Him than God. They tell us [in Sunday school] He's the same as God, but He was down here with us, and I can imagine Him — from all the pictures of Him — and I can talk with Him. No, it's not the same as praying. It's different. It's Him being a friend, and He's like your folks, only He's not there all the time, telling you things, and getting all upset because your room is a mess. Maybe they got all upset with Him, when He was a kid, His folks! Didn't they tell us that He was just like any other kid, and it was when He got older that He showed He was wise — maybe twelve or thirteen, a little older than I am? So He'd be easy to talk with, I think.

"Sometimes I'll say something, and I talk back to myself, and it's me talking back, but it sounds better than me; I mean, smarter. It could be Jesus, saying something to me — I mean, using my own voice!

"You shouldn't be too sure of yourself! I don't like it when people say they know what God is like and they know what He wants us to be like! I want to say that God isn't like that! He isn't a person who wants people fighting over Him! I guess He's *not* a person! But for a while He was, and maybe he still is; I mean, partly. When I pray, or when I picture Him and talk with Him, it's a person I'm seeing, and He has a voice, and I hear it. No, it's not completely mine; it sounds different. No, it's not my dad's or my mom's or anybody else's. It might be my mind, making up the voice. I mean, it's my mind, yes, but when I hear what He's said to me, I think it's Him, Jesus; I believe it is. I hope I'm right.

"Some things I could never bring up, even if God came and gave me some food and slapped me on the back, the way my cousin does when he comes and visits us. He's a great guy. I like him better than any of my friends. He's sixteen. But if you look up to someone — I guess you feel real ashamed if you think of telling him that sometimes you're selfish; I mean you think of yourself first. (That's what my mom will say to us: 'Stop thinking of yourself first!') I don't mind confessing [to God], but some things, I just can't say them. I don't have the words."

With those poignant and candid words he broke off; he looked down at the floor; and then a phone call for him saved him from the silence. As I sat there, hearing his lighthearted telephone voice in the background — such a contrast with the gravity of our recent subject matter — I began to think of the meaning of God a bit differently. This boy's God was a supernatural friend who could materialize out of nowhere and offer a kind of psychological sanctuary. When others — perhaps even his parents — let the boy down, Jesus was approachable, and often, it seems, on call. Though this boy got on rather well with his parents, no parents are perfect, nor any child. At times Jesus became a stand-in for those parents, enlarging the well-known "Oedipal triangle" into a square. Yet even Jesus had to be distanced on occasion, seen as a kindly judge, but a judge nevertheless. As the boy himself observed once to me, "If you can help it, you spare yourself a bawling-out; or you give it to yourself." Often Jesus was the opposite of a scold — the one who offered forgiveness, a moral refuge. On the other hand, He was no fool; He was a serious judge, rather, whose high-mindedness could be fearfully hard for even this friendly, trusting, decent boy. God as a potential critic, if not a major fault-finder, had a life in the child's mind.

As I looked again at the interviews I'd had with children here and abroad, I began to realize that psychologically God can take almost any shape for children. He can be a friend or a potential enemy; an admirer or a critic; an ally or an interference; a source of encouragement or a source of anxiety, fear, even panic. Obviously, religious tenets, reinforcing a child's ongoing spiritual reflection, can become an integral and persuasive part of a conscience, either its self-critical side or its friendlier aspect, the so-called ego-ideal of psychoanalytic theory. Often, children whose sternly Christian, Jewish, or Moslem parents don't hesitate to threaten them with the most severe of religious strictures (and thus who do likewise with respect to themselves), can construct in their thoughts or dreams a God who is exemplary yet lenient, forgiving, encouraging, capable of confessing a moment's weakness or exhaustion now and then.

One of the children I worked with most intensively for this research project kept dreaming that he was in an airplane flying to Ireland (where all four of his grandparents were born). The plane runs into trouble, goes down toward a crash landing over the Atlantic. But he miraculously stays up in the air, and while doing so, floating, as it were, amid the clouds, he sees Jesus walking there. They meet and talk. Jesus reassures the boy convincingly — even tells him that he, too, has felt lost and confused. The boy is surprised, doubly: he has yet, in the dream, to become anxious, even though the plane in which he was traveling has just plunged earthward with his parents and sister aboard; and he has never thought of Jesus as being in any way limited or vulnerable. At this point — not only startled but puzzled and with anxiety at last rising in him — sleep ends, and the boy has suddenly moved from the clouds to his bed. "I've had this dream a couple of times, maybe more," he told me, and when asked for his explanation he was decidedly brief: "Maybe the Lord wanted to talk with me, and so He did."

We will never know the Lord's intentions, but the boy's aren't too hard to discern. A boy finds God's company preferable to that of his parents, at least for a moment. In this august company, he learns that he is far from alone in his sense of being directionless. He has had a short, powerful encounter that he keeps calling to mind, days later, when he feels himself making the small mistakes of everyday life. He has worked at finding his own voice through a middle-of-the-night evocation of Someone Else's. He calls such a dream a "visit," and why not? At a minimum it is a psychological event which a child holds on to as significant, as a guiding moment of spiritual reflection, as an assist in settling a few uncertainties, in feeling less peculiar and alone.

When I was learning to do psychiatric work with boys of his

age, eleven, I kept being told by them, once we got to know each other, how lonely they felt — not because they were without friends or, of course, loving family members, but because they were troubled by some of their "impulses," their lusty moments, their combative or envious or frustrated moments. No wonder such children turned to God, to Jesus, to Mary, to Mary Magdalene, to Martha of the New Testament, to such Old Testament figures or pairs as Moses, Samson and Delilah, David and Goliath, in order to gain some perspective on their solitary selves. Girls have told me that Mary, the mother of Jesus, appears in their dreams: "She was smiling, and she told me you have to know when to laugh, even if it's trouble you're facing" — this from a ten-year-old whose father was gravely ill with a malignant melanoma and whose psychological life seemed to be shored up by Mary's appearance in her dream.

Biblical stories, or lessons in the Koran, have a way of being used by children to look inward as well as upward. It should come as no surprise that the stories of Adam and Eve, Abraham and Isaac, Noah and the Ark, Abel and Cain, Samson and Delilah, David and Goliath, get linked in the minds of millions of children to their own personal stories as they explore the nature of sexuality and regard with awe, envy, or anger the power of their parents, as they wonder how solid and lasting their world is, as they struggle with brothers and sisters, as they imagine themselves as actual or potential lovers, or as actual or potential antagonists. The stories are not mere symbolism, giving expression to what people go through emotionally. Rather, I hear children embracing religious stories because they are quite literally inspiring — exciting their minds to further thought and fantasy and helping them become more grown, more contemplative and sure of themselves.

A nine-year-old boy, Timmy, the son of devoutly Catholic parents (they live in West Roxbury, an almost all-white, middle-class enclave in Boston), was having a terrible time at school — constant struggles with one teacher after another. I got to see him because I knew his family's parish priest, whom I accompanied one day on a home visit. Timmy's shyness with both the priest and me masked his everyday combativeness at school and in fact, I gradually realized, showed the other side of the same coin. The boy's father was a tough man, a police lieutenant, fiercely moralistic and not unwilling to use his belt as a strap to exact discipline, enforce punishment. Timmy's mother, on the other hand, was easygoing, if not indulgent. Her husband argued with her about that, even accused her of "permissiveness" — a serious charge in this socially and culturally conservative home. Caught in between was a boy who adored his father and relied upon his mother for nurturance and encouragement. I had my psychiatric guesses about the causes of Timmy's school behavior, but I kept my hunches to myself. I wasn't sure I was right and I wasn't being asked for an opinion; I was just beginning my neighborhood visits. My friend, the parish priest, was a wonderfully intuitive person yet wasn't sure himself what to make of this apparently solid, stable family. (Timmy was the oldest boy, a second child; he had an older sister, three younger sisters, and a baby brother.)

Just as I got going on my own — having weekly meetings with Timmy and, separately, his older sister, Kathleen — I realized that Timmy's troubles were beginning to disappear. His dad told me, "The boy is fine now," and his mother gave me a similar report. I was reminded of Anna Freud's wonderful advice for parents worried about their child's psychological troubles: "Time wins all the contests." His parents had the confidence, I decided, to stay the course, and now their son was the stronger for it. His teachers wrote home saying that the boy was "calmer" and "much more cooperative." Timmy, who had been quick to take offense, was no longer trying to turn each teacher into a monstrous tyrant whom he, at nine, must fight.

Eventually I would learn that Timmy did indeed deserve credit for his own growing mastery of himself, but that he had also been the recipient of someone's active intervention — that of his father's mother. An unlikely psychological scenario, I remember thinking — but in time I got to know the grandmother and heard her analysis of what ailed her grandson: "For a while, when Timmy was younger, I thought he was a chip off the old block. His father was always ready to stand up and fight for what he thought was right. The trouble was, we tried to tell him (my husband and me), you can mistake your *idea* of right for what *is* right, and then you're really in trouble! I do believe our son

Tim could have been one of those kids that become a delinquent if it hadn't been for that young priest who told him once — I'll never forget it: anyone can go shouting what he's thinking and try to make others agree, but a wise person spends his life trying to find out what he believes, and when he does find out, he's grateful, *quietly* grateful! I remember his every word — and now he's still our priest, and he wears his age well!

"He rescued our son. It wasn't dramatic. He had no tricks. He just came and went for a walk with the boy. They'd go to Brigham's and have their ice cream sodas. Tim's father had two jobs, to keep us going, and he came home dead tired and ate and went right to bed. The priest lived up to being a 'father'! He told Tim that Jesus was stronger than a lot of people who were strong. They were strong because they had weapons and they could scare people and kill them; Jesus was strong because he could stand up for what He believed, even if it meant dying. The priest got to our Tim. Don't ask me how — he just did. It's true, they were friends. But the priest was more than a friend. He was someone Tim respected, and he earned the respect. He taught him about Jesus, without force-feeding him a lot of Sunday school sermons. Tim hated Sunday school. He was not one who would listen to preaching — at home, at school, at church! I guess it was my fault. I had to be two parents, and I'm a very religious Catholic, and I'm afraid I used to get carried away, you know! Father O'Brien would never order Tim to do anything. He'd tell him stories from the Bible when they'd have their sodas, and I could see he got my son to thinking. He didn't give him a Bible to read, either. He gave him a book that had those stories in it, from the Bible, and then they'd talk — they'd talk about a lot of things, but mainly they'd talk about why Jesus acted the way He did and not some other way.

"When you have a priest who coaches basketball, and he's a regular fellow, and he'll take the time to be with you, then you'll learn from him — that's how I see it, and so when my grandson, little Timmy, only eight or nine, started having all this trouble with his fights, and worse than his father, because he was taking on the teachers, mind you, I thought of going right to Father O'Brien, and you must know what I mean, because he's a friend of yours, right? But he's been sick; he had an operation to clean his heart vessels, and I just couldn't burden him, so I said to myself: you're the boy's grandma, and you know the father from day one, and for heaven's sake, you could try to help out, and he does like you and trust you! So I started! I'd take him to Brigham's, the same place my own son would go with the priest! I didn't lift my voice to preach. I just talked with him and watched him eat those huge sundaes! Oh, how I wish I didn't have diabetes! Diet Cokes at Brigham's! Timmy felt sorry for me, because he knows I can't eat a lot of sweets, and he knows I have a terrible sweet tooth. It was *that*: he'd stop and pity me, and then I'd have my say. I'd tell him that you have to pick and choose your fights, and you don't fight diabetes, because it's just too strong for you, so you find a way of making peace with it, even if it's frustrating. He'd listen — but it didn't much sink in, I mean not the way I wanted it [to sink in]. But I tried!

"I don't even know if the priest ever tried to change Tim. He just spoke to him from his heart, and of course he had Jesus in his heart! I tried to be like Father O'Brien. I knew I'd get nowhere with preaching! When you get to be over seventy, you either have learned from your mistakes, or you haven't! I'm not saying I *have* learned, but I'm trying. I sat with that boy, and I tried to show him I was a sick old lady but I had strength and will power: I could settle for a diet Coke and be happy. I told him; I said, 'Timmy, *you're* here with me, and that's better than a sundae!' I don't think he believed me! But I'd tell him how I prayed, so I could be a good patient. My husband is sick, and I have to take care of him. If I got sick, he'd die, I know he would. The doctor says so. You have to think of others! I guess that was my 'message' to the boy. He began to listen — maybe it was because I was confiding in him. I was talking about my illness, and his grandfather's. After a while I did bring in Jesus — look, He could have been out only for himself. He could have done what would have given Him pleasure, but instead He had His mission, and He stuck to it.

"I was trying to tell the boy to quiet down and stop losing control of himself, but I wasn't being very smart! That's because I'm *not* very smart! Would you believe it — I went to see Father O'Brien, and I said, 'Now, father, what did you ever do to have to hear all the troubles of our family, two generations of them?'

He laughed and said, 'It's a real privilege!' 'Now, father,' I said, 'I don't want to be responsible for turning you into a liar!' He laughed! I told him about young Timmy and all I'd been saying, and he said, 'You're doing fine!' He said I should tell Timmy about David and Goliath: 'You let him know that David didn't just pick a fight! You let him know that David knew why he was taking on Goliath, and he prepared himself, and he was grown up and had become strong in his body and in his soul.' Well, that sounded good coming out of *his* mouth, but how was *I* going to talk like that?

"I wasn't very good at saying what our priest said I should say. He'd have done so much better! But he was sick and he's older than me, and I wanted to try, I think. It may have taken me a few months, and lots of temptation — if I'd have gone alone to Brigham's all those times, I'd have broken down one out of two times — but in the end my grandson did begin to grow up a bit. I don't know if it was the ice cream or my stories from the Bible or me, or all three. My son said, 'Ma, you're so good, you should get a job as a school psychologist.' That'll be the day! I wouldn't know what to think or say — not to this younger generation! But Timmy did tell me that he thinks he might bring one of his friends along some day when we go to Brigham's, and I got really scared. Two of them to try to talk into being better behaved in school! He's never mentioned that again, thank God!"

I thought of Anna Freud yet again as I tried to understand exactly what this grandmother had done. "When we look back and try to figure out what has worked," Miss Freud once commented, "we run the risk of imposing our idea of what *should* have worked, and we may never know the truth, the complex truth, of what actually happened." As I myself listened to this elderly woman (and her priest, who was such a good friend), I found my own sense of life shift a bit. "Don't be in such a hurry to win everything all the time," Timmy's grandmother had softly remarked one day as Timmy ran so fast to pick up a coin he had spotted in the street that he had trouble stopping himself in time to avoid being hit by a car. Her words came to my mind a couple of days later as I pressed the gas pedal of my car angrily, intent on passing a "provocatively slow" driver ahead (the dreary rationalizations we find for ourselves!), only to miss narrowly an oncoming car whose driver had every right to wish someone would talk sense into me.

A year after Timmy had ceased being a "school problem" (the principal's phrase) — he was now ten and thinking ahead to adolescence and beyond — he told me: "I learned one thing from my grandma: David was way smaller than Goliath, but he was all grown up when he said, 'Hey, I'll take him on!' Two things, actually — that you have to watch yourself, or you'll be a fool, and then people will laugh. No, she didn't say it like that; she told me about Jesus. I've been learning my religion every week: I go to Sunday school. But when Grandma told me [about Jesus] she got me thinking. You know something? My dad says if there was a real small Bible, he'd carry it with him at work, because someday he'll meet a guy they've arrested, and he'll want to hit him one, the guy's such a mean, dirty 'low-life.' A 'low-life' is the worst crook you can imagine. Some of them deserve the chair. In this state there's no death penalty, though. Dad walks away from them. You've got to keep your cool. If I became a cop, I'd find that Bible, a real small one, and keep it in my back pocket. Then, if I was ready to blow, I'd sneak off somewhere and read from one of those pages my grandma likes."

I heard more along those lines for a few months, and then, as he gradually "settled down," in his teachers' words, the Bible was no longer such a pressing matter for him. (At this writing he is an honors student at Boston Latin School, headed for college.) As I sit and think of Timmy's childhood, I recognize its psychological contours — the way, in a family of Irish background, race and class and religion and cultural values combine to work their influence on a boy's life. Moreover, he was growing up in 1980s Boston, with plenty of troubles in the school system as the city struggled to achieve desegregation amid many pressures from many quarters. Timmy's father, a leader among policemen, is often in the thick of those pressures, and his son was for a while creating a few pressures himself, both at school and at home. But if Timmy's family had its private vulnerabilities and tensions, it also had sources of strength all its own: the grandmother's informal, unpretentious spirituality, for example, which she knew how to summon at just the right moment.

In a telling discussion one day, Timmy told me how much he loved his grandmother. At first he emphasized the "treats" she offered him — all that ice cream and buttercrunch. Then he mentioned, almost casually, another kind of treat: "She's good at screwing my head on tight, and she sure gives me something to think about!" He had heard his teachers, at the height of his rebelliousness, exhort him to "screw your head on tight," and at the time he would in his mind give their own verb back to them: "Screw you." Now he could look back calmly at his earlier self, abandoned for the one he had assembled with his grandmother's considerable help; and now that "head" of his not only held tight, but held an abundance of stories.

In some homes where religion is more explicitly and constantly evoked — rituals practiced, mandates and rules enforced — spiritual values become for children part and parcel of the emotional life they struggle to consolidate for themselves. Timmy's family was devoutly Catholic but was also, in important ways, a secular, bourgeois late-twentieth-century American family. In American families that are committed to the evangelical tradition, to fundamentalist religion[3] (and, of course, in the Orthodox Jewish families I met in Israel, and in the passionately Moslem families in Tunisia), religion and psychology in a sense merge — for instance, those children in their rebelliousness have to contend not merely with schoolteachers, as Timmy did, but with the full everyday force of their families' beliefs. Children are rewarded and punished in the name of God, told what to do and when. "God is my parents' parent, and mine, too," an eastern Tennessee girl of nine told my son and me one day. She talked about the minute-by-minute watch the Lord had on her life. "He's always looking down on us, I know that for sure." Such a child's passions, ardent and angry, will engage with that parent of all parents, will make a complete psychological engagement. The child will love God, spurn God, fight for God, obey God, angrily disobey God. It is hard, I think, for those of us whose religious life is merely a part of what we do, one of many commitments, to put ourselves in the shoes of people for whom the phrase "God's presence" has an utter, rock-bottom psychological reality that gives meaning to the phrase "my parents' parent, and mine, too." In such people, I have felt, spirituality makes up the very warp and woof of psychology; the integration is as complete as that described for me by the Tennessee girl. She and others like her feel God's parenthood so deeply and continuously that their every emotional moment seems God-connected, if not God-haunted. No wonder such children ask so many favors of Him; turn to Him with passion and disappointment alike; beseech Him openly and in the secrecy of their private moments (not to mention their half-forgotten dreams); rail against Him or, more consciously, obliterate Him with doubt. When that same girl, that same afternoon, told my son and me that "God is in heaven, but He is in my mind, too," she was perhaps making the definitive analysis of the relationship between young spirituality and young psychology — a fusion. Let others visit God on Sunday for an hour, or have their discreet moments of engagement with Him, spiritual in content, psychologically significant; for her, God is just what she once characterized Him as being, "a companion who won't leave."

6

Young Spirituality:
Philosophical Reflections

THE NINE-YEAR-OLD, who refers often to God as her "parents' parent," a girl from the eastern part of Tennessee, told my son one morning — he had been interviewing her and others every day for several weeks — that she kept "dreaming the same dream about Jesus." He was not shy about inquiring, and he soon heard her dream: "It seems I'm walking in the woods, not too far from my house, but I get lost. Funny, though — I'm not scared. I just keep walking. But I see the sun has been moving across the sky, and I realize in a few hours it'll be dark, and then I'll be in trouble if I don't find a way home. So I start walking faster. The faster I walk, the more tired I get, and my stomach starts telling me I'm hungry. I don't know what to do. My daddy has told me never to drink water in the woods — you could catch all these bad germs. My mom says, 'Don't eat the berries you see, even if they look "friendly," and like the ones you buy in the store.' So I gave my stomach the 'big lecture,' but it didn't pay me any mind. I prayed for my stomach to stop pulling on me, but it just wouldn't.

"I started running. Then I got tired, so I slowed down. I was getting really worried. I was crying. I'd even forgotten about God, I was so scared. I think I was imagining lions and tigers — in our woods here near Chattanooga! I tried to calm myself down. Just as I was ready to stop and take a drink from some water in a stream, I looked ahead, and I saw a house. I got real excited and I started running toward it. There must be a phone

there — I thought that. The place wasn't as near as it seemed.
I kept running, and it kept moving back from me. It was like in
the desert, you know — when you see something, but it might
not be real, you begin to realize. Yes, a mirage. [My son had
suggested the word.] I got scared, even more, because never
before had I seen something, and then it kept slipping from me,
just as I thought I was getting to it. But I kept up my walking,
and all of a sudden — it was real strange — the house was right
in front of me. I couldn't believe my eyes: it was that gingerbread
house like in the story. I was standing there — I was dreaming,
you know — and I was asking myself if this was some silly dream.
But it felt like it was real; I mean, it *was* real then. I wanted to
go inside and see who was there and ask if I could call my folks.
I was remembering our phone number, and I was wondering if
I should use our area code, 615, or if I was in another area code
by then. I was also wondering if there'd be any of that cake, that
gingerbread, inside: like the stuff on the side of the house and
the roof. I saw the bell, the button, and I rang it, and that's when
this man came to the door — it wasn't like in the story — and
he was young, and he looked like, maybe, Elvis Presley. My uncle
collects pictures of him, and he has a lot. (He works in a music
store; he runs it.)

"This man had a banjo, and it was in his hand; he was just
holding it. I didn't know what to say to him. He didn't say a
word to me; no, not even hello. I was tongue-tied, I guess. Then
I heard a dog barking, and this dog came up close, and I was
really afraid. That was when I started crying, and the man told
the dog to sit, sit, and the dog did. What kind of dog? It was a
big dog, a hunting dog; it was dark, it was black. I don't know
the breed. After the dog stopped barking, the man asked me if
I wanted anything, and I said I did; I wanted to call home if
he'd let me. But he said he didn't have a phone. I guess I didn't
believe him! I said, 'You *don't?*' He said, 'No.' I just stood there.
I didn't know what I should do next! It was then that he said I
could have a glass of milk if I wanted; and he had a box of Milky
Ways, my favorite when I go to buy candy. He said I could eat
all I want! My mom always says, 'Never more than one in a day!'
He said he could play a song while I eat the Milky Ways. He said
he'd call it 'Milky Way,' the song.

"It was his smile I remember the most. He was standing there, and he had his banjo in his right hand, and his left hand — he was leaning with it against a wall. It was like — well, he was chuckling, that's what he was doing, that's what got me nervous, real nervous. I had picked up a Milky Way, but I didn't want to eat it. I started looking around the room. I walked around and around. He asked me, 'Whatsamatter, little girl?' I told him, 'Nothing' — but I really wanted to call my mom and my dad, and would he please, please, let me call them, then I'd leave. But he kept saying no, he didn't have a phone, not a real one. I didn't know what he meant, so I told him I didn't, and then he went over to a cabinet, and he opened the door, and he took out this telephone (it looked like one) and he brought it over to me and showed me it, and I could see, it was made of cake, just like the walls of the house, and I think those silver Hershey Kisses, there was a circle of them — maybe to look like the numbers you dial, or something.

"I was feeling real scared, real upset. I just wanted to be back in the woods. I'd rather be lost, there, than in this house — that's what I thought! So I decided to go. I started walking; I walked toward the door, and that's when he started playing the banjo, and the lights were on, and they went off, and I got so scared I started crying, and then, all of a sudden, I saw the door open, and there was a flash of light outside; it was like lightning, and I think it was Jesus. He'd come to help me, and I had this handkerchief in my hand, and I was going to clean my face — wipe my tears away, maybe — and then I don't remember much. I mean, I was walking with Jesus, maybe following Him, and I think He was telling me something; I think He was saying you should be careful where you go, or you can get lost, or you can slip and fall, or you just go around and around in the woods, and you don't find the right way to get you home. And then I woke up, and I was shaking. I went to see my parents. I went to their bedroom, I had to; I had to wake them up. I didn't actually wake them; I stood there, and maybe I did touch my mom a little, but she woke up fast, and she was upset for me, she told me, and she got up and she made me some hot cocoa, and I felt better, so I went back to bed.

"I was just lying there on the bed, on my back. I think I was still afraid — I was afraid to go back to sleep. I thought I'd have the same dream again! I've had a dream, and then I've dreamt the same dream twice. Our minister told Mom that can happen. But this [dream] was so scary. I thought I'd just lie there until it was morning, and then I'd get up and have some orange juice, and I could make some instant oatmeal for myself, and toast from Mom's banana bread. But then I fell asleep. No, no sir, I never did have that dream a second time."

In this tight-knit fundamentalist community, such a dream was not taken lightly. The girl told the dream to her mother and then, with her mother nearby, to the minister. He was reassuring: God had come to save her from "temptation." She had been "lost," and He had "saved" her. I didn't take the dream lightly, either; I was tempted to make a psychological "federal case" out of that dream, with its florid sexual imagery, its banal, fairy-tale character. I had my job to do, my training to remember. Here was a girl lost temporarily to her instincts, hungry and thirsty, tempted by a musical man — but in the nick of time delivered to the safety of Jesus' company. He strengthens her already firm moral resolve. He gives her a psychoanalytic lesson or two in how to negotiate her way through impasses. She emerges unscathed: id erupts; superego rallies, with a boost from the Lord; ego becomes more flexible and robust, also with the Lord's assistance. Yet the way this girl viewed her dream in retrospect over the subsequent weeks became more interesting to Bob and me than the substance of her dream.

Her name was Mary, and she had told us several times she didn't like her name "too much," because "so many people have it." But after that dream she reconsidered her attitude toward her name: "I was thinking, Jesus came to Mary, and she didn't know He was coming, so she was really surprised, and she must have wondered why He chose her; I mean, why God chose her to carry His son. My mom told me that now I know, just a little, how Mary felt! I sure was surprised, afterwards, when I realized I'd been dreaming of Jesus, and He'd been walking with me! Since then I'll be having some trouble at school, or I'll be disappointed, because I bought something and I didn't like it — and I think of Jesus, and what He said, that I should remember what's important, and not let every little thing that goes wrong bother me. It's true, He didn't say a lot to me in the dream. [I had asked her about that — what she remembered Him saying to her.] But since then, I'll go to church, and they'll say what Jesus thought, and I'll think of Him talking to me there in the woods. He was telling me — I do remember, I think — that you have to ask yourself what's important and what's not important. When the minister the other day said that Peter didn't think he was worthy to die the way Jesus did, to be crucified, I thought: How do you die so that God, so that Jesus will say, 'You've been a good person, Mary, and thank you! — you've been worthy'? Our minister says we have to try every day to be worthy. I try sometimes; but I don't always remember to try. I should remember harder!

"Maybe — this is a strange idea, but I've had it a lot — maybe when I was having that dream, it was me, trying to be with Jesus, trying to be worthy, to prove I'm worthy, like they'll tell you in church. Maybe He was just being Himself, and He knew I was having this scary dream, and He decided that I was trying to be worthy, but maybe I'd never get home, and that man, he'd capture me; so Jesus decided to send me a message, and He did: He showed up, and He pointed out how I should be careful when I go for a walk, and now I feel closer to Him. It was — it was like a gift, and I was given it, and maybe I didn't deserve it, but now that I have it, I keep remembering, and I think I've been better, in school and with my friends. My best friend (she's named Mary, too!) — she told me yesterday that I was nicer, and that I'm not so jumpy anymore. In church, they talk of the 'peace of Jesus,' and I think I was given some of it that night. I'll never know until I meet Him, and I'm hoping I will! My aunt said Jesus gave us our minds so we can think of Him and honor Him. Maybe He lets us have dreams for the same reason, so He'll come and visit us, and we'll have Him with us when we remember the dream, and Him in it."

A girl not yet ten, from a region of the country not rarely called backward, and from a region of Tennessee also not rarely, by some who live in its more cosmopolitan areas, called backward, experienced a vivid, memorable dream, and then found her life rather notably affected. She became more inward-thinking, more reflective. She seemed to have a longer perspective on things. She lost her impatient, petulant inclinations, at least some of the time. She was still in elementary school, still an American girl of the late twentieth century, and so she had her eyes on "cute" dresses, on "religious rock music," on a bracelet she saw a girl wear and very much wished she might one day own, and yes, on one of her male cousins, whom everyone in the family called "cute" and whom she, also, regarded as "really cute." She thought of becoming a nurse: "I've wanted to be a nurse, because in Sunday school they told us you should choose what to do with Jesus advising you. But He may advise me differently when I'm older. Maybe it wasn't Him advising me when I thought I'd be a nurse — when I first decided that — but it was me hearing the teacher talk. Maybe at just the right time, I'll have another dream! He could do that! He can come and teach us what to do, tell us [in] any way He wants! For a few nights I'd go to bed and I'd wonder what would happen — whether I'd have another dream like it, with Jesus there. Mostly I don't dream anything at all. I just fall asleep, most nights, and nothing happens all night. But some nights, I just lie in bed, and I think of Jesus, and I try to talk with Him, and ask Him how it's best to behave, and I think of His disciples — Peter and Mark and Matthew and Luke and John, and the others."

At certain points in this young girl's life, psychological turmoil yielded to philosophical reflection, both perhaps aspects of her spiritual life. Her life was an unremarkable or ordinary one, her mind was quite normal. Her personal struggles were those of a child who was trying hard to be decent, kind, sensitive, and "God-fearing," a term her parents and grandparents used all the time. Every once in a while, of course, she stumbled, felt a surge of irritation or anger, or a surge of emotionality which she expressed in a shy and delicate and gentle manner: "I do like that boy Mark, I'll admit it." Most of her life was impressively conscientious, and most of her affectionate side and her competitive side, as well as the frequent traces of anger she rarely acknowledged, got worked into dreams like the one she told my son, or her music, into which she poured her heart and soul: singing in a church's "children's chorus" and playing the piano. She also used drawings and paintings to give vent to a good deal of resentment she felt toward a cousin who was five years her elder —

an extremely troubled adolescent girl who had run away from home twice, and who swore, smoked cigarettes and marijuana, drank beer illegally obtained, and in general scandalized her family and community. An occasional drawing of Jesus as a man of obvious energy and power showed, too, her interest in strong men: her father, whose beard and brawn made him look a bit like Mary's pictures of Jesus; and another cousin, also older, a teenage high school boy, head of his church's "youth group," whom she clearly regarded as an ideal. As I listened to her talk about those people, those activities, I heard not only reportage or expressions of approval and disapproval, but comments about life's meaning — comments not specifically religious in nature, yet very interconnected with her ongoing religious life.

She wondered, as do all children, about her future, but the way she did so told a good deal about her spiritual and philosophical life.[1] "I don't want to waste my time here on this earth," she once said to me, a surprising statement for such a young girl. When I tried to be reassuring, which is my usual course when a child seems to be a bit overconscientious, she deftly let me know, without apparent displeasure, that she wanted or needed no consolation — quite the contrary: "I'm so happy I've been given this time here! Think of all the people the Lord hasn't sent here!"

She was intending to continue, but a look of alarm and confusion crossed my face. She stopped. I was speechless. What should I say — tell her that she had just evoked an image of billions and billions of sperm and eggs uniting to populate the earth? Tell her that I don't usually hear children speak about their lives with such perspective or with such openly asserted gratitude? That her self-consciousness was notably lacking in egotism? I managed this: "Mary, I was a little startled to hear you think of all those unborn people."

She quickly resumed her remarks, with the air of one who had every intention of sharing her ideas fully with me: "When you're put here, it's for a reason. The Lord wants you to do something. If you don't know what, then you've got to try hard to find out what. It may take time. You may make mistakes. But if you pray, He'll lead you to your direction. He won't hand you a piece of paper with a map on it, no sir. He'll whisper something, and at first you may not even hear, but if you have trust in Him and you keep turning to Him, it will be all right.

"I was singing in church last Sunday, and I thought that God must be enjoying us, because we were hitting all the notes right! Then, when we were through, and we were just sitting there, and the minister was talking, I wasn't hearing him too good, because I kept having my thoughts — I was thinking that maybe God put me here so I could sing like I just did. No, I don't want to be a singer. [I had asked.] I'll wait to see what He thinks I should do when I'm older. But it could be there's only one thing He really wants for you to do, and the rest is up to you.

"I listen when the wind gets strong — if He wants to speak to me. I don't hear His voice, no. It's my own voice I'll hear — but He's got it going! When I'm asking myself what I think about things, and what I should do, then I know it's God saying, 'Mary, you're down there, and you're nearly ten, and you can do a lot now, and you just go ahead, and I'll be there, helping out.'

"I heard a minister, a visitor, tell us God can be 'hidden.' I don't agree. Just because you don't see Him doesn't mean He's hidden. He's all over the place! I was trying to sing, and my sore throat wasn't *all* the way over, and I almost asked the [choir] director for an excuse, a sickness excuse, but I held on, and then I heard myself doing everything, *everything* right. I knew why! I said a thank-you prayer later, and I promised God I'll sing until my voice begins to give out, and then I'll know He's found others to make music for Him!

"Last week I was walking, and I saw a squirrel, and it was chasing its tail, I thought. Then it saw me, and it decided to do something: it went over and got an acorn that had fallen from the big oak tree near us, and it scurried up the tree and put it in the hole it has up there. I thought: I might be a big person, a god, to that squirrel — and I reminded him that he should keep on the track and not get caught wasting time. Maybe the Lord wants us to get down to business, like the squirrel did. We're here for *something!*"

In that last, brief sentence, spoken with such conviction, I heard an unpretentious child affirming her conviction that her stay on earth was far from senseless; that her existence, which she was capable of looking at as if outside herself, was no random accident. I chalked up her declarations to a rural, fundamentalist culture (though she doesn't really talk with the literal-minded subservience, the overworked confidence, that I heard from others who live near her, including a relative or two). However, there were occasions when her thoughtful examination of this life was virtually free of explicit religious references — as if, like many children from the secular world, she was quite capable of asking herself the same questions existentialist philosophers pose, the eternal why's of this life: "I saw our neighbor, and he'd been in an accident, and he told my dad that he'd just as soon die now as later, because of all the pain he has. His stomach hurts all the time. He's got the worst back pain you can imagine. I wondered what it would be like to have all that pain — to be hurting by day and by night. I don't know if I'd want to live. I might just be hoping I'd die. I'd not pray to God that I die, no — because He's the one who decides; it's not up to you.

"The funny thing — our neighbor, he smiles, despite his troubles. He's glad he can see the sun come up in the morning, my mom says. Today I saw the sun coming up, and I was glad, and I thought, I should be double glad, because I can see it, and I love the way the whole sky becomes lit up, presto, and I don't have any pain. I had a cavity, and I didn't have pain with it, a few weeks ago. I'm not sure I've ever had the least bit of pain, other than a fall I took [riding a pony] back last year, and I've told you of that.

"I saw a tree fall last week. Some serious wind came blowing, and *crack*, it went: sounded like someone shooting his rifle off yonder! When a tree goes — that's life, too. You don't want to cry for people and forget the rest of the world! My mother says I asked her when I was real little if a tree hurts, or a rock. She said no, they don't. She said I came back at her with: 'Mommy, God must hurt when a tree is in trouble.' She told our minister what I said, and he said I was going to be a 'good one' for Sunday school! I like going there, but the teacher this year isn't my favorite of all time. I'd just as soon think about God by myself, and do my singing!"

Her assertions to me about nature, about pain, about death, about what stretches ahead, often sent my mind reeling — and reminded me of other children: a boy in Brookline, for instance,

Jewish, her age (three months older), and headed for a professional life already (he is the son of a lawyer). Gil went along with the Hebrew school education he was getting, but was willing to announce some grave doubts about his religion, about all religion: "How can you prove it's right? My father is a real Jew! He loves Shabbat — all week he's thinking ahead to Shabbat. My mother likes the food we eat then — she makes a lot of it, the challah, always — but she says, 'It's all a big mystery!' Sounds right to me — I think we could just be here, and when you go, you just go.

"I wonder every once in a while if we're the only ones who think. I guess our dog does, a little. I guess the flowers my mom plants, they don't. The trees, they don't. The ants, they don't. The birds, they might. My kid brother was throwing rocks the other day, and I told him, 'Look at it from the rocks' view — they don't like being thrown around and around for no reason!' Daddy told me I'm becoming a 'naturalist.' (He heard me.) I asked him, 'What's that?' He said, 'You love nature.' I don't, I don't think. I don't love all the stuff in the woods — but when we take a walk, my little sister asks if the trees notice us, like we do them. They don't, I know they don't. But if you see a squirrel staring at you, maybe it's saying: hurry up and get away, so I won't be scared!

"When I look up at the sky, I wonder if there are people up there, looking down at us. No, my daddy says no. But how can you know? Maybe God put us Jews on other places up there. He could have — right?"

Gil noticed my unwillingness to take a stand. He put it to me directly: "What do you think?"

I replied, right away, "I don't think there's any human life on the planets or the stars." I'm surprised by the unequivocal nature of my response. Why have I been so quick to shut the door?

Gil insists on the wisdom of qualification: "I heard on television [the public broadcasting program *Nova*] that it would take years and years for our satellites to explore a star. They might find people up there! Maybe there's someone up in one of those stars who thinks this planet is empty [of people] — that no Jews are here! Maybe God lives on one of those stars!"

I am delighted with Gil's imaginative leap and gentle rebuke, but I hear myself (with condescension?) thinking: Gil is a solid boy whose exuberant flights of fancy are — well, just that. He's not a prepsychotic child about whom I should be quite worried. Meanwhile, I smile at his comment and tell him he is right — we don't know, and anything is possible.

A pause, and I expect us to move on, to talk, maybe, about the Jewish high holidays, which are nearing: a week to Rosh Hashanah. But he has his own thoughts to pursue, this boy whose father taught American history before becoming a corporate lawyer: "Thousands of years ago, the Jews were in the desert, and they were a tribe, and they wanted to keep together, and they had to defend themselves. I'll bet they looked up at the sky, just like we do! I'll bet they wondered who was up there — and then they heard God, I think they did. I don't know the Bible, the way a lot of us do; my folks will be very religious one day, and the next they say if you're Jewish, it means you 'belong to a people,' and you have these customs and your favorite food — like the Italians. But they took us [him and his sister, two years older] to Israel, and I could picture those people — my ancestors! — staring up there at the sky, and then they heard God talk. I asked our rabbi how He talked — I mean, how God sounded — and he said it was a voice the people who were listening heard, the Jews of way back in time. That was when I had this idea: Jews shouted across the whole universe, the stars, to other Jews! I told my dad of my idea, and he laughed: 'It's as good a story as any!' " Did he really say that, I asked. "Yes, he said that."

In the course of two days, we discussed the Bible as a series of stories. Gil asserted his faith and his doubts, his Jewishness and his lapses from Judaism: "They were tough folks [the ancient Jews]. They fought, and they wanted to win. They figured, I think, that if you hold on to God, you won't disappear. I wonder where they got that idea. Why didn't some of the other people, the tribes over there [in the Middle East], do the same? Maybe they did; I don't know. To me, the Jews were a really religious tribe, and the other tribes, they just wanted to conquer. I have a friend, he's not Jewish, and you know what he told me? He said, 'The Jews conquered the world.' I said, 'Yeah, yeah.' He said, 'No fooling.' He said, 'Look, this guy Jesus, a Jewish guy, became the God of all the people.' He's wrong, though — don't forget the Arabs, the Asians and their Buddha. But I know what he means. Jesus *was* a Jew, and all his friends were Jews. In Jerusalem, you sure stop and think when you see that [Wailing] Wall — all the Jews before you! I wondered what they looked like a long time ago. My dad said he didn't know — not blue jeans, though! I wondered if Abraham and Isaac, and Moses, all those people, know about the Wall, and I wondered if they pray now. I guess we don't know if they are around. Where's 'around' — that's the big question, right? When I wake up early, and our dog really wants to go out, and he leaps on my bed, and I know he won't let me go back to sleep, I just know it — he'll lick my face, and he'll whine, and he'll lean against me hard, real hard — and when I give up and take him out, and I just stand there, and it's still dark, and you can hear your dog sniffing, it's that quiet: it's then I know there's someone up there, maybe God, maybe lots of people, too, the souls of all the dead folks. It's too big for you to figure out. My dad tells me that when I ask him about God and where heaven is and if there's a soul. He says there is *definitely* a soul, but it's not 'physical,' so I shouldn't keep asking him, 'Where is it?'

"He's right; you can ask too many questions! That's me — always trying to find out answers to everything! I wish you *could* find them. In the last year or so, I've sort of slowed down asking! I just look up there and say, 'Maybe!' I was walking our dog in the park, and it was real quiet, and you just wonder if there aren't people out there — *souls* out there — and they must want to talk with someone. I guess they talk with each other. But how? Where are they? Dad says he thinks when you die, your soul dies with you. But then, it's not a soul, it's your mind he's talking about, isn't it? It's probably best just to forget everything except what you have to do today; and the same thing with tomorrow. The only thing is, when you go to Hebrew school and *shul* [synagogue], they tell you God is with us, the Jews, and your soul is His gift to you, that's what the rabbi told us kids when he visited our classroom, and I was going to ask him where in your body God puts the soul He gives you, but I decided that I'd be getting myself into real trouble, because the Hebrew school teacher says I ask too many questions, and I should just learn Hebrew and read from Torah and stop trying to be a 'philosopher-king.' Well, what's that? Yes, I asked. The teacher didn't think it was funny, my question [as he and I did!]. He said: 'No more of your questions!' If I'd raised my hand like that, when the rabbi came to visit our class, I think that teacher would have taken that [blackboard] pointer of his and charged me with it, like in the Middle Ages, when the knights went after each other with swords or spears.

"They tell you one week you've got to listen carefully for God's advice, and every word [in the Torah] counts. The next week, if I start wondering out loud what [language] they speak in heaven, something like that, they'll tell me I'm going 'too deep' into things! I wish they'd make up their minds! I know I can be a pain, though. I don't just ask, I keep asking! I should know when to stop, my mom tells me. She says, 'Gil, if you don't learn when to stop asking questions, people will start ignoring you.' But in school, the teacher likes us to ask lots of questions. It's when I ask about religion, about God, questions like the ones we've been talking about — then is the time everyone tells me to cut it out! Dad took me to his big dictionary in his study, and he showed me the word 'discretion.' I didn't know what it meant; I read the definition, and then he said I should remember the word and use it a lot. So I say 'discretion' when I take our pup out for a walk!

"Dad was trying to be nice — but he was telling me to think of other people when I want to know something, and 'behave with discretion'; that means be careful not to offend someone, and don't shoot your mouth off, but think first! I asked Dad if Moses showed 'discretion' when he asked the Pharaoh to 'let the Jews go,' and Dad said, 'Gil, you'll be a lawyer one of these days!' I don't want to be a lawyer. I think I'd like to be an astronomer, maybe, or an astronaut. By the time I'm grown up, people will be flying all over the place, to the planets and into the space beyond the planets. We'll explore, and we might be surprised by what we find!

"I don't know what I'd like to find. [I had asked him.] Yes, actually, I do: I'd like to find God! But He wouldn't just be there, waiting for some spaceship to land! He's not a person, you know! He's a spirit. He's like the fog and the mist. Maybe He's like something — something we've never seen here. So how can we know? You can't imagine Him, because He's so different — you've never seen anything like Him! I guess I *should* try to 'use discretion'; I should remember that God is God, and we're us. I guess I'm trying to get from me, from us, to Him with my ideas when I'm looking up at the sky!"

It struck me as unusual, his use of "ideas" as a mode of connecting with a Lord way beyond the reach of eyes, even telescopes — but not beyond the reach of imagination. Gil was searching for God even as he was not sure there was, in fact, a God. Often he'd make reference to the Jews as "scattered" and suggest that perhaps they are "more scattered" than most of us think. I felt that he was speaking facetiously when he made such comments — I saw a twinkle in his eyes, the faintest smile possible, but a smile. When I pressed him, asked whether he *really* believed some Jews might populate a "part of the heavens," he was marvelously clever and knowing with me: "Well, we're here, and this planet is 'part of the heavens'!" A smile from me connected to his slightly triumphant smile, and I began to get irritated: enough of this smart talk.

I decided that his banter was telling me that he himself didn't know how seriously to take some of his serious ideas. But after a few more months of visits, I began to change my mind. Gil's spiritual speculations, delivered in wry language, were, again, not unlike those of Kierkegaard — he had a kind of ironic seriousness, a theological and philosophical attitude that did not take itself unduly seriously. At one point, when I least expected it, Gil became poignantly inward-looking: "I was taking our pup for a walk and doing my thinking. That's when I'm most me! I'm not listening to anyone, and I'm not talking to anyone! I ask all these questions, and I'm not sure God hears me. Why should He? How could He ever hear everything everyone decides to say to Him? It must be hard for Him not to be nearer to us. No, I don't mean that He doesn't 'live nearer.' [I had asked.] I mean that He's in hiding, a little, and we're trying to find Him. We play hide-and-seek — us kids do — and once, the other day, we were playing, and I thought of the times you and I have talked, and what I say, and what you ask, and I thought: you know, Gil, you do that when you think about God and you talk about Him, and maybe *He* does it with us.

"I don't mean to say something bad about God! I don't think He's hiding from us because He's spying on us, or He doesn't like us, so He stays away. I've wondered if it might be true, yes I have — that we're so bad He doesn't want to come near us! [I had asked.] My dad says, 'God must cry because of all the bad things that happen, especially Hitler and the Holocaust.' He says that sometimes on Friday night, when we have our Shabbat supper. We had a guest; he is a lawyer, and he was in a concentration camp. He looks old. He is very smart. He has the numbers on his arm; it's like a tattoo. He showed it to me. He told us he didn't believe in God. He said he's a Jew, and he believes in the Jewish people, and he'd die for Israel, but he can't see how there is a God, because Hitler almost won the war back then. He and Dad had a friendly argument. We all just sat and listened. I was on his [the guest's] side a lot of the time. I was loyal to my dad; I wanted him to win the argument. But I was really impressed with that guy!"

He stopped, and I could see him reflecting on the discussion he heard at home — the problem of evil and of God's response to it. He shifted in his chair as he got ready to talk about a painful subject: "While they were talking I was going to raise my hand, like in school, and ask what if Hitler was going to succeed in killing every single Jew, then would God have stopped him? I guess not. I guess He never interferes; that's what our Hebrew teacher says, that God doesn't ever try to stop something or start something. I don't see how He could have sat up there and not stopped Hitler! If the Jews are His people, then He could have lost us. I asked my father, 'Then would God have cried, if all the Jews had died in those concentration camps?' Dad said he doesn't know; he doesn't know if God cries or He smiles, or what He does. But He'd be unhappy, wouldn't He, if the people He's loved for thousands of years, if we all had gone to the camps, and they killed us?

"It's best not to try to figure out the answers to all those questions — Dad and the rabbi and everyone say so. I've stopped trying, most of the time. It's just that you can't stop completely! See what I mean — if you have a head on you, it'll work sometimes! You'll say something, and you hope God is listening, or you wonder if He's listening!"

The word "listening" prompted Gil to stop talking. He sat

across from me in the teachers' room of his school and seemed not so much at a loss for words as desirous of doing some listening himself. The silence lengthened, and I wondered whether to end our meeting, which had lasted almost an hour. Finally Gil spoke: "It's all too much for me! Maybe when I grow up I'll be an astronomer, and then they'll have telescopes that can see so far into space that we'll know what's going on there. A kid in school told me his grandmother said God holds the whole world — the planets and everything — in His hand. I thought that was funny! The kid didn't like me laughing. I wasn't making fun of him; I was just trying to picture the scene! The kid asked me what I thought, how God looked. I told him I don't know. If you're Jewish, you don't think of what God looks like. I can't help trying, but I can't come up with anyone who looks like God might look! I see Him as, maybe, a huge, big giant; I see Him as an old man with a beard and a long white robe or something; or I see Him as sitting on a throne, with a stick, a staff, holding on to it. Then I say: He's not anything like what we think. For a while, when I saw pictures of Jesus, I thought God looked like Him, or He looked like God. But that's foolish — Jesus isn't our [Jews'] God, and even if Jesus is the son of God, even if the Christians are right, He's not God. They must look different! Anyway, it's not looks that count. It's who God *is*, not what He looks like. God is love, you hear people say that. My sister does; she's in high school, and she has love on her mind!"

He stopped there. Again I was impressed with this boy's lively sense of humor, his capacity to be pointedly sardonic yet also quite serious. No doubt he was being the prematurely wise younger brother, pretending to know the score whenever possible. But he was also able to indicate, through humor, his sense that our spiritual life is very much connected to the rest of our life. In a sense, his comment was both a psychological and a philosophical statement: I am aware that someone's description of God is also — to a certain extent, at least — someone's description of himself or herself. True, Gil doesn't explicate his asides or turn them into general pronouncements. He simply offers his thoughts, attributing them, often, to his parents, his teachers, the rabbi, and the Hebrew school teacher, or now and then daring to acknowledge his own daydreaming self as the original author of a speculation.

"At Shabbat," he once told me, "we try to get serious." His father was the one who occasionally prompted such turns in the table talk. The boy knew full well why: "He decides that we're not being *Jews*, so we have to stop kidding around, and try to be serious. We've got to talk about our [Jews'] history; or we've got to talk about Israel; or we've got to talk about religion — what God wants you to be like. I shrug my shoulders and say '*Dad*' when he'll ask me something, his serious questions. He knows the Bible better, way better, than I do! My grandfather wanted to make sure that Dad knew Hebrew, and knew the history of our Jewish people. I go to Hebrew school, but it's just once a week, and I forget a lot. My father doesn't try to push religion on us, the way his father did on him. It's different. But Dad has told me he used to ask himself a lot of the questions I do, and he couldn't find the answers, and probably I won't. I don't ask questions anymore. I just try to listen, and some of what I hear I believe, and the rest I don't believe! I think there's a God somewhere, but He's not like we might think He is; I mean, He may be different — and that's about all I know! Maybe it's fun for God to keep us all guessing! It's probably better for us, too. We're on our toes, and we're not falling asleep. God wouldn't want all His people dozing half the time!

"When I heard the noise of the *shofar* [trumpet] last week in *shul* I wondered if somehow God heard it, and if the people you read about [in the Bible], like Moses or even Adam and Eve, if they're around, their souls. Look at all the people who came after Adam and Eve! We asked our [Hebrew school] teacher about that — whether you could trace people back that far. He thought we were trying to be wise guys, but we weren't! A lot of your thoughts on religion — they can get you dizzy. You have to remember that no one really knows for sure who God is and what He's got in mind! We'd like to have a hotline to Him, but I don't think we'll get one. If you go to *shul*, you're probably hoping for that hotline, or else you're just showing up to be seen by the neighbors!

"I was riding on my bike, and I could hear the sound of the *shofar* in my head. Maybe God is nearest you when you think of Him, and talk with Him, and remember the sound of the *shofar*, and remember what you've memorized in [Hebrew] school, the prayers, and what Moses said, and Isaiah. This is an 'experiment,' here on earth. My grandfather told me that a couple of years ago, and I think he was right! He meant [I had asked] that God decided to try out making human beings, and letting us have this planet, and giving us the freedom to live as best we can, or to be as bad as possible. That's what has happened — we've been good and we've been terrible. The experiment has given us lots of trouble, but there are nice people, too. You have experiments in science in school — you see how you can create things. Well, we've been created, and we're in an experiment, and one day God will try to figure out what the answer is to the experiment. I don't know how He'll do it. How could He *ever* decide? I asked Grandpa, and he said, 'Look, Gil, these things are too big for you and me. All you can do is try to be good, and let God take care of the rest!' I asked him some other questions, but he said if you think too much you get 'brain exhaustion,' so we went in his car and got some ice cream. I joked with him: this is part of God's 'experiment,' too [their getting ice cream]!"

Gil was trying to comprehend the universe and the religion of his ancestors. He had called upon family members, teachers, his experiences, his imagination, and, not least, his mind's intellectual, contemplative capacity: the ability he has, with the rest of us, to learn symbols and use them, to borrow metaphors or similes or images used by others, to create some of his own — all for the purpose of doing what philosophers have traditionally done over the centuries. Like them, the boy was searching for an explanation of what is, of reality as he saw it, heard it, felt it, both palpably and within his mind. Like them, he pursued wisdom with his mind's energy and in hopes for moral answers, a clue or two about how this life ought to be lived. Like philosophers, he examined the beliefs of others and was becoming an analyst and critic of ideas. Like them, he was trying to pull together what he had observed, learned, read, heard others espouse — to make, thereby, his own "system," his own set of principles. He had yet to (and may never) write articles for journals of philosophy, but he most certainly was trying to assemble what he had learned in a narrative of his own, which he could offer to others: a description of the perceived world; a discussion of the views of others with respect to that world; an enunciation of his own manner of making sense of that world; and, not least, an affirmation of the moral principles he had constructed for himself. As I listened to him and to other boys and girls making similar intellectual and ethical struggles, I often found myself remembering their sometimes urgent determination to define God, to locate Him in time and place, to know Him as precisely as possible, to explain (to themselves and others) who and what He is; and I found myself wondering whether the children themselves aren't the very treasure they so obviously seek: God as children pondering, musing, ruminating, brooding on Him, young minds bending and applying themselves in His image.

✳ ✳ ✳

7

Young Spirituality: Visionary Moments

SOME YOUNG PEOPLE go through intense visionary moments. I often remember a boy or girl looking, looking with eager passion, toward a spiritual horizon that has escaped my eyes and maybe everyone else's. These intensely personal visionary moments, as I think of them, sometimes conveyed softly or tersely, sometimes rendered with eloquence and compelling power, are times when a mix of psychological surrender and philosophical transcendence offers the nearest thing to Kierkegaard's "leap of faith" I can expect to see.

I start with the Hopis, whose extraordinary spiritual life had my wife and me enthralled during the years we spent in New Mexico and Arizona. When I started this process of asking children about their religious beliefs, learning from them about the spiritual side of their inner lives, I knew I should go back to the Hopis. Indeed, I did get to know (in the late 1980s) the children of those onetime children I had seen almost a generation earlier and had described in *Eskimos, Chicanos, Indians.*[1]

Upon my return to New Mexico and with the help of an old friend who is a schoolteacher, I met and began to learn from Natalie, aged eight, whose mother I remembered from my early days out West. Natalie, an oldest child, had two sisters and a baby brother. She was an "average" student and inclined to be "moody" at times, various school officials told me. She was not troublesome, however. Rather, in the words of the school nurse, she was "a typical Hopi girl who is much closer to the customs of her people than [to] our Anglo world" — an understatement. When I began to know Natalie well enough to sit with her for an hour or so at a stretch and talk about not only her life but life in general, I started realizing how probing a naturalist she is (which is not unusual among Hopi children) and (more extraordinary) how preoccupied she could become: her mind seemed almost lost in thought, so engrossed was she with the land and sky, the sun, moon, and stars, the flowers her mother grew, the animals, the changes of light that came with clouds.

On that first afternoon when we really talked, we were sitting on chairs in front of her house. For miles beyond us stretched the flat desert — and then, abruptly, a mesa. The sky was everywhere, noticeably so to me because I'd just arrived from "back East." By that time of day the sun was beginning to lose its tight grip on things. Natalie touched her left arm with her right palm and fingers and noted a diminished heat, a relative coolness. She was sipping some orange soda, and was anxious that I try a bottle. I said no, that I didn't like soft drinks. She remembered — her mother had told her I liked iced tea, iced coffee. She offered to go make some, but I'd had more than enough for the day. We continued along such tentative, impersonal lines for another minute or two, and then the flow of our exchanges stopped because she had spotted a pair of hawks circling above us. She watched them carefully. She was attentive enough to me to point them out, and relaxed enough not to feel the need to say anything. I was glad our small talk had ended, but after two or three minutes, a long time under such circumstances, I began to wonder how long we'd sit like this, our heads up, our eyes following the circling birds. Finally, as the hawks, in their ever widening sweeps, departed from our visual field, Natalie lowered her eyes first and then her head. She looked straight at me, seeming sad, and said, "I guess they'll find something [to eat]. I wish they were just going on a ride and not really hungry. I love when they glide, then stop, flap their wings, and continue gliding."

I realized, at those words, how watchful she had been, how carefully heedful of details I had not noticed. We went back for a while to pleasantries. She was looking right at me all the while, and I was getting ready to ask her some questions about her religious and spiritual life, her beliefs, when in midsentence she broke off. Her head turned about forty-five degrees to the left, she looked up — the hawks had returned. How had she known? Rather, how had she known where to look? I was ready to inquire, but I had to wait once more until she returned to me, as it were. Another several minutes. I didn't consult my watch, but my legs, crossing and uncrossing, told of my impatience. I was now irritated enough to call her, silently, rude. Then I felt ashamed at my presumptuousness. This was her life, her place, her afternoon. I was the rude one, coming here to pose questions, request drawings and paintings. Because I had done so many times was no reason for me to feel I had a right to do so whenever I felt like it. No sooner had I settled that matter with myself than I heard another word sound in my head, "anxious" — Natalie was made anxious by my interests as they got translated into questions, and thus she was only too happy to greet those hawks, so high and mighty, in preference to me, with my own manner of being high and mighty.

Eventually the hawks again retreated from our portion of the sky. Natalie returned to me, to her orange soda, to her chair, whose warmth caused her to lift herself up for a few seconds so that the utterly arid air could welcome whatever moisture had accumulated on the seat of her khaki pants. She decided to say something about those hawks. She decided to tell me a story, as she had heard her parents do and as she had done during prior visits. "Those hawks," she began, "were looking at us." She saw my face form the lines of doubt, of polite reticence. She did not wait for my tactfully stated skepticism, if not opposition. She lifted her voice a bit and began to explain and exhort, in a gentle but insinuating singsong, "The birds are watching us. Two birds watching two birds. Don't you think?"

I thought otherwise, actually. I decided not to say what I thought. I was there to hear what she thought, not to participate in a two-person ornithological seminar. I wondered aloud — since she had posed her opinion as a question, expecting yes for an answer — whether the birds were really paying attention to us.

She brushed aside my implied objection. "It is in them to know we are here. They see everything — better than radar, my dad says. What is radar? [I had asked.] You don't know?"

I felt accused, correctly, of being mischievous. I told her that I did "know" what radar "does," but I had no idea what it "is."

She was amused, understanding: "Like with the birds — they see, I know, because they fly and fly, so high up, then they swoop, and they never miss. They head for what they want, and they get it!"

We were enjoying our agreement. We talked, mostly, about the desert world stretched out before us; it was simmering down by then, at five o'clock in the afternoon. I nudged us along with questions and comments, but afterward I was left with memories of what she said as if it were an extended, uninterrupted aria: "The hawks are pointed for what is there. A rabbit would try to hide, but his chances aren't good. The rabbit will soon be flying! The hawk will feel jumpy for a minute. Dad says we go from one life to another. Mother says, 'Live this one, and stop asking about the next one in line!'

"She tries to be patient with me. She listens while I talk, and then she tells me I'm her daughter, because I say what she used to say. What? [I had asked what she used to say.] Everything! I think of the mesa a lot; it is where our people live, who are gone, and my mother was taken there when she was little, and she has taken me there, and so I think a lot about the mesa, a lot. I visit it [in my thoughts], and I meet our ancestors. They give me a blanket, and they hold me, and they point to the sky and say there are more up there — our ancestors. Only some of them come to the mesa, and then they leave. Do you see birds on trees, how they leave, to get a drink or a bite to eat, fly away, and others follow, and the whole day goes by, birds and more birds? We become birds when we die. We fly away, but we come back. I know because [I had asked] I feel myself sometimes wanting to lift off, go right to the mesa and have a feast: eat our bread, stand in a circle, and hear my grandmother talk about our people.

"She is sick. She is between here and there [the mesa]. She will leave us for there, and then she'll prepare for us to come there. I woke up yesterday, and I realized I'd been there myself [in a dream] to visit her. Later [in the day] I saw her here, and I wiped her forehead, I gave her water. She gave me her hand, and I held it. She told me she prays to be taken there soon. I heard her, later, talking to *her* grandmother. They'll be together there, and we'll go visit!

"Toward night the sun does its tricks before it dies. The moon waits politely. Never try to get in the way of the sun! I love seeing the sun leave. The mesa is where our people have lived from the beginning of our memory. My uncle said we once lived inside the earth, but there was an explosion, and we were pushed up to the mesa, and we first saw this land from the mesa. We decided not to live there, but keep it the way it was, so if we're called back, we'll just walk in a line across the desert; we'll climb the mesa; we'll wave goodbye to the sky, and we'll go back inside the earth. But my grandmother says my uncle is all wrong. We came from the sky to the mesa. We were put there so we could always see for miles and miles, and we'd be nearer to the clouds and the sun and the stars and the moon. All of us come from them — the sky moved closer to the earth, and the wind brought us down. I don't know how. The wind helps the birds, and it helps us. It brings the spirits of our ancestors from here to the mesa and back. When the wind shifts, that's the time to stop what you are doing and listen very carefully. That is when you hear what will happen. I have seen my ancestors and others lifted toward us by the wind. They come here and whisper to our old people, and then they [the old people] talk to us [about what they have heard and learned]."

I asked her whether she was awake or asleep when she saw her ancestors. I knew she was not psychotic, and having worked for years with Hopis, I understood their vivid, metaphoric language. Still, what did she mean, *exactly?* I decided to press the question as insistently as I knew how: "Natalie, what do you mean you have *seen* your ancestors being *lifted* toward all of you here?"

"I mean that I will be sitting near the window, and I pray to our ancestors. I see them."

"How do you pray — on your knees?"

"No, I sit. I close my eyes. I let myself join our people. I ask them to include me in their number. I talk to them. Then I see them."

"Are your eyes now open?"

"No, they are closed. [I judge them only half-closed.] My thoughts cross our land and they are heard on the mesa. They are like the birds. They rise and circle and circle, and then they gradually head for the mesa, and our ancestors wait there for news of us. Then I hear news of them. They are expecting my grandmother any day now."

I thanked her for taking the trouble to explain, but I wasn't sure I fully understood what was happening in her mind. I failed to pick up much that the Hopis, adults and children alike, had to say to each other: their winks and nods, the raising and lowering of their arms, the sudden furrowing and then relaxation of their brows, their many naturalist allusions, their apparently simple stories or their very fanciful ones — people turning into aspects of nature, and vice versa. "Magical thinking," a phrase that I learned to use a lot during my residency in child psychiatry, descended on my mind rather often while Natalie talked, yet at the same time I was taken by her simplicity, her lack of pretentiousness, her apparent lack of interest in whether her visions were credible by my psychological or cultural standards. I decided, finally, to keep encouraging her to tell me what she "saw" and believed to be happening in her world, to observe her as discreetly yet carefully as I could, to accept her as she was — and to learn as much as I could of her thoughts, without feeling the repeated, almost automatic need to submit them to the muster of *my* thoughts.

The words of Natalie's that follow were drawn from various conversations: "When I wake up I look at Blackie, our dog. I stare at her, and she stares at me. We know it's time to start another day. The light has summoned us! We know we'll keep doing this [getting up, going to sleep] until she goes and then I go, and we'll be together: to the mesa, and then — who knows where? My grandmother told me a long time ago that we travel from one place to another; we move through people, and maybe we move through animals, I don't know. Blackie has a soul, I know. She looks at me and I know she is ready to live for me and die for me! She cries when I cry. She barks, to laugh, when I laugh. When I slow down — the sun's heat — she sits still. When I run, she's ahead of me, and her tail is dancing!

"I took Blackie with me on a walk toward the mesa. She was excited. I was, too. I wondered if we'd ever come back — I mean, as me and Blackie. I mean, I wondered if I'd wave to another part of the world, and Blackie, too. I look at those birds, and I think I might be one someday. Blackie, too — then we'd be together still. When I look in Blackie's eyes, she cries a little: she is telling me of her love, and I tell her I love her. We'll always be part of our people — I tell her that my grandmother knows what happens to us, and when Blackie hears, she's excited. On the way to the mesa I talked with Blackie, and I talked with all of our people there — we belong to them: we come from them, and we're here now, and we'll go back to them. I don't know how to explain this: the Hopis are there on the mesa, their spirits. Each spirit is a soul. You can't see them, not the way you see me and I see you. But they are there — and when we go there, we sit, and they talk to us. The wind sweeps across the mesa, and [that way we know] we've been noticed and welcomed! I say 'mesa' to Blackie, and she jumps and dances and cries: the Hopi are calling her back! I jump and dance, too. Some days I wake up, and I know I've already been there [in a dream] with Blackie, and I think to myself: we've already had the most excitement — now to get up and do the chores!

"Sometimes I'll get upset. I don't know why. My spirit may want to leave me — go to the mesa, or go flying high toward the sun! The sun draws sweat from you, and it heats you up. Your mind gets drowsy, but your spirit wants to take off! But I'll look at Blackie. She is lying on the floor; all of her legs are hidden underneath her. She is staring at me. I know what she is thinking! Here eyes are speaking to me: 'Natalie, quiet down! Go through the day! Remember, the hours go by, and when it's night, you can go anywhere you want! It won't take long — and you'll be over this life, and in the middle of another one! So be patient, and enjoy yourself until the end!' I look into her eyes, and tell her 'Thanks a lot,' and her tail goes back and forth a few times — she thanks me!

"I was walking with Blackie, and I saw some smoke in the sky, a trail of smoke. I realized it was a plane. I wondered who was in the plane. I've never been to an airport. They showed us pictures of one at school. I pictured Blackie and me in that plane: we'd point it toward the sun, and keep going! I know the plane would melt; they told us in school everything would melt if it came near the sun. But the sun doesn't melt your spirit! We'd

1 · Heaven and Hell

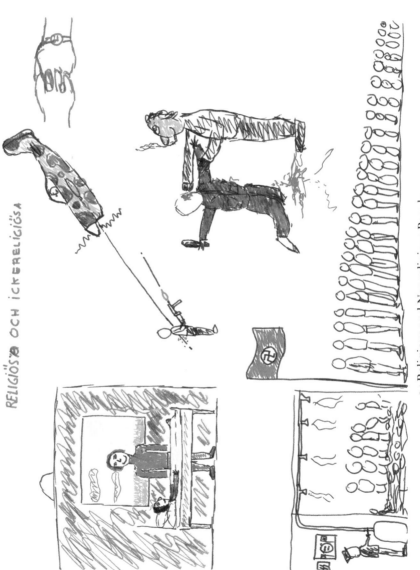

RELIGIÖSA OCH ICKERELIGIÖSA

2 • Religious and Nonreligious People

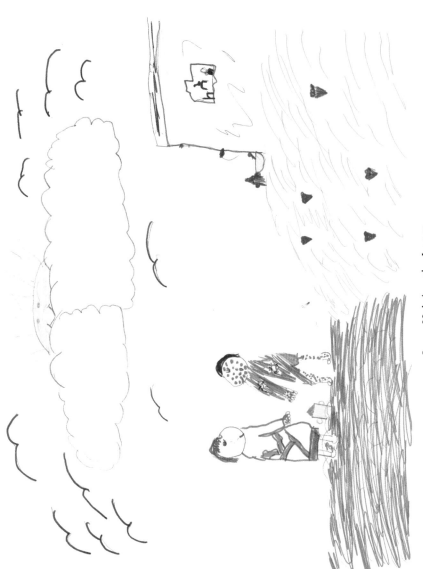

3 • Jesus Helping the Leper

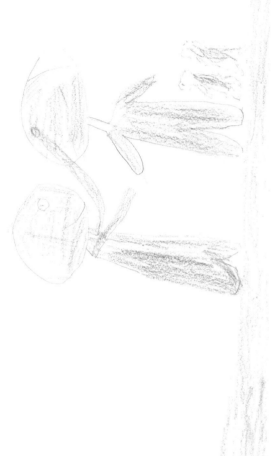

4 · Jesus Helping the Blind Man

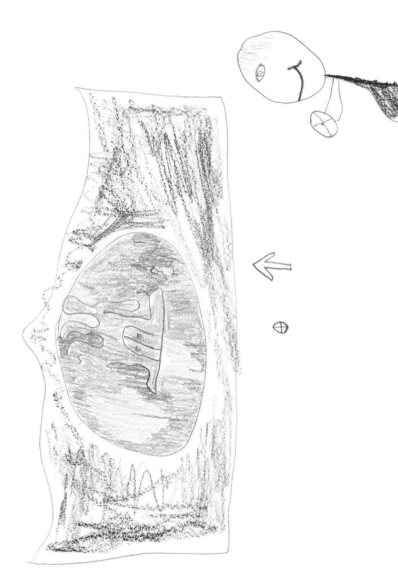

5 · The Planet Where God Lives

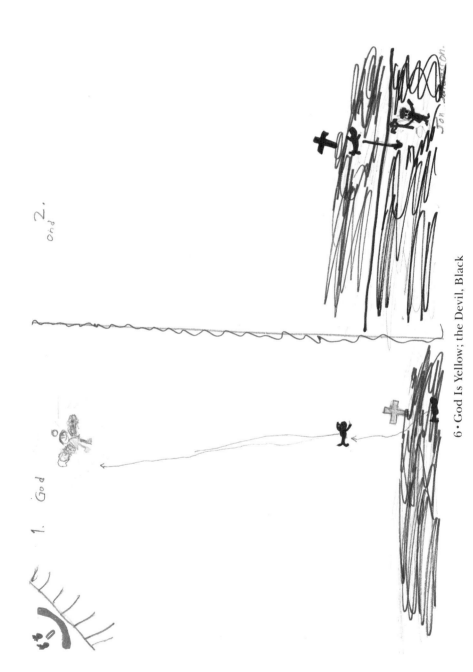

1. God
2. God

6 · God Is Yellow; the Devil, Black

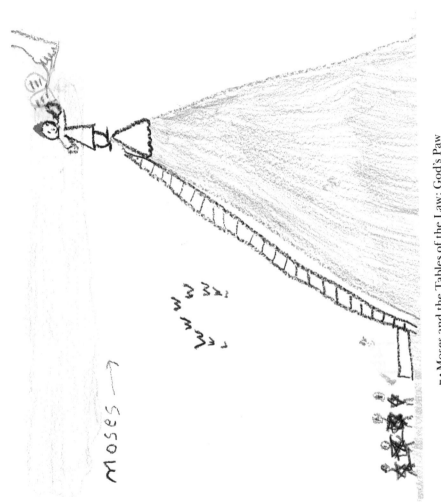

Moses →

7 • Moses and the Tables of the Law; God's Paw

8 · The Crucifixion

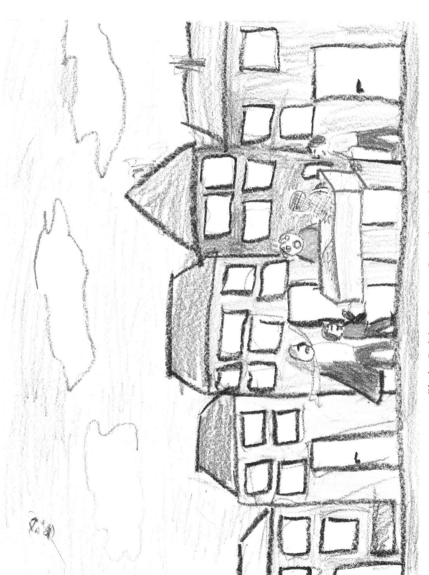

9 · Christ Raising Lazarus from the Dead

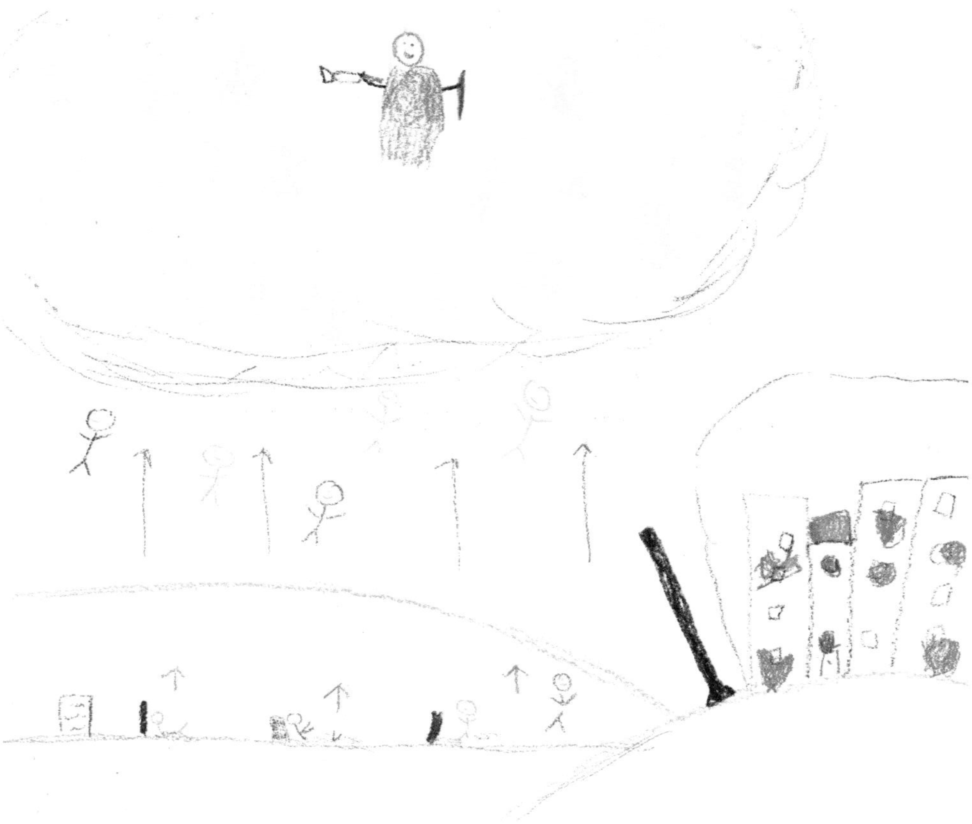

10 • The Saved and the Damned

11 · The Second Coming

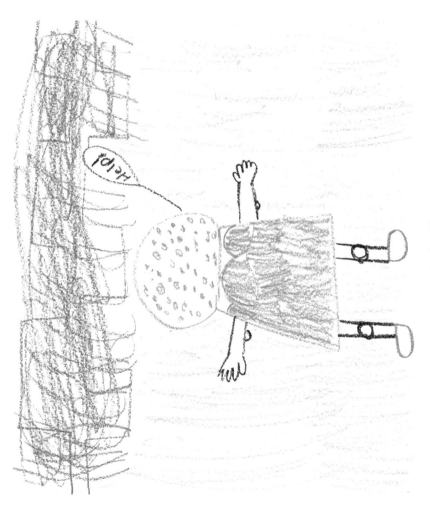

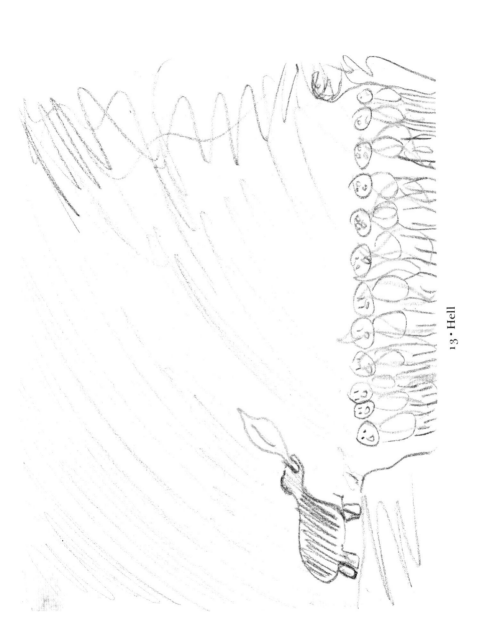

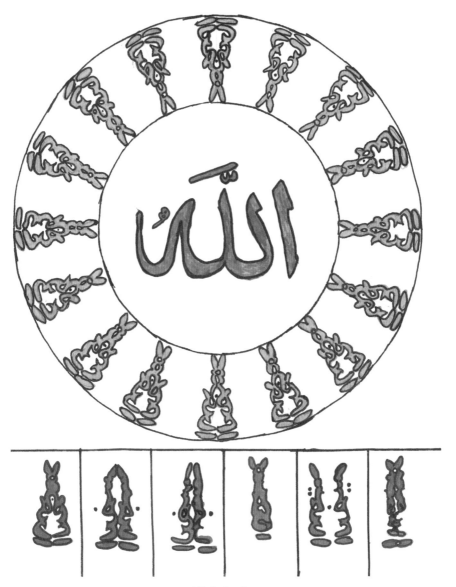

14 · Allah the Supreme

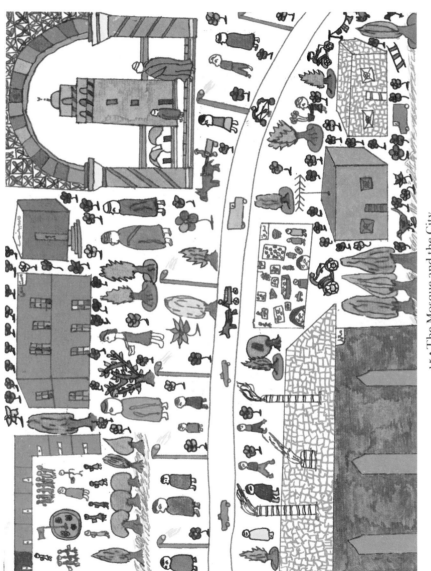

15 · The Mosque and the City

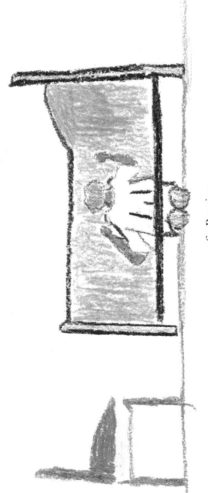

16 · Praying

wave to the sun and the stars! They send us light, and it is a gift to us, and they sent it a long time ago, and now we have it.

"I'm just [day]dreaming, I know! I dream of meeting our Hopi ancestors, and we sit together and talk about the time that will come — the time when all of us are together, and the waters of the rivers are full, and the sun has warmed the cold part of the world, and it has given the really hot part a break, and all the people are sitting in a huge circle, and they are brothers and sisters, *everyone!* That's when all the spirits will dance and dance, and the stars will dance, and the sun and the moon will dance, and the birds will swoop down and they'll dance, and all the people, everywhere, will stand up and dance, and then they'll sit down again in a big circle, so huge you can't see where it goes, how far, if you're standing on the mesa and looking into the horizon, and everyone is happy. No more fights. Fights are a sign that we have gotten lost, and forgotten our ancestors, and are in the worst trouble. When the day comes that we're all holding hands in the big circle — no, not just us Hopis, every-one — then that's what the word 'good' means. The teacher asked us to say what is good, give an example. Blackie is good; she is never going to hurt anyone; and the whole world will be good when we're all in our big, big circle. We're going around and around until we all get to be there!"

This vision of an ultimate circular harmony — an amalgam of lessons told by elders and a child's embellishment of them, her private journey — has stayed with me as I have tried to under-stand the nature of spirituality in children. The Hopis taught Natalie that one day her people would be united in a large circle of amity atop the sacred mesa she had learned to regard as a tribal shrine of sorts. But Natalie went further, on her own and with no particular ideological purpose in mind. She was not preachy or interested in establishing herself as a leader. Her mind wandered across the barren, much-loved tribal land of her people; but her mind also raced across clouds and planetary bodies toward the sun, with its great, life-giving heat, with its light that extends over eons of time. Her mind embraced the stars, too. She was dazzled by the sight of them — they were often her last glimpse before sleep claimed her. Her mother once said, "I hear Natalie saying good night to Blackie. She hugs her and pats her and kisses her. Then she says good night to the stars. Then she falls asleep. The stars are her friends."

She wanted very much to see human beings linked to one another and to the world around them, and in a visionary way she constructed a circle of inclusion. Her vision stood in sharp contrast with the confrontation and opposition that orders most of human society as it divides itself into various clans and tribes and countries, classes and races, neighborhoods, even religions. Natalie's vision was one in which edges and corners give way to a final roundness that would pull us all together in a celebratory union that surely resembles the more prophetic moments of both our Old and New Testaments: "For you shall go out with joy, and be led forth with peace: the mountains and the hills shall break forth before you into singing, and all the trees of the field shall clap their hands" (Isaiah 55:12).

Natalie shook her head when I asked her about God, who He is, what the word means. Neither she nor her parents were comfortable with that word. Rather, she responded to the word "spirit," the collective spirit of her Hopi ancestors, the particular spirit that was hers, that was the dog Blackie's. (I was about to write, by the way, "*her* dog Blackie's," but how out of keeping that would be with her spirit and, she would say, Blackie's as well! Natalie, like so many Hopis, is not possessive so much as eager to be possessed. Her body is not an owner of what she regards as the spirit, now housed there. Her body is a link in a chain of life, even as all those links are part of a universe of life. I am fairly sure that these words do justice to Natalie's spiritual vision, yet I am unable to understand them fully or to feel at home with them.)

Once I tried to link arms, so to speak, with Natalie and her Hopi people in my own way: "What is the 'spirit' you often mention?" She looked at me with worry on her face. Was I all right? Did I need some water, some food? Her silence made me realize that I was never going to succeed on *my* terms with this interview.

But she did, at last, speak — after glancing at the omnipresent Blackie for reassurance. "I don't know what to say," she began. Then there was silence. I had expected as much! Suddenly she stood up; so did Blackie. Natalie walked a few steps away from where we were sitting on our folding chairs, in the direction of the mesa. Now what? I hoped not a walk for the three of us: it was terribly hot, and I was tired. She looked up at the sky. The dog looked up at her — she is Blackie's sky. Abruptly Natalie raised her right arm and whirled it around and around, making circle after circle — a discus thrower, I thought, readying for a climactic heave; and then *it*, the last big exertion. The dog didn't wait. Blackie knew. She was off and running, furiously running, despite the early afternoon heat. When would that dog stop? At the mesa? No, she'd die before she got there if she didn't slow down. What was the meaning of all this, anyway? I asked those questions of myself while Natalie stood staring at Blackie, who seemed to be pursuing some mirage or other. In about fifteen or twenty seconds Blackie stopped, faced about, looked at Natalie, started running toward her, kneeled at her feet, received an affectionate hug, and heard the words "thank you."

What did this pantomime have to do with what had been (or so I thought) an attempt at rational discussion? When Natalie returned to her chair she was quick to help me out: "The 'spirit' is when you go running for someone. It is when you try to send signals to someone. It is when you are being as much you as you can be. When Blackie ran, her spirit was there for me and you to see! When I used my arm with her, it was my spirit talking to her spirit! Every time I look into her eyes, and think of her, and all she does, and all she has been for us, I am trying to see her spirit, I think."

I was ready to forgo further questions. Natalie's spirituality was lived in the everyday, in the various acts of getting through time. Natalie's sense of "spirit" involved a visionary affirmation: the sight of others going through their appointed rounds and rhythms, and the sight of herself doing likewise. Death for Natalie meant a shift in the universe, a spirit moving on to new territory. No wonder she laughed wryly as we talked about American power and Navaho power: "People don't feel at home near their mesa, so they want all the mesas in the world! Then they have so many, they'll never be able to choose which one to call their home! Their ancestors must go from one mesa to the next, and they must cry, because they don't know where they can stay and be together, and they don't know if they'll ever be seen by the people [alive] in America, or on the Navaho land." An interesting notion: we are lost without the kinds of enduring attachments to a place, to a scene, that Natalie and her Hopi people still possess. It is that fight — the struggle for a spiritual homeland — which the Hopis have waged long and hard, and so far with success.

Sometimes as I watched Natalie leading and being led by her dog — by Hopi standards, a spiritual marriage — my mind wandered back to South Boston, where for a long time I observed school desegregation through the eyes of white children.[2] In Boston's Roxbury neighborhoods, where I talked with black children, the experience was regarded as full of promise, if tough — to be bused all over the city, with hostility awaiting, for sure, at the end of the bus ride. In South Boston, however, the experience was constantly infuriating: why us, why this massive federal intrusion upon our turf, our life? These children of machinists, police officers, civil servants, office workers, had learned to think and talk as if the world would soon come to an end. In one South Boston family, however, fear of blacks seemed notably absent. The father, a devoutly Catholic policeman, had worked for years in Roxbury, and though he knew of the black gangs there, firsthand, he also knew South Boston's white gangs intimately. He saw in both communities vulnerable, hard-pressed families, families burdened by poverty and illness and all the anxieties that go with a marginal life. His populist outbursts moved me; often I quoted them to my well-to-do, well-intentioned friends who lived elsewhere and worried out loud about the "racists" of South Boston or about the "culturally disadvantaged" blacks of Roxbury. His decency and capacity to put himself in the shoes of others was not an abstract, intellectual matter but rather a drama lived out — an everyday effort to befriend the white children of Andrew Square in South Boston and the black children of Grove Hall in Roxbury.

The patrolman relied morally and psychologically upon his wife. She had told him when they married that she wanted all the children the Lord would let them have. They had eight — five girls, three boys — and lost two more, one at birth, one at three months of age, a "crib death." Eileen and Jack Corrigan were brave supporters of the decision of a federal judge (who lived in Wellesley, an upper-class, almost all-white town, whose children were never ordered bused anywhere). "One of these days, in this country we'll really talk about what keeps people apart," Jack told me many times, and always these words followed: "Class is there, a big part of it, not just race." Sometimes he got more specific, pointing out to me that "in the fancy suburbs no one's compassion and tolerance is being tested by a federal judge" and that smug and arrogant people who lived there went unnoticed by reporters, while in his neighborhood "plenty of hate and meanness" were being duly recorded by newspapers and the television stations.

"Class determines your reputation," he once told me and one of his police friends as we sat in a bar and wondered when, if ever, Boston's schools would "return to normal," a phrase he used often and occasionally regarded critically, as he did that afternoon: "I guess we'll never have 'normal' again, if by 'normal' you mean the way it was — 'us' here, and 'them' over there, and our kids never seeing one another in school or anyplace else." He stopped, thought things over, then added: "Wouldn't it be nice if some of the kids who live in the rich suburban towns could be challenged the way our kids are." He wasn't being sarcastic — a touch ironic, yes, but also quite earnest: "The only chance for the nation to be united is that way, for kids to learn about other kids, for *all* kids to have that chance."

Later that afternoon his wife was rushed to St. Margaret's Hospital in Dorchester and gave birth to Meaghan, their youngest daughter. The hospital, run by Catholic nuns, is situated "on the frontier," some say — between a white and a black section of Boston. Years later, as Meaghan became very much interested in the racial crisis in Boston, her mother wondered "whether it was where she was born that got her so concerned with the troubles of other people." She was joking, of course, but she was also attributing, modestly, her child's largeness of heart to the location of her arrival rather than to her upbringing.

Now Meaghan approached adolescence — a lively, studious girl of twelve whom her mother briefly described this way: "If she didn't like boys so, I'd think she'll be a nun when she's older!" Religion did indeed play a large part in Meaghan's life. She went to church several times a week, usually with her mother. But so did her older sisters; even her brothers, robust athletes, boisterous and cynical at times, were frequent churchgoers. "The Catholic Church is not dead in this house," Eileen said occasionally. In their house, hanging on their living room wall, a "bleeding heart of Jesus" picture reminded me of what I saw as a child in some of my friends' homes, to my childhood bewilderment and even apprehension. But Meaghan's ruminations about God and Jesus, about South Boston and Roxbury, about people rich and not at all rich and quite poor, ranged beyond the realm of the traditional religious teachings she and her brothers and sisters and friends heard almost every day, and certainly on Sunday in church. When I tried to figure out where her prophetic, articulate, strong-minded voice came from, I recalled her grandfather, her dad's dad. Now retired, he was a policeman once, and he was also a populist with a strongly rhetorical manner of speech. *His* father was a longshoreman and a labor organizer, "fresh off the boat from the old country," and "a speaker who could sing the birds off the trees right to his hand," as Meaghan put it. She had a touch of that persuasive intensity, that credibility of being as well as of word. She also could dream out loud — not only at night about the past, but by day about the future, hers and everyone else's, and often with a lilt and with speech mannerisms that revealed a lingering nostalgia for the old country.

"I was sitting on our swing [on the porch of her family's home] and I wondered if God thinks about *us*" — with those words she had responded to my open-ended inquiry, put to her when she was nearing her twelfth birthday, "Do you think much about God?" (Some children have answered yes or no, and that is that. Other children have qualified it — one day a lot, another day briefly. A few children have had the strength, maybe the quick wit, to ask me about myself — you tell me before I'll tell you! Because of the nature of the research I'm doing, I've told them, I can't help but think about God almost every day. Few children have ever turned the question around as quickly as Meaghan did, and none have used it so promptly as a provocation for a wide-ranging spiritual polemic.) "When Jesus died, He was really in pain," Meaghan told me, "and He was wondering if it was worth it, all the trouble He'd had. But then He went to heaven. Since then, we're supposed to remember: He saved us. But we forget! I asked our nun [in Sunday school] how you can be saved and still be bad every day. She told me I was being naughty and bad right then and there, because I was confusing what she'd said! So she explained again to us: if we believe in Him, we'll be saved and go to heaven. But while we're here, we make mistakes."

She stopped to catch her breath and let her theologically aroused mind take a short rest. We discussed the possible destination of an ambulance whose urgent siren we heard. Her friend's dad was very sick with lung cancer. He lived a couple of blocks away. "They" could be coming to take him to the hospital yet again. He was near the end, only forty-five. This seeming detour offered her an opportunity to go full speed ahead: "He is the nicest person you'll ever meet. Our priest says he's a saint! He's ready to help everyone. Even now, he'll call people up if they're in trouble, and he'll give you the shirt off his back, my dad says. And he's dying! We can pray, but he'll die soon! My dad says it's just not fair — but you know, sure enough, it's not fair to us, but it could be fair to him! Maybe he'll be better off away from here — all the trouble. His son's bicycle was stolen, and he's had his radio in his car stolen, and because he told the kids to stop shouting at the colored kids, the blacks, he had a threat: a guy phoned him up and told him he'll 'get it.' My friend [his daughter] said her father never heard such bad words in his life. Maybe God heard them, too! Maybe He's up there, and He's sitting someplace, and He's saying: Francis Boyle is a good man, and he has suffered enough, and I'm going to call him right up here, and he can have a long, long rest, and no one will swear at him, and he won't have that cancer anymore, and it's very painful, and he's suffered enough."

She not only stopped speaking but breathed deeply, as if the working of her lungs had suddenly become part of her consciousness, or as if she were struggling for breath, as she had heard Mr. Boyle do. Then she became aware of what she was doing. She asked me questions about lung cancer, medically astute questions — where it spreads, what course it takes with respect to symptoms, approximately how long someone "in pain like Mr. Boyle" has to live. She wondered out loud how in the world a "God in heaven" can find the time to take note of each and every Mr. Boyle in this world of "billions and billions of people." (I have often wanted to ask that of children who've rather too reflexively told me that God watches over them and everyone else, but have kept my mouth shut and duly recorded yet another spoken piety.) Meaghan now turned the tables on me, to my great surprise: "I don't understand all this. How do you explain it? Tell me — answer me this: where [do] God and Jesus get the time to look after Mr. Boyle, and all the other people in every city and every country — people who are sick? How do they [God and Jesus] do it?"

Immediately I said, without thought, "I don't know."

I was preparing to think more seriously about a possible reply when she made it clear that she had no intention of accepting such an evasion: "Have you ever wondered?"

"Yes, lots of times."

"Well, what did you think?"

"I've never been able to answer the question. I really don't know."

"But it's really important — because God is up there waiting for us, and we want Him to know what's happening [to us]. So there must be a way He can look after each of us." She pushed aside the hair that had fallen over her forehead. She stopped swinging, by putting her two feet firmly on the porch floor. She looked up toward the cloudy sky and reminded me that we were going to get rain soon and asked if I had left my car windows open, the way I had a couple of weeks before when a long thunderstorm gave me a wet ride home. I told her the car was securely closed while continuing to wonder what in the world to say to her.

She spared me, however: "I guess He's not one of us! He *was*, but then He went back to being God. I guess if you're God you know everything, but you're not like us, so the way you know everything — it's different. In church they say we should say our prayers a lot, and I try to remember. I try to think about God a lot. When I do, I close my eyes, and I try to have nothing on my mind but Him; that's what my mom and dad say you should do. I think of Him, and I try to talk with Him. I ask Him the same questions, like how He remembers everything. You know what He says: 'I just do!' That's simple! A lot of times it's hard to tell Him what I want to say! I just can't find the words. I'll picture Him — He looks like He does on the windows in church — and I want to tell Him what's on my mind, but I don't have anything there, just these feelings."

I wanted to know about them — those "feelings," a trigger word for a psychiatrist. She was vague about them. She talked of being sad that her father got tired easily. (The family had been told he had high blood pressure.) She talked of being sad that her mother had so much work to do. Her mother loved the movies but could find practically no time to go to one — even to sit and watch one on television. Meaghan wondered why her family was of modest means, barely getting by, while other families were so well off. To be sure, she knew the answers; yet she wondered about fate in its various forms: "When you're born, God has decided to put you where you are, and not somewhere else. I was wondering why. It's the throw of the dice; that's what my dad says about almost everything."

I was relieved that she quoted her father rather than asking me for an answer to the question, to the riddle that she had been examining in her mind. But she was not totally ready to pass me by, helpless though I felt and helpless though she knew I felt. "What do you think — is there some plan God has when He makes all His decisions?"

I shook my head and shrugged. For some reason I was withholding my words. Why? She seemed not to mind. Maybe she didn't notice, was less self-conscious than I. A blessing, I thought.

Suddenly it began to rain. She watched closely as the grass below received its welcome refreshment. She listened to the roof register the change in the weather. "They told us a long time ago [in Sunday school] that Jesus wept during His life," she said. "My mom says sometimes when it rains that it could be Jesus is crying. Maybe He knows Mr. Boyle will die soon. Maybe He worries about the schools, all the trouble we have. He could be crying for them, in Roxbury, and for us here, because Daddy says we just get by, that's all, and there are lots of poor families here. He could be crying because He wishes everything is better — but it isn't.

"Last weekend we had the best weather you could want. I rode my bike to the beach [the part of South Boston that borders on Boston Harbor]. I could see way out to sea. I saw those waves — the ones far away, not the ones that land on the sand. I just stared. As far as you could see there was water, and then there was the sky. I wished with all my might that I could say a prayer and mention the people [who need God's intervention] and He'd come from up there and say, 'Meaghan, I'll help out!' He didn't come and talk with me. Why should He? But I got close to Him. I stood still and I looked out as far as I could see, and I thought I could see His face. I mean, I *didn't*, but I did: He was smiling. Then I realized *I* was smiling — so it wasn't Him, it was me. Where would we be if He wasn't around to help? When my mom asks that, I know He's already helped her! My mom doesn't say anything; she just closes her eyes. That's her way of praying: close your eyes and be still, and hope your heart speaks to His heart. She learned it from her mom. Her mom died having a baby, my aunt."

She closed her eyes to pray for her grandmother's soul. She remembered that beach again. She told me that the sight of the ocean brought her closer to God. I asked why, and she answered with marvelous originality: "There's no one there, no one to talk with, just Him, way off — and remember how He walked on water! Maybe one day He'll just walk up to Southie [South Boston] from Carson Beach or City Point!"

Her silence thereafter had a special quality. She was thinking about God, holding on to the image she had just evoked. She closed her eyes, held them shut a few seconds, opened them, and resumed where she had left off: "He *could* come back here, right here! This is as good a place as any! Dad says that about Southie: 'It's as good a place as any — you have your bad, but you have your good. It's a little more in the open here, now.' That's what he says. Maybe Jesus will come here, and then He would heal all the people. But you can't know what He'll do — I know that! When I was looking at some of those waves I thought: He could just rise up, out of the ocean! He could walk over the water. He could walk down towards our home. Maybe people wouldn't pay any attention to Him! You know, He might not tell them [who He is]. He might test them. That's how He might come — and boy, we'll be sorry if we ignore Him! He might be walking, and people would say, 'Look at that bum, he's all wet; he must be a no-good drifter; he must be from somewhere else.' "

This intense, imaginative, bright, compassionate girl had said all she wanted to say now. She turned silent in a way that I knew meant we were finished talking about God. She made one final gesture: she opened both hands, curved her palms a little into two cups, collected a bit of rainwater in them, looked at her hands, and emptied them by flipping the rainwater onto her knees. Soon she was standing, ready to go check on the house's open windows, in case her mother, making supper, had forgotten. That act of consideration for her tired, overworked, warmly decent mother struck me as a child's quite touching epiphany: seeing prayer and the search for God not as a fleeting vision, isolated from the events of this world, but as a means of connecting oneself to the ordinary moments of living.

So often, as Meaghan tried to speak her mind, only to retire into silence without embarrassment or disappointment, I realized the virtues of a quietly visual spirituality, expressed in her various images of God, and especially Jesus, in her head, and her delight in drawing or painting Jesus for her Sunday school teachers and for me. Not that she didn't crave to find the words that would reach Jesus, prompt Him to take notice, to respond with words of His own, with a gesture that would show He had heard, He was indeed moved. But at only twelve years of age she had learned of His inscrutability; she had also learned that "His ways are not ours." Though such knowledge was not formally assembled in her mind, it informed her spiritual life — hence her calm awareness, a lot of the time, that Jesus is no magician, switched on by rituals or words. He lives beyond the eyes and the ears, she told me, beyond the human mind — and she struggled to bridge that infinite distance with her imagined scenes, her provocative questions (which could border on or trespass over to radical doubt). Her wish for Him to arrive, to take charge of a troubled world, to right the wrongs she knew existed tells us a good deal about what was most distinctive about her; but also tells us what she shared with so many others, a wish somehow to escape the bounds of the flesh and soar to that place where the ocean meets the sky, that point of light, that spot in the infinity of space, where He may well be.

I left Meaghan's home that day and drove back toward mine.

The child's keen desire to be in touch with the eternal stayed with me as I held the steering wheel and pushed on the gas pedal. I compared her with Natalie, from such a different world — yet they are two American girls of about the same age, each of whom is going to be very much a part of the new century, and each of whom looks backward as well as forward, back to the time of the Jesus who walked Galilee, living such an exemplary life, or back to the time of the Hopis who lived with an almost apocryphal (I suspect) freedom and spontaneity — "before the Anglos, before there was this country."

Both girls, however, strive every once in a while to break the confines of self, of society, of time and space, even of faith; they look within themselves for the strength to leave themselves, to pursue a vision — of the mesa, the Christ risen yet again. They look within themselves for the words (a kind of strength, a *human* kind of strength) to give expression to that vision, connect the seen to what can be shared with others by speaking. Their visionary moments can, of course, be rendered silently on paper — and in the next chapter they appear. Still, words make us what we are, and define our never-ending struggle, as Flaubert knew. Often I have thought of his words in *Madame Bovary*: "Human speech is like a cracked kettle on which we tap crude rhythms for bears to dance to, while we long to make music that will melt the stars." To remember this while hearing Natalie's or Meaghan's words, to watch them set aside language to do a chore, to do a favor for another, is to be a lucky reader of several texts, at once different and similar — the great storyteller lamenting his inadequacy, and the child gazing with her own kind of ambition at those same stars and acknowledging no less candidly her inability to comprehend their significance, let alone "melt" them. In young spirituality that passion to reach and affect the entire universe is constantly given expression as children yearn to catch a moment's flicker or glimmer of recognition from even one star, it being left to others, grown and inspired, to attempt more.

8

Representations

FOR MANY CHILDREN moments and stretches of silence can be the means for important statements, an irony not lost on them. William Carlos Williams, no stranger to the challenges of language,[1] also could take note of its prolonged absence: "I am with a child, and I want some information — and he'll clam up, or she'll stare at me stonily. I'll get impatient. I'll get angry. On a good day, though, I'll remember what I shouldn't have forgotten — what I've learned after hundreds and hundreds of house calls: when a kid falls silent I should keep my eyes open." In his own terse, aphoristic way he had offered a young medical student a clinical wisdom gained after years of work with the young — to pay attention to the wordless narration that can take place as a child uses his or her face, arms, or legs, or, as child psychiatrists have learned, a paintbrush, some crayons.

We adults have our own way of silently making statements — recalling dreams. "Often a child will tell me about a dream — that it has taken place the night before — and then say nothing," Anna Freud once remarked. Then a pause, with its dramatic power — it was an invitation to share with her those times of perplexity when I had hungered for information, for words, yet somehow sensed I had best respect a child's preference for taciturnity. Silence on my part, so she continued: "I will ask the child what he *saw* last night — and that word can move us away from what otherwise might be a stalemate." Another pause, and then, without an explicit request from me that she elaborate, she described the spells of edifying wordlessness she had so often experienced in her psychoanalytic work with children: "Some children know right off what I mean. They will tell me that 'this picture came at night,' meaning they had a dream; or that they caught a glimpse of so-and-so, and then so-and-so appeared, and next thing there was 'no more picture.' Other children require me to be the teacher who explains something carefully — and that was my first wish, to teach school, before I decided to become a psychoanalyst! I will say something like this: 'When we *dream* we *see*.' I've often compared some dreams to silent movies — and only when we wake up do we connect words to the picture or pictures that have appeared in our heads."

Another pause; she seemed lost in her memories of dreams described to her, of particular encounters with one or another child. Soon, however, we were discussing the visual side of human communication — in dreams, in facial expressions, in bodily postures, in actions taken, in drawings and paintings attempted or completed. She, whose work so much depended upon the remarks made by her patients, was ready to admit her occasional frustration with words, with spoken narration: "I have experienced moments in analytic work with certain children when I am grateful for silence in the room! You must know the feeling — we all do: words are leading us round and round! The other day a twelve-year-old girl let me know, fifteen minutes into our session, that she had nothing more to tell me. I didn't say anything. Nor did she thereafter — until she announced that she wanted to draw a picture. I didn't even have to speak; I smiled! She went about her business [of drawing], and when she was done I knew a lot more about her than I'd have known if I'd pressed her for more talk!"

Often, as I've talked with children about their religious beliefs, their spiritual interests or concerns, I've thought of that conversation with Anna Freud and of the writings of Shakespeare and Chekhov and Beckett, all of whom knew the futility and inadequacy, the impasses, that the use of language can present to both speaker and listener. Again and again, children have thought long and hard about who God is, about what God might be like, only to find refuge in the stillness of a room, the stillness of their own minds or souls, as they struggled to express what might well be, for them, the inexpressible. Let fingers work at the matter, with crayons or paintbrushes or a lone pencil; let the fingers supply a contrapuntal reality of asserted action that belies tellingly, even stunningly, an earlier avowal of baffled inadequacy, the hush that precedes the resort to portraiture.[2]

"I can't tell you about heaven, what it's like, or hell, what it's like," remarked young Martin, a Swedish boy of twelve who seemed bored, then aggressively indifferent, then visibly annoyed as questions about his faith — or lack of it — were put to him. Yes, his parents were nominally Christian (Lutheran), but the boy realized full well that they had a habitual inattentiveness to religion, as well as a cosmopolitan materialism that informed their way of thinking about life. Yes, he was baptized, and even sent to Sunday school, but so were his parents, and that is that — empty rituals, a mere nod to a nation's, a family's, history. God? Who can say anything about Him? — not Martin: "No one I know has seen Him." The Bible? A book more praised and quoted than really contemplated: "I see Bibles in homes [of friends], but there is dust on them" — a wry statement all the more astringent for the clipped Swedish accent given to words spoken in English. "I hear people speak of heaven and hell, but I've never heard someone describe them." A three- or four-second lull was ended by an interesting qualification: "I mean, someone who has been there, to heaven or to hell." (So much for all the descriptions that humankind has produced.)

Several days of such brief but pointed exchanges persuaded my family and me to seek other, more talkative children — but then, at the last minute, I found myself thinking of all the crayons and paints I had lugged across the ocean. "Martin, would you like to paint or draw — anything? Martin smiled, and his visitor expected, maybe, a Stockholm scene, a soccer game, a summer's triumphant sun, even a self-portrait. (He seemed so neat, so self-possessed — surely he would want to show us himself in all his Scandinavian urbanity.) He was soon busily engaged with many crayons, while his former questioner, at last silenced, pretended an interest in other matters — the arrangement and rearrangement of notes, tapes, maps. In time a drawing was done. The silence of a drawing session gave way to the silence of a Swedish boy who had finished doing something and was now staring resolutely at an American man who was, for his part, staring at a drawing (Figure 1) — and drawing a complete blank.

"It is heaven and hell." The hint was not enough. "In heaven you're way beyond everything; you're not you anymore — light as a wisp of a cloud, or like the wind going through a meadow. In hell it is very intense. You're stuck — you're stuck with yourself, and with all that's weighing you down, from your life: very tough!"

That commentary having been offered, the boy surveyed his picture and decided to help the viewer. He took a ruler and a pencil, drew a line: heaven is here, to the left; hell is there, to the right. "I may have made a mistake just then." What did he mean? "I made the difference [the distinction] too clear — too final!" He had originally, in fact, let his "heaven" gradually merge with his "hell," and then had drawn the pencil line as a teacher does: to teach. He decided to erase the pencil line but had immediate second thoughts: "It is all guessing, so I won't worry!"

Later, we talked about his picture, with words that could be spoken only after the picture was done and there before us, on a table, with its own palpable reality — utterly abstract, yet with plenty of suggestive immediacy. A boy who had sounded like a skeptic, supremely wedded to the here and now, let crayons create the basis for a spoken theology as sophisticated as it was unpretentious: he saw heaven as the loss of the self into an almost unimaginable lightness (crayons hesitantly applied to the paper); and hell as a condition of overbearing self-involvement (the heavy wear of those crayons on the right side of the paper). Not for this boy devils or angels. Not for him Jesus or Satan. Not for him the Lord in any form — or humanity either, after death.

Martin said no more, and my visit seemed about to end. Suddenly, however, the world of representation through illustration required another try. A boy notably terse, if shrewd, with words didn't even speak; he did not ask for permission, as some children would, to do another drawing, but took a piece of paper from a nearby pad and got to work, this time using felt-tip pens rather than crayons.

When Martin was through, he glanced at me, picked up a brown felt-tip pen, and used it to give his picture (Figure 2) a title, rendered in Swedish: "Religious and Nonreligious People."

The boy had, of course, been asked about the rights and wrongs of this world, as he had learned of them at home, in school, in church, only to reply with bland and pious alternatives: "Some people seem good; others aren't good at all, and they might even get in trouble with the law. You are good if you obey the law and are nice to your family and you do the work you should." No wonder I didn't mind when the subject had changed to Martin's travels abroad: to Norway and Denmark, to West Germany.

Yet if I had held out little hope that Martin wanted to share his spiritual reflections with me, a surprise was in store. He constructed a vivid picture, full of eloquent ethical distinctions, provocatively represented and suggestively placed on what turned out to be a child's moral canvas showing starkly the rights and wrongs of this world, and juxtaposed in a way that told a lot about Martin's capacity for ambiguity: "Sometimes we're good, sometimes we're bad. People will fight — then with their friends, they hold hands. It's what you *mostly* do that counts, I guess. If you take care of people or you kill them! My uncle is a doctor, and even if he makes mistakes — I know he has, my dad told me — he tries to help people. He's got a temper, but he tries to help people. When people fight, they're hurting each other. The Nazis hurt more people than anyone knows exactly — millions. They had concentration camps. They killed people all the time. If you like people, you're doing what Jesus said [you should]. If you fight and kill people, you're doing what Jesus said you shouldn't do. We like to play cops and robbers, and play war, but I hope we don't get serious and become crooks and murderers! It's important to respect people and shake their hands and be a gentleman! If you remember what you learned from your mother and father, and from your minister, then you'll try to be good — unless they are bad people, and they teach you [the] bad. My father says in Germany, while the Nazis ruled, there were ministers who obeyed them, and they were on their side, so you can be religious and bad, and even if a doctor doesn't go to church, he can be religious, because he's doing what's right to do."

Here was a morality based on everyday deeds — the simple handshake, for instance, rather than church attendance on Sundays. Martin, who had spoken candidly, even bluntly, of the dislike he felt for those "who brag of their Christianity," had made his point. We next asked, "Please show us whatever you wish about the subject of religion: what you believe or don't believe; how you picture God; what really matters to you as you think of what you've learned from the Bible, or about the Bible." The invitation was open-ended, but of course he might have refused it, had he desired to do so; or he might have asked for further clarification, followed, maybe, by an all too obliging and literal-minded response on his part. ("Tell me what to draw," some children eagerly say, "and I'll do it.") In contrast, Martin made a statement rooted in his family's life and values and in his continent's history: "My grandfather fought the Nazis. He didn't have to. Sweden was neutral. But he wanted to. He was a scientist. He never went to church. He told my father, 'Jesus didn't go to church — and if He came back [to earth] and saw people boasting that they're good because they go to church, He'd want to leave!' My father told us many times the story of his father — how he slipped into Norway, and fought with the resistance there, and the Nazis captured him, and they were going to kill him, but they were trying to get Sweden to do things for them, so he became a hostage. They sent him to a concentration camp, and he nearly died. The Americans came and rescued everyone just in time. The Nazis were trying to kill all the people in the camp. They shot my grandfather, but he didn't die. He lost his right leg. A [German] tank ran over people, and then they [the Nazis] shot them; but still, he lived. I remember him walking with crutches. He died three years ago. He told me, 'God is in your heart and your conscience, not in a church.' He said that to me many times. He said, 'Martin, you must pay your respects to God, not the church. It may cost you [to do so], but that is what makes a Christian.' I hope I'll remember his words always."

The Swedish boy's English was impeccable, if a bit formal and arch, though he had other than linguistic matters on his mind as he spoke: he was struggling to retain the dignity of self-control, and struggling, too, for a certain stoicism and reserve, qualities he clearly regarded as manly. Light-haired, with blue eyes, slightly stocky, round-faced, he might for all the world have been the boy Dietrich Bonhoeffer as he spoke to us of his family and national history and as he tried to sort out how formal religious life makes connections to one's moral and spiritual values. Several times, in response to questions aimed at a further discussion of his religious habits, his spiritual thoughts, he held himself silent, seemed to demur, tilted his head toward the drawing he had done, with its version of an earthly heaven of human relatedness, an earthly hell of violence and killing — his picture being the only statement he felt it necessary or desirable to make.

Other boys and many girls in Sweden were as talkative as American children had been. But one Swedish child was very much like Martin in her relatively taciturn manner and in her wish to offer drawings and paintings as the mainstay of her spiritual reflection. Josephine was nine when she met us and had a chance to respond to our inquiries. When asked, one day (six weeks after involvement with this study), what Biblical story meant the most to her, she responded not with words but simply by reaching for some pencils and crayons. In time, she offered (with a look that was grave, yet full of pride) what she had accomplished (Figure 3). Quickly she realized my perplexity — hence the terse explanatory title, "Jesus Helping the Leper," which she spoke first in Swedish (*"Jesus botar den spetelska de Manen"*) and then in English.

After I had a chance to reflect on what I had been shown, I asked Josephine why she had chosen this subject, what the event meant to her. She was not initially forthcoming. She was in fact silent. Tall for her age, brown-haired, with hazel eyes and long arms, long fingers, long legs, she sat quite still, both palms planted on the outer margins of her picture. At first she looked at it; then she looked away toward the window, the sky. When she was again asked about the drawing — asked to say anything about it she thought important — she did so, but with an economy of words: "If you are really remembering Jesus, you remember the people he wanted to help."

A school bell interrupted us. With a class calling, Josephine made a point of letting go of her work right away (not all children do so), even suggesting forthrightly, "It is yours to keep." So I did, though two days later the drawing was with me as I talked with Josephine in the schoolroom where she had done her Biblical scene. My questions were the same — a request that this thoughtful, poised, introspective girl share any thinking that may have informed her earlier artwork. "I don't like hypocrites," she suddenly announced. I asked her if she knew many. "Lots," she replied. I asked her next, whether "they" tended to congregate, principally, in the neighborhood where she lived, or in the school where we sat, or in playgrounds or places elsewhere which she frequented. She was unresponsive, then suddenly asked this: "You are a doctor — have you ever treated a leper?"

"No."

"Would you?"

"Yes."

"Have you ever treated someone you don't like?"

"Yes."

"Did you want to treat that person?"

"I don't follow you — are you asking whether I didn't want to treat the person because I didn't like him?"

"Yes."

"I tried to distinguish in my mind between the man's personality, his character, and his disease, his illness."

"What if you were wrong about the man?"

I was even more perplexed by that question, to the point that I was silent for five or six seconds. Just as I was getting ready to say that I didn't quite know how to answer, Josephine began talking as she hadn't ever before — more expansively. "If we are to be Christians we should try to find lepers and go be with them and help them. There aren't any lepers here in Sweden, and in your country either, I don't think. When Jesus lived, I think there were lepers around[3] — and people would have nothing to do with them, the respectable people. My cousin [a college student] says you should use your imagination when you read; so I have tried with the Bible. There are lepers here, but they don't look like the lepers did back then [when Jesus lived]; I mean, they're not lepers, but they are treated like lepers. Do you see what I mean?"

A pause, and I nodded. She resumed right away: "Jesus had a lot of trouble to face when he went to a leper and was friendly and tried to make him better. People said lepers weren't people! That's what happens! If you're a Christian, you try to be like

Jesus. It's good to pray to Him, but if you don't follow Him, then you're not being a Christian; you're praying and going to church. There's a difference."

Rather too quickly I heard myself categorizing Josephine — one more modern Swedish child with a noticeable animus toward ordinary churchgoing and ordinary attempts to communicate with God. But I looked at the picture Josephine had drawn, noted the care she had lavished on both Jesus and the leper, the garb of the healer, the ravaged skin of the wounded man. I observed the two clouds above them — joined, with a smiling sun beaming above. I looked at the brown earth, the grass-covered earth adjoining it, with its house and nearby flowers. I looked, finally, at Josephine: she was not flaunting secular doubt of established Christianity — rather, she seemed awakened and touched by what had come from her energetic right hand. I asked for Josephine's help: "Would you tell me what is happening there [in the drawing]?"

"Oh, yes." She hesitated — perhaps to tell herself, first, what she had meant to convey. "The leper was there, in the desert. Jesus was tired. He was carrying a candle. He'd walked a long way through the night. He was hoping He could find a place to rest — but then He saw the leper, and his heart went out to him, and then He stopped and spoke with the man, and He healed him. Then He could go and rest, and maybe get something to eat. Probably the leper felt much better. Maybe he went and ate with Jesus. I don't know. I'm sure He wouldn't be afraid to eat with the leper. I'll bet lots of people were afraid, though, and they probably said bad things about him, and probably they thought he was going to die and go to hell — *but not Jesus.*"

I italicize those last three words to echo Josephine's spoken emphasis. But even as pictures can offer their own silent testimony to a child's inner life, her spiritual wakefulness, so do her facial expression and the gestures she uses as she talks. As she spoke those last words Josephine looked hard at her drawing. With her left hand she gave a gentle but noticeable thump on the table, as if to remind both herself and me of the singular moral stand Jesus took during his healing ministry, his Galilean journey. With her right hand she briefly touched the Jesus she had created, then the sun. In a moment both hands were at her side, and she reminded me that an important meeting was soon to begin elsewhere. As the shy, soft-spoken girl got up, she curtsied, smiled, thanked me, said goodbye to me, and then, with a smile on her face, looked at her picture a final time and waved goodbye to it — exhibiting a relaxed formality that I kept remembering for a long time. She was a child who meant, I felt, not only what she said, but what she had drawn.

Josephine's portrayal of Jesus as an iconoclastic healer reminded me of work I had done, six months earlier, in a Boston ghetto with black elementary school children — especially with a black girl, Henrietta, scarcely three weeks Josephine's elder. Henrietta could be voluble at home and in her neighborhood but was loath to say much in the classroom. Once, as I tried to converse with her, only to encounter long stretches of silence or, at best, monosyllabic replies to my increasingly coaxing questions, she decided abruptly to set me straight: "I'm not a good student, so I keep my mouth shut here in school!"

"But your comments at home have been very helpful," I insisted, "and they have taught me a lot."

"Oh, thank you. If you told the teachers that, they'd not believe you!"

"Should I try?"

"No! The more you say what's good about me, the more they'll disbelieve you!"

"Are you sure?"

"Yes, I'm as sure as I can be!"

"I really wonder, Henrietta, if those teachers are so completely convinced that you can't do well."

"I know they are! They're blind when it comes to us. They are."

"I'm sorry to hear that!"

We stopped at that moment because of a fire alarm. We all trooped out, stood on the street outside the school building, and laughed and laughed because there was no fire, only an alarm that had summoned help. (Such an occurrence was no rarity.) Later that day, however, Henrietta and I had a chance to chat again, and at that time she was quite upset; she had received a poor grade for a composition she had written for her "least favorite teacher." She was "counting the minutes" (ninety) left until school would be out, and looking further ahead — counting the days left until Christmas. She would drop out soon, she told me, and my obvious chagrin didn't faze her. Rather, she reprimanded me — with a smile, yes, but with every intention, I sensed, of making again the serious point she'd several times conveyed to me: school is not congenial territory for her.

I mostly sat silently and read some notes on other interviews with Henrietta as she drew in response to my request that she try to picture her favorite Biblical scene. She worked carefully at the job, stopping several times to close her eyes and lower her head, as if she were praying. Once, after she'd done that, she must have seen the curiosity on my face. With a smile of recognition and of toleration, even friendship (I later realized), she answered my unspoken question: "I was just trying to picture Jesus in my mind, and someone he was trying to help."

I soon saw the results of that leap of her moral imagination (Figure 4). Initially I was puzzled. This girl, called "rude" repeatedly by one of her teachers, showed herself to be eagerly sensitive to my slowness of mind, maybe even ignorance: "Do you remember Jesus trying to help the blind man?"

"No, I guess I don't."

"Well, He did."

"Oh, yes — now I do; He tried to help lots of people, 'the lame and the halt and the blind,' I seem to remember my mother saying."

"She was right!"

I still didn't quite get what Henrietta was intending — and so, without saying a word, she sweetly and tactfully took my right hand and put it near her drawing, and then took my right forefinger and moved it toward the upper part of the left arm of the person on the left in her drawing, and then moved it along that arm until it came to rest at the end of the arm, which (I then began to understand) merged with the eye of the second person, on the picture's right. Henrietta saw by my expression that she was helping me see, even as she had tried to show me Jesus healing a blind person. By now she knew me well enough to speak without being spoken to, and as she talked I couldn't help but notice how powerfully and compellingly she spoke (in contrast with the judgment on her capacity for language made an hour earlier by an English teacher down the corridor): "When Jesus was with the people, He tried to be good with them. He worried over them. He didn't just walk into someplace and expect everyone to come rushing over and say 'Ooh' and 'Aah' and 'Ain't He the tops.' They show that circle [halo] over Him in some pictures, but my grammy said it's the church folks trying to make Him into someone so different, that He was God. But when He was here, talking with his friends and [others] like [them], He didn't look as if He'd just fallen out of the sky. He was this guy who built houses (wasn't He? a carpenter), and there was this secret in Him, that God had picked Him — and maybe He [Jesus] didn't know Himself [that] He'd been picked. I mean, God could have kept it from Him, couldn't He?"

I said nothing because her question was obviously rhetorical and she was quickly continuing on her way — leaving me intrigued theologically, even stunned, by the notion that God's will had been exerted arbitrarily through a Jesus not yet aware of His destiny. Henrietta continued her exposition this way: "There must have been a lot of people who thought He was dumb and stupid. Don't you think?" There she stopped and looked at me.

I said, "I'm not sure. I know He was unpopular with some. I don't remember whether He was regarded as dumb and stupid."

"Well, the words were different, maybe — but you know how people say bad things about other people, and He didn't [do so], and that's why they were glad when He kept moving, and didn't stop and live in their villages. He just visited them, and then there were more places to visit, because He wanted to meet a lot of folks." A slight pause, a glance at me, and a decision on her part — because I seemed blank — to call upon authority: "Our minister says you should think of Jesus as a champion walker! He kept on His feet all day, and He went from place to place, and He'd have to rest, but not for too long, because there was more to do, more people to see, and He wasn't going to sit back and take long naps, no sir!"

I smiled, thinking of an athletic, vigorous Jesus in top shape, moving, always moving. But now Henrietta wanted to stop Jesus in His tracks, and as she did so, I began to think of Him as more fragile, more tentative in His manner: "When He saw someone

in trouble, His heart skipped a beat. A lot of folks, they have
hearts of stone, our minister says. Mommy says she thinks the
minister is tough, and he has a girlfriend, besides his wife, everyone knows. Jesus wasn't no minister, talking one way and being
different in real life, not like that at all, no way. He'd mix with
the people — I mean: He'd see someone, and he's stumbling
and he might be blind, and Jesus could feel just the way the man
felt, blind Himself, and He'd get right in there, try to get the
man back to seeing."

I was touched by the energy she put into her remarks, and by
her directness in describing a moment of therapeutic and ethical
action, just as the picture had. Something in me, however, didn't
want the matter to rest there. I didn't reflect before I heard
myself saying, "How do you think Jesus brought that man 'back
to seeing,' Henrietta?"

"I don't know," she immediately offered — and I thought:
What did I expect this child to say? What could I expect any
reader of the Bible, upon reading of Jesus' miracles, to think,
to say? The girl has taken her usual careful measure of me. She
is far less upset with me than I am beginning to be with myself —
or maybe she is disposed toward pity, rather than annoyance.

She began to amplify: "I guess He touched the man's eye, and
that made a big difference. He must have had the Lord inside
Him. If you do, then things can happen — I've heard people
say so. You pray that God will be with you; that's what we say
in church. I don't know how He gets with you. I guess that's up
to Him, if He'll choose you to be with! I know you'd like to figure
out more — me to figure out more — but I don't think I can.
When we 'pass,' that's when we meet Him, and He'll tell us the
answers — or we'll never see Him, that could happen, too. If
you go 'downstairs,' you're ruined, and you'll just be left out and
it's a bad place, hell. Some say it's hot as can be there, and others
say no, it's cold, cold. I hope I don't find out! I hope I find my
spot 'upstairs,' where God stays!"

She had let me know that she could understand only so much,
go only so far, at least with words. Yet I sat there with her, looked
at her as she looked at her drawing, took note of the satisfaction
her face and body were registering — the eyes concentrated on
the paper, her seriousness still apparent in the way she kept

holding the paper with both hands — and all of a sudden her vision, which I'd only partly comprehended, settled on me. At last I saw the unselfconscious balance of this picture, its gentle, subtle evocation of intimacy, its natural unobtrusive symmetry, and, not least, its wordless story — much of that story, ironically, achieved through the artist's use of two lines to convey two mouths and so much more: Jesus as the One of confidence and hope (His upbeat mouth) who reaches out to a blind man, who is somber, even dejected (his downcast mouth).

The two lines, the two of them — Jesus and the blind man — become one, each with a piece of the sky, and behind the blind man are others, all the children who await Him, "all God's children." The two of them, their brown skin, the brown earth under them: a black child making her claim upon divinity. When Henrietta noticed me looking at the blue door with its window to the outermost left of the picture she missed not a beat in answering my unasked question: "That's other folks, their house." The world of blue, of blue eyes, the world that has given her and her people so many reasons to feel and to sing the blues, as Toni Morrison has reminded us in *The Bluest Eye,* for instance.

I asked Henrietta one last time for a comment on her picture: "Is there any talk going on? Do you think Jesus was saying something to that man as He healed him?"

The girl sat still, stared intently at her work of art, let her right hand go over it gently, a caressing act, an attempt, perhaps, to get closer to the heart of the matter. Finally, all she could say was: "Maybe He said something." Then she herself said nothing more. While I searched for words to utter, she continued to look at her picture as if it would tell her a further truth. At last she came to a conclusion: "I don't think He said anything, no — He touched him, and that was everything, and the man could see, and look who was there, God, and He was the best friend in the world to the man."

She looked away. Her eyes were on me. What to say to this man who wants not only a picture, but words? I decided, at long last, to put no more inquiries to Henrietta. My eyes fell on her picture, staying with it — but I could feel her continuing to look at me. The silence was at last broken by her: "Maybe Jesus sang while He healed." I was surprised. I forgot my vow. I quickly —

the old psychiatric reflex, ever ready — came back with the obvious: "What kind of song?"

"I don't know," she told me. But in a second she did know something: "My cousin, he plays the sax[ophone]. He likes to play for us. He's great. Maybe Jesus could make music like my cousin plays, even if He didn't have a sax." In my mind I heard "Bird" or John Coltrane, the yearning sadness of their music, its low, low notes, hitting bottom, and suddenly the full rise, the high mellow notes that sing of release, an arrival after that down time: this bittersweet world, this bittersweet life. A little later, Henrietta slowly moved her drawing toward me, let go of it as it touched my hands. I looked at her; our eyes met. She was smiling, and only then did I smile — to acknowledge her gift. I realized that for a few seconds I had been lost in reverie, my face far from beaming. Maybe this girl found my face in need of what her face offered, saw my eyes in need of what her hands were slowly offering me, the picture, yes, of course, but something else too.

In another part of Boston, where white, working-class families live, I heard music connected to God and His life in a different manner, by a ten-year-old boy, Andy, of mixed Irish and Lithuanian background, who had on previous occasions indicated no great religious interests, no strong inclination to look inward spiritually: "I go to [a Catholic] church sometimes. My mother used to like to go, but she doesn't now. She thinks a lot of the priests are dishonest — they say one thing and they do another, that's what Dad says about them. He likes them one Sunday, and gets communion; but the next he laughs and says he'd rather starve to death! We always go when my grandma comes to visit, because she likes to go — she says there's a heaven, but we can't see it, because it's so far away."

I asked Andy whether he'd ever had any thoughts about heaven, and he said, "No, no thoughts." I asked him whether he had any thoughts about God — what He wanted of us, what He looked like, where He was. "No, no thoughts," said Andy one more time. I told him again (as I had several times before) that I'd welcome any drawings he chose to make — pictures that might help him convey what was on his mind with respect to religious and spiritual subjects. That afternoon Andy was ready to take me up on the suggestion. While I reviewed some notes and transcripts, he sat busily at work. First he depicted a boy with blond hair, like his own, at a wheel, and then he moved to the construction of a wide rectangle, whose inside he gradually decorated with an assortment of colors. He had me quite puzzled. I really had no idea what to make of his effort. At last he seemed done, after devoting much time to the use of the red, purple, orange, yellow, blue, green, and brown crayons — it looked like an Easter egg, I thought for a moment, placed on a black background. Just before he announced that he was finished, Andy put down the crayons, picked up his pencil, and drew a small figure of a man, filling up a white space I began to realize he had deliberately left intact amid all his up-and-down motion with the crayons; and he drew a direction sign, pointing up, and a plus sign, surrounded by a circle. Now the picture (Figure 5) was mine — he handed it to me with a broad smile.

I looked carefully, wasn't sure what to think, said to Andy, "I can't quite figure out what you've done here!"

"Oh, I've taken a trip!"

"You have?"

"Yup."

"Where did you go?"

"Up in space."

"What did you see?"

"Well, I didn't see anything for a while — just the sky, and it is huge, millions of miles! First there were clouds, and then there was 'space,' and you can sleep, and when you wake up, it's the same as it was before. But after a long time, you'll see the other planets — and this [pointing at his picture] is one of them, only it's different than the others."

"How come?"

"Well, it's a planet, but it's not the usual one."

"Which one is it?"

"It's where God lives."

"Oh!"

"Do you see Him?"

"Yes, I think so, now that you've explained what you've done!"

We were both silent. I stared intently at the drawing and was still a bit perplexed. Was that building God's home? Why the black around the multicolored oval form? It had to be the smallest God I'd ever seen drawn! Meanwhile, Andy was also looking at what he had done. He interrupted the stillness with a question for me: "Do you recognize me?"

"Yes, I guess so — your blond hair, there. But you don't have a potbelly!"

"That's part of the seat I'm on — it's a spaceship I'm in, that's taking me through the sky! I'm steering. We're going up and up, and we're headed for heaven. We're listening to music — Billy Joel or the Stones! I've punched 'heaven'; if I punched a 'minus,' we'd go down, right through the earth! Then we'd see 'hell'!"

"I see! But what's happening in heaven?"

"Oh, there's a big gingerbread house, and that's where people go, if they're going to heaven; and God is outside, and He's the one who decides if you get in!"

"I see!"

"The black," he said, just as I was on the point of asking, "is the space around God and His house. I heard on television that it's dark way up there. 'Space is black,' our teacher said, so that's why."

"Are there many people in that house?"

"Yes, I guess so."

"What are they doing?"

"I don't know. You only find out if you get there, and you don't know whether you will until you do!"

"Why is God so small?"

"Oh, it's because He's really invisible to me!"

"I don't follow you."

"I mean, I'm bigger than God because I'm alive. God isn't alive like we are, though. Right? You don't see Him, right? I mean, when He became Jesus people saw Him, but that was only once, that it happened. I guess if I was really drawing the right kind of picture, there'd be no God there; maybe I'd just *tell* you He's inside His house!"

"Why did you use all the colors, Andy?"

"Well, it's pretty up in heaven, I think; and people are enjoying themselves."

"Why is the house made of gingerbread?"

"I don't know — maybe because it tastes good. When you're in heaven, you have lots of good things to eat!"

"Would you want to draw a picture of hell now?"

"No!"

"What would hell look like?"

"It would be a room, and there'd be no windows, and no doors, and no music, no sound, and a fire, a big fire would be going on inside!" As I contemplated such a scene, though I said nothing, I was thinking of the Sartre play *No Exit*. Andy broke into my reverie, my memories of a college teacher giving us an explication of that play, with a final smiling comment: "It's all make-believe." Now I had even more to think about! I didn't dare ask Andy what he meant by "it."

As I left Andy's house that day, I remembered many children's drawings on the themes of heaven and hell, of God's upwardness and the devil's subterranean existence — the geography is no surprise, of course, in view of what children learn in Hebrew schools, Sunday schools, synagogues, churches. I remembered, especially, a Swedish boy's lecture on heaven and hell — the ascent, the descent: "When you die, there are two directions you can travel: you can go way up or deep, deep down! It's all decided right away. How could it be otherwise? You can't start going up and then go down; and you can't go down and suddenly reverse directions!"

I decided to be a bit difficult. "Why not?"

The boy, Jon, almost ten, dismissed my question with one word: "Because."

I waited for more and got only his quiet, satisfied look. Finally, with a slight air of condescension, he decided to explain: "God would not allow there to be confusion. He makes up His mind; He is decisive. He waits until you're near death, and then He says 'Up' or 'Down.' That's what our godfather tells us: 'You'll go up or down — so you'd better decide which direction you want!' "

Then he showed me God (Figure 6) and said he was convinced God looks like the sun, though He does have wings and "maybe a face." As for the devil, he is black (God is shown in yellow), and he carries his stick, and he tries to pull people toward hell, but he can be only as successful as the Lord allows: "He will say no to someone, and then the devil gets him. If He wants you, He pulls you up, and you get there — fast."

I noted the slight hesitation before that last word and decided to ask another question; I wanted to learn the rock-bottom details of the boy's cosmology. "How fast?"

He had no trouble with my insistent curiosity. "A snap of the fingers."

"Whose?"

"God's, naturally." As the last word was spoken Jon looked right into my eyes — trying to figure out, perhaps, whether I was plain dumb or just provocative and skeptical beyond the bounds of politeness. I thanked him for his answer, hearing in my lowered voice an edge of shame.

I remember another picture in which going up and going down figured prominently, a picture drawn for me by a ten-year-old Jewish boy who lived north of Boston in Swampscott. I had gone to a Hebrew school to talk with a group of children. Morton was not especially forthcoming as we talked about Judaism, its tenets and values. But he saw my stack of crayon boxes and looked at them hard enough for me to offer them to the eight children in the room for their use. I suggested that they draw a scene from the Bible, and soon Morton was constructing a sky, then a figure of a person on top of a hill, holding the familiar tablets, the Commandments (Figure 7). Eventually he would do something interesting and original — put some people at the foot of the hill, their torsos shaped like Stars of David. Near them stands the metallic calf venerated by the Jews — a symbol of their lapse into idolatry — while Moses and his God are carrying on their conversation. Morton's reserve, his constraint with language, yielded to his pride of artistic accomplishment: "The Jews had been led from Egypt, but they forgot about God. Moses went up — he climbed up the mountain, to the top, and he spoke with God. You know, my aunt is a psychologist, and she said Moses was a leader of the Jews, and he was also a friend of God, and he soothed Him."

The boy saw something cross my face and, unsurprised, said

no more. I was the one who asked for amplification: "What do you mean, 'soothe Him'? Soothe *God?*"

"Yes, soothe God."

Not a word more until I asked, more aggressively, "Morton, do you mean it's your understanding that Moses soothed God?"

"Oh, yes. God was very upset with the Jews. We're His people, but we built that calf, and we were worshipping it. God got very angry, but Moses kept talking to Him; he did it so God wouldn't just get so angry He'd punish the Jewish people, and we could have been destroyed — He can do it! Moses soothed God; he told Him the Jewish people made a mistake, but he'd go talk with them, and so he did; he climbed down and he had the Commandments and he explained things to them, and they changed their tune! They became Jews again! You can always lose your religion — that's the danger."

Morton went back, then, to his drawing. He decided to put a hand in the extreme upper right corner of the paper — a paw, God's paw! When he'd finished that, he turned his attention to the two tablets and to their recipient. He used red to make lines on the blue tablets, used it to cover the head of Moses, used it to connect the Lord's hand with the words He had offered His chosen people. Moses the therapist became Moses the messenger way up there in the sky. The blue sky touched the blue tablets, which were suffused by the yellow sun, some of which seemed to be emanating from God's lower hand.

I wanted to know more about all that from Morton, whose apparently casual work with a few crayons seemed to be culminating in a representation of the ultimate mystery of God's language (spoken in what tongue?) as it was supposedly conveyed to a great leader. How to ask a boy to talk about a mystery he seemed to have depicted with great suggestive intelligence? I decided to begin with a detail, Moses' red hat, a yarmulke, I assumed: "Morton, the red on the head of Moses —?"

I needed to go no further. "He is prayerful before God — maybe I should have made it [the yarmulke] black!"

The boy gazed not at his drawing then but across the room, where a single wide window allowed a view of a cloudy sky. When the eyes returned, they focused on the drawing briefly, then me: "I shouldn't have drawn the hand there. We shouldn't think of God that way!"

I was quick, perhaps too quick, to reassure the child. I told
him that a number of Jewish children had been more than
tempted, in the course of drawing sessions with me, to render
God in a human form: to draw an arm, a face, even a part of
the body. I told him of some Islamic children and their wish, at
times, to envision Allah.

He interrupted me. "Did you stop them before they did?"

"No. One stopped herself; the other was drawing a picture of
a mosque, then drew a picture of a face, a neck, shoulders, and
two arms, but stopped himself and told me it [the picture he was
doing] 'could be Mohammed, maybe, or Allah,' but it was 'wrong'
for him to be trying to imagine what they looked like."

"Do you have the picture?"

"No. The boy told me he was going to tear it up. I'll admit —
I said nothing, but I was sorry."

We both held our tongues. I was aware of having confessed
to a researcher's greedy annoyance at the everyday course of his
work: the small moments that tell a lot. Suddenly I thought of
these drawing sessions as sinful — a Pakistani boy in London,
learning the religion of Islam daily, for a moment tempted
sorely, wrongfully. Morton was reading my mind with great subtlety — the initial greed I felt, and the later contrition: "If you
were sorry, then it was OK. When I pray to God, I'll see Him;
I mean, I'll think of Him as looking like an old man — a little
like my grandpa! He doesn't look like anyone, I guess!"

Morton became quite thoughtful, staring at what he had just
done with his crayons. His right forefinger moved slowly up the
ladder on the paper, and when the finger reached Moses and
the tablets and God's hand and the sky and the sun, the boy
spoke: "I wonder whether God wrote what He told us [in the
Commandments]. Did He chisel the words [on stone]? Did He
speak Hebrew to Moses? If Moses spoke to Him, he must have
spoken Hebrew!"

We were both, by then, sitting in hushed contemplation of a
singular and ineffable mystery — the means by which Moses and
God communicated to each other. Morton's picture did justice
to that mystery, I began to realize, better than a ton of words,
even a weighty theological discussion. With his red crayon, he
had linked the mind of Moses with the words of the Commandments and the hand of God — all this amid the sun's rays, bril-

liant, penetrating light that unites God and man and the words that would command, instruct, inspire a people. The yellow earthly transgression is redeemed by the sun in heaven; the yellow of a golden calf becomes the yellow of spiritual exchange. No wonder the black arrow that tells us of Moses is given the shape of a flight skyward of birds, their wings of faith showing a direction to the people below.

My mind noticed something, and I heard its watchfulness being given voice: "Morton, I notice you made the bodies of the Jews there [at the foot of the mountain] look a little like the Star of David — do you see? — but not [the body of] Moses."

The boy peered intently both at the Jews on the ground and at the one perched high up, his right hand in the midst of radiance. "Well, I guess Moses was different than the others." A few seconds of silence were followed by an afterthought: "Today the Ten Commandments are for everyone, not just us."

After that last remark, Morton reminded me that Moses went up the mountain twice, that in anger he broke the tablets he brought down when he saw the golden calf his people had built, that he ascended again to converse with God — and was told by Him that he'd not see His face. Morton also pointed out the triangle on the top of the mountain, aware that I, having been attentive to just about everything else on that piece of paper, had paid it no heed. He explained, "God made a place for Moses where he could stand and they could talk. I think Moses calmed down God, and then God calmed down Moses, because he was really upset by what his people did [the making of the golden calf]."

At that point my mind left Swampscott, Massachusetts, and recalled Freud in London in the last year of his life as he revised the manuscript of his book on Moses, originally titled *The Man Moses: A Novel,* then becoming a long psychoanalytic essay, *Moses and Monotheism.* I remember reading the book; I remember hearing Erik H. Erikson talk about it. Freud was determined to find out who Moses was (an Egyptian?), and what kind of leader he was, and what that leadership had meant, psychologically, over the centuries. How ironic that the founder of psychoanalysis was less interested in what took place between Moses and God — their important effect on one another, the shifts in mood and attitude that each prompted in the other — than was this boy, scarcely a decade old, planning by his own declaration a future as a businessman (in his dad's firm) rather than as a psychiatrist.

Then Morton said, "Doctor, I've wondered whether — when God comes to us [the Jews] again, whether He'll speak Hebrew, or what."

"I don't know."

"No one knows, I'm sure. How could anyone?"

"No way."

The boy smiled at my choice of words, and I did too. I wondered why I spoke in such a manner — perhaps to get us back, through a colloquialism, to our everyday lives, there being no point to further speculation on the unnamable and the unknowable. Two months later, in another conversation, Morton added, "Moses really suffered when he came down from the mountain and saw his people worshipping the calf. He was angry, but I think he probably cried, too. Then God healed him, I think." This child had a sense of a prophetic figure as someone exquisitely balanced between charismatic power and exceptional vulnerability. I had never before thought of Moses as weeping — rather, I had seen him as a man of tremendous moral indignation in response to that terrible moment of disappointment and betrayal by his own people.

Months later, as I looked at a drawing (Figure 8) made for my son Bob by an eleven-year-old Catholic girl in Hungary whose mother had recently died of cancer, I found myself remembering Morton's Moses, Morton's sense of Moses as weeping as well as inflamed with outrage and anger. Maybe my mind was connecting these two children because of what Anna, the child from Budapest, had to say to Bob after she had finished her Crucifixion scene: "It's a sad day, Good Friday. Jesus was there [on the cross], and He must have cried. I asked my mother [a year earlier] if He'd cried, and she said she didn't know, but she thought He was brave and He didn't weep. He just kept thinking of God, and [that] He'd be there [in heaven] to welcome Him [Jesus]. But I still think He *did* cry — maybe."

She then asked Bob what *he* thought. Bob quoted the famous Biblical sentence "Jesus wept" and said that he found it entirely reasonable to imagine Jesus crying — He was in terrible pain, and He felt (and said that He felt) quite abandoned. Young Anna agreed, and they both looked, after that exchange, at the picture she had made, using crayons and a pencil. Atop a hill of green Jesus hangs on a cross. Beside him four flowers stand, their heads bowed, nature's acknowledgment of mourning — the landscape as a pietà. Above is an air of darkness; it is indeed a black time. Yet there is light, free-floating light, light from on high, light cutting its way through the sky, through the blue (the blues?) of the hovering world. This light, though, is contained. Anna carefully encloses with her black crayon all the yellow: an atmosphere of gloom, yet a statement of possibility as well — a dramatic, electrically charged moment in the world's history. As for Jesus, blood pours from both His feet, both His hands. His heart is shown, and it, too, seems to be bleeding, and His mouth as well. With a pencil the artist shows tears, hard to notice except on close inspection, but definitely there. "He will soon be gone," Anna announced when she was done with showing Jesus at approximately the moment when He "cried with a loud voice and died."

As Bob and Anna talked about her picture, she told him that she had wondered, from time to time, what Jesus thought as He hung on the cross. When Bob asked her what *she* thought He might have thought, she was not shy in replying: "He must have been really upset to be dying. He told God that He'd been 'forsaken,' so that proves it. He must have been in the worst pain, and there was no doctor to help Him, and they didn't have the medicines we have today. He could have been groaning, and I wonder if some of the people nearby heard Him, and what they thought. They punished people then by crucifying them, and they didn't seem to worry that the person really suffered. I'm sure Jesus wanted to forgive the bad people nearby, but He must have wanted to punch them hard, get back at them."

She stopped, caught her breath, sipped some water, but needed no prompting to go on. "Do you think God was crying, too?" She did not await Bob's answer. "How could He not cry? His son was dying! The priest told us God knew before [the Crucifixion took place] that it would happen; and He could see into the future. Even if He knew [the events of] Easter would happen, He must have cried, because of the way His son died.

It was a form of torture — that is what the priest said. The whole world shook, I think, while Jesus was on the cross. His mother must have cried until she had no more tears. I think the sun stopped shining for a while. All the world was sad, except for the people who wanted Jesus to die."

She and Bob next turned their attention to the life of Jesus, in contrast to His death. Anna stated her knowledge of her Savior's magical powers, the healing He did. Then she mentioned His capacity to take on death itself — the story of Jesus resurrecting Lazarus. She volunteered to draw that scene and then drew it with great industry and enthusiasm, placing the miracle against the backdrop of a city street, with houses of various colors crowded together (Figure 9). "I wonder what He said to Lazarus," Anna said as she put the finishing touches on Jesus, on Lazarus. "I know He called him, and he awoke, but He must have explained to Lazarus what happened. Our priest told us the Bible doesn't tell us everything — not every word! When Lazarus rose, that must have convinced everyone! People must have been happy, but they could have been scared, too. Even your Superman doesn't do that!"

A big laugh from Bob, and a beaming look of self-congratulation on Anna's face: she had let this young American know what she knew about his country, and she had somehow connected the Biblical past with the twentieth century in a way that delighted both parties — each now mindful of the persistence, over the centuries, of our desire for supernatural transformations, whether they are attributed to God or conjured as fantasies in comic books and movies. Bob noted, after Anna's reference to Superman, the dark cape she had given Jesus, and His outstretched arms. A little later Anna mentioned not the death of her mother but that of her favorite aunt, and told him she had wondered, at the funeral, whether she ought to pray to Jesus that He come to the church, lift open the casket, and bring life to her aunt, only forty-five when she died: "I thought that He could do it, if He came here. He's supposed to come back, sometime. We don't know when. My mother said you can't ask for miracles; they just happen. She said she's never had one happen, but some people have. My aunt deserved a miracle. She was the nicest person in the world. The priest came and told us Jesus is weeping for her. I was going to ask him if we all could pray for Him to come and make her live again, but my mother said no, no, it would be terrible to ask that. The Bible tells of the past, not now — that's what my mother told me. [Bob had asked her what her mother's reaction was to her idea of beseeching God for that miracle.] She told me Jesus would be insulted because He calls us when He wants — and we shouldn't tell Him He made a mistake! But we were all sad!"

No doubt Anna's interest in the story of Lazarus' revival at the hands of Jesus was prompted by her attachment to her aunt, not to mention her mother's more recent death. Anna was, in general, quite fascinated by stories of magic, of the supernatural; and she loved not only Superman but the space explorations in the *Star Trek* television series, which had made their way to Hungary. Children do not easily forget that side of Jesus' life — His ability, as described by His followers, to perform a host of miracles. Again and again, in nation after nation, I have heard boys and girls echo Anna's interest in those miracles, her curiosity as to why they aren't now available to us. No matter how parents or the clergy speak of the miracles, children persist in wondering whether somehow, through someone's intercession, those miracles might return. "When my aunt died, I stared at the sky all the time," Anna said. "I thought that if I really concentrated on Jesus — prayed to Him a lot and begged Him to hear me — then He'd notice us here, and He might decide to help out. The other day I saw a cloud, and it looked like Him — His face! I stood still and watched, but pretty soon the cloud was gone. I know: a cloud is a cloud. I just wish there was some way Jesus would visit us, the way He did those people long ago. They were lucky, and we're not so lucky!"

Nor was Anna altogether selfless in her yearning for a Second Coming of Jesus. Chicken pox had blemished her face. In private moments of self-scrutiny she wished for a better complexion, and, through prayer, she asked for a transformation she knew she was unlikely to receive. A number of American children have confided similar yearnings as we have discussed the life of Jesus. Not that some of those children haven't been told of later miracles, of the long list of them recorded in the Vatican; still, the stories of Jesus as someone who raised the dead, healed the lame, gave sight to the blind, appeal powerfully to children who have not yet acquired the everyday realism of their elders.

Meanwhile, miracles being unavailable, some children dream of the time when praying for them will be unnecessary — the Second Coming. Child after child,[4] in the United States and abroad, given a chance to draw whatever he or she wished with respect to a religious or spiritual subject, turned his or her attention to that Biblically promised moment when the Lord will appear, when the dead will rise, amidst great celebration. Even as Anna concentrated her energy on the past resurrection of Lazarus, two other Hungarian girls, Sophia and Vera (all introduced to my son, Bob, by the same priest), were anxious to show what lies ahead on that day of days. When the two girls (both ten) had finished their work, they smiled, even joked with their guest from abroad, Vera especially: "Maybe we'll live to see the Second Coming! I have no memory of my grandmother, so I'd be truly happy to meet her when the dead become alive; and maybe that'll happen soon, so I won't have to die first and then wait."

She stopped and gave some thought to what she had said, then continued, half declaring her anticipations, and half asking by implication how that utterly extraordinary transformation of dead bodies into live ones would be accomplished: "I guess it'll just happen — God will come, and He'll wake everyone up, in all the cemeteries. There will be music — trumpets, I think — and people will sing. I've wanted to ask [the priest] how it happens. What about people who are cremated — will they be awakened, too? My father told me not to try to explain it [the resurrection of the dead]. He said it'll just happen. It's the souls that'll go to meet God — except for the bad people: they'll be separated, and they'll never go to heaven. God will call the good folks with His trumpet; and the bad folks, they'll be cut down with His scythe. I wouldn't want to live in the bad places — in that city, Babylon, I think, or any place where there have been lots of people who do wrong, and they don't care, they just keep on doing wrong."

Vera had made clear in her drawing (Figure 10) the world of the saved and the world of the damned — she had drawn a thick black wall between the two. When asked for more detail about those who live in the morally condemned city, in the buildings she had drawn, Vera was at first nonplused. She repeated herself, talked of "bad folks," of "bad places." When asked once more what was going on that was "bad" in the "bad places," she shrugged and disclaimed any specific knowledge. When asked again, in another way ("How are the people in the cemetery or aboveground different from those in the buildings?"), she pondered the matter for a number of seconds and then repeated her analysis but also expanded on it: "The good people will go up to be with God; the bad won't get near Him. The bad people swear, and they are mean, and they lie and steal, and they don't think of anyone except themselves. Maybe they cheat on their wives. Maybe they don't obey the laws. Maybe they don't go to church and they don't pray. God knows them, who they are. We can fool people, people can fool people; but God, no one tricks Him."

Vera had heard the priest talk of the Second Coming, heard him read from the Revelation of St. John the Divine, though she could remember no particular passage. Like Vera, Sophia supplied the Lord with a scythe in addition to a trumpet (Figure 11), but it was the spirit of the latter that engrossed her. She asked her American friend what someone would say in English, were he or she suddenly "reborn." Bob wrote "Yeah!" on a piece of paper, and she copied it first with a crayon, then with a pencil. She was proud to know the word, and used it whenever possible after that. She was a musical child — she played the piano — and wondered what the Lord would play on the trumpet. Like Vera, she wanted the viewer to understand the upward thrust of things (for the saved). Both girls used arrows and markers to help any observer who might not realize the momentous nature of the occasion, but also maybe to help the girls themselves, who several times returned to the mystery of the promised resurrection. Sophia, a generally hopeful and happy child, had a doubt or two: "If we turn to dust — I think it says we do in the Bible — I don't know how we become alive after that! It's in God's power, I know that. My mother says you should never try to understand how God does His work, because you cannot. He's a magician! He's not like the magicians you have at your birthday party; He's the best magician who ever was! Someone I know asked our priest to tell us how Jesus did His miracles, and how God would do His, when He came here and sent people to heaven and others to hell, and in the graves, He'd send people both ways, not just living people. The priest laughed and said it's foolish for us to try to steal God's thunder! If you keep trying, he said, you'll get into real trouble. You mustn't be too curious, anyway! You should do what's right, and then everything will happen the way it should."

Vera was listening carefully, and Bob could see she was eager to join the discussion. When Sophia had finished her homily — her assertion of faith, mingled with a warning about the dangers of at least some kinds of curiosity — Vera quickly joined in: "If you go looking for trouble, you'll find it!" Bob had certainly heard that observation before, though not in Hungarian. He told the translator to say as much to Vera. She smiled and made her point yet again: "Remember what happened to Lot's wife!"

Bob did remember, but he wanted to hear Vera remember, and so he asked her what exactly had happened to Lot's wife. Vera told him, "She wouldn't just leave that bad city [Sodom]; she kept looking and looking, and so she was turned into salt by God." The girl wanted to know if Bob would like her to draw a picture of Lot's wife. Yes, of course. But suddenly she changed her mind: "I wouldn't know how to draw her. Should she look like a person, or should she be a pile of salt?" Bob suggested she draw her whatever way seemed desirable — but no, Vera could only shudder: "It must have been terrible! I'd rather just die than end up like the salt you see in the market." As they prepared to move on and discuss some of Vera's other drawings, she herself looked back, as it were, and asked Bob to look back as well: "Has anyone drawn Lot's wife for you?"

"Yes."

"Many people?"

"No."

"How many?"

"I'm not sure, one or two people — one [drawing] that I clearly remember."

"Who drew it?"

"A girl in America, about a year or so ago."

"Do you have it here?"

"No — I left it in the States."

"Oh. What did the picture look like?"

"Well, actually, it's one my dad and I will never forget, because it's really clever, we thought. Lot's wife is standing on some grass, with her arms outstretched, but she's already turning to salt — I mean her face is a circle of salt crystals, and her body hasn't quite turned to salt, but if you look at the picture, the body and the face together look like a salt shaker, with arms and legs attached to it, and the salt shaker (I mean, Lot's wife) is saying 'Help!' "

Vera looked puzzled, so Bob tried to copy on a piece of paper what he remembered of the picture, done by a girl of ten who lived in East Tennessee, her parents quite fundamentalist in their Protestantism. Vera was intrigued and interested enough to speculate. "I suppose the arms and legs turned into salt after a while, didn't they?"

"Yes, I guess so."

"And then the person couldn't say 'Help!' Isn't that true?"

"Yes."

"Then she wasn't Lot's wife anymore?"

"Yes."

"She wasn't anyone — just salt!"

"Yes."

"What was her name — I mean, before she turned into salt?"

"I don't know."

"Was she only called 'Lot's wife'?"

"Yes, I think so."

"That's too bad."

Then complete silence. Bob described it to me later: "She sat as still as I've ever seen her sit. She looked down at the floor. I looked at the drawing I'd made for her, my version of the one done by Joy Marie in Tennessee (Figure 12). I don't know what she was thinking, because I didn't feel comfortable asking. She seemed lost in thought. I was too, a little: I was thinking about what Vera had suggested — that 'Lot's wife' was in trouble before she looked back, because she was only 'Lot's wife' and not herself, someone with a name, someone who belonged to herself. Before I knew it, though, Vera had come out of herself, and she started talking about the ballet lessons they were giving in school — how she loved learning to dance, learning to have control over her body."

Children, who so often seek to exert control over their unfolding lives, are frank to wonder how it is possible even for an omnipotent and omniscient God to exert control over everyone's life, in the sense that He is supposed to choose who goes where after death. In a classroom in Kasserine, Tunisia, boys and girls brought up in devout Moslem families kept telling my son Bob how much they worried about hell; it was a real presence generating great fear in their lives. Fire is what they believed awaits the ill-fated ones, the transgressors, those who do not adhere to Islam's rules, principles, values. A twelve-year-old boy, Habib, made quite clear the grim fate in store for those who fail in life, as it were — he has a nameless beast spitting eternal fire and a horde of sinners doomed to an endless spell of consuming heat (Figure 13). "If you could die in hell," the boy pointed out, "you would be glad, but you don't." The prospect of suffering forever aroused in him a fervent wish to be a good Moslem, a loyal and devoted son, a conscientious student at school. He talked of his "will" to improve his life, to get through school, to "prove" himself before his family, his teachers, and Allah.

One morning he wrote the word "Allah" and surrounded it by a word meaning "the supreme" (Figure 14). On the bottom he offered six figures representing mirrorlike permutations of "the supreme." (He chose the leftmost one for his circular band around Allah's name.) This same boy, so straight in his posture, so careful in his choice of words, so earnestly anxious to be correct and polite, told Bob one day, a month into their acquaintance, about "the dangers" of the world: "I pray a lot. I hope I am heard. Allah hears us, I know — but I worry some days that my voice is missed because so many others are stronger! My father says the quiet voice is the loudest, but I hear voices that keep me from hearing my own! What does Allah do [when such voices come His way]? I do not know! We cannot imagine Him [what He looks like, how He makes His decisions]; we can only be His servants! He will be with us if we are with Him." Yet Habib *had* tried to "imagine Him," had let his mind think of Allah more concretely than the phrase "Allah the supreme" allows: "When the wind picks up, I think Allah has come near. The wind goes right through our house, and I think of Him. When the sky turns red [at sunrise or sunset] I think of Him — He is waking up or going to sleep, and the entire world says so!"

Even as the boy struggled on behalf of his soul, lest it go to hell, he also opened his soul to a religion's mysteries. Desert winds and desert light affected him deeply, made him ponder Allah's nature and purposes. Islam for him was a demanding religion of conscience, and his moral imagination tried to keep pace with the jeopardy he knew could lie in wait, not only in the form of hell's eternity but in each day's potential pitfalls: "I must walk straight from the first moment the sun shows, to the time [when] it leaves us here. We pray many times [a day], and always it [the prayer] is the same — to follow Allah and do what He wants, to keep clean, and eat right, and respect my mother and my father and my grandparents and my uncles and my aunts and my teachers, all the elders." As for the naive American's apologetic question about why so many prayers each day: "Don't you see — we can forget!" Then an important afterthought: "We love Allah and His prophet Mohammed; we pray out of love. It's a chance to show it [our love]!"

Love and fear alike find in prayer a daily opportunity for expression with children the world over — Moslems, children of other religions, and children attached to no religion at all but with minds no less eager to understand the nature of things and speculate on rights and wrongs, on what the future holds, if anything. Habib was wary of specifically religious depiction, even apart from his obvious constraint with respect to Allah. In one drawing the boy would depict a large mosque and show warriors confronting one another in struggles between legions of the good and legions of the bad: here was a child growing up and trying to find an honorable, law-abiding way for himself. In another drawing the boy would let his mind wander (Figure 15) to produce in rich detail a utopian notion of a busy, productive community, one at peace with itself, in which people pursue their various daily activities, with the green mosque (green is the color of Islam's Paradise) integrated into those activities but not dominating them. (He had visited the capital city of Tunis.) Habib was most free, however, when he connected his Islamic passions to the desert world of Kasserine. Then his work was very much like that of Hopi children, a naturalistic religion of sky and land whose vastness becomes a metaphor for eternity, for the inscrutable mysteries of the universe, for the Lord, for Allah.

Even in London, where Islamic children had no desert nearby to stimulate their imaginative life, and where the sky was not so easily seen in its vastness, the boys and girls we met tried hard for their own kind of pictorial and meditative freedom. They drew huge suns with large features, skies choked with stars arranged in such a way that the viewer thinks of the human form. Their minds were intent, clearly, on making the outside world do the work of the voices within, as in these observations Habib made after he'd painstakingly rendered Allah's name and then sketched a sunrise over his village: "Somewhere Allah is waking up, and He is stretching Himself. You can catch a look at the sun very early [in the day] and very late. When I see it I think — there He is! It's wrong to think you can see Allah. No one here [who is alive] ever does. No one. That is the sun, my father says — no more [than that]. But maybe Allah is there [in the sun]. They told us in school that if the sun dies, the earth does, too — everything here, alive. Allah gives us life; it is His sun."

It was not hard to fathom the boy's logic, his vigorous interest in how the world around him works, an interest aided by teachers and prompted by a desire to integrate school knowledge with his parents' passion for a hidden, awesome deity, the Supreme, who eludes visual definition yet gets addressed daily in the morning, at midday, in the afternoon, in the evening. "When I hear the call to prayer," the boy said, "I stop everything. Before I pray, I tell Allah, 'I'm only this one boy, but I believe in you.' Sometimes the wind is strong, and I think I'll be picked up and carried away! He [Allah] hears our prayers, and He speaks back [through the wind]." To see such children halted by the fervent singing of the muezzin summoning people to prayer is to see a young spirituality frozen silently in time: "I hold myself as still as possible while I hear it [the call, through word and song]; then I go." That private moment of utter bodily restraint, with the heart beating faster, no doubt, and the mind both stopped still and racing away — so does a child's basic soulfulness become affirmed without words or ritual, in anticipation of words and ritual.

I close with a black girl's picture: "Praying," she called it (Figure 16). She was twelve when she drew it, a daughter of one of the black children my wife, Jane, and I came to know in the 1960s in Georgia when we talked to participants in the school desegregation struggle. The girl, Leola, became a paraplegic in a terrible car accident that took her father's life. She is not an especially bright child; school tests have warned of her "borderline" intelligence. She has spent a lot of time with her grandmother and has struggled to "keep on the move," as she put it: "from my favorite chair to my bed, and back." How she loves to crawl! "It makes me feel like a baby again," she once exulted — and she loves those times when young kin come over, when babies are brought to her, and with them she crawls and crawls. She also loves to pray: "I pray sitting [in the chair], and I pray lying [on the bed], but most of all, I pray on the floor, holding on to the bed, my poor knees doing the best they can to bend." It is hard for her to get in that position, one that most of us take for granted: we bend, we extend our arms. Leola's torso and arms are strong, though; their powerful musculature, harnessed to her mind's eager yearning, enables her to leave her chair, move across the floor, reach the bed, and arrange herself so that she holds on to it in a kneeling position. Such an effort, minutes in its accomplishment, enacts her passion pursued, her pilgrimage. Then she collapses into a prayerfulness that starts slow and ends up big, real big, in its glow, its ecstasy: "I hums to the Lord, and I sings to Him. There'll be a day, I just tells Him of my 'down-and-out blues' — Gramma told me to say. I tries to be grateful that He sent me here, and if He can see that Leola is 'deceptifyin',' then He'll forgive me, because if you try to be good, and you can't get there, not all the way, then that's only making you one of His folks, and He can't expect more of you than He gave you, and He sure knows that by now, what with all of us He's put up with!

"There will be times when I honestly don't know what happens: the praying goes to my head, and I gets lost, I think — it's like, well, He comes and takes me, and I'm no longer thinking and talking, I'm just someplace else, I don't know where. I can even look down from there, and I see poor little me, Leola and her bed, and the chair is there, too. Then I come back to me, and I'll try singing a song to Him, and I'll feel my hands letting go [from their grip on the bed], and I'm ready to be the slump on the floor that moves — and then I get up on the chair, and I can be me again, sitting, and if someone will bring me the Cheerios, they're my favorite."

I remember Leola and her pink bedspread, knitted by her grandmother; Leola and her red and yellow pillow on her favorite chair; Leola's stark room in an inadequate house: "Things are broken-down hereabouts," her mother said, looking at an entire neighborhood whose people, mostly, do menial work for low wages. What bleak prospects — intellectual, educational, occupational! What a struggle with her body: "Oh, I talk to my legs. I tell them I'm sorry it happened to them, I'm real sorry! I tell them I won't forget them! I tell them we'll take up the slack — my arms and all I can get me to do from the waist up! I pray for them! If I'd been there, when Jesus was down here with us folks, maybe He'd have caught sight of me and fixed me up good, real good. But He's watching, and I'm waiting, and I just hope I can have a second with Him, and He might touch my legs then, or He might not: it's all the same to me, because it's the soul that counts, I know! I mean, I forget sometimes — but mostly I know, I *do* know! When I'm praying, I know: that's when I know. Praying is when I walk like I used to walk — to meet Him!"

Then she looked at what she had drawn — the colors, her colors, her color, her body, both halved and suggestively complete in its intense and committed holding, its mix of self-affirmation and self-effacement, its spread of white and black and brown, its back turned in a goodbye to itself, a hello to the Other One, who is beyond all skies and clouds, even suns and moons and stars — who is the great blank of the infinite receiving one child's picture of devotion: a rendering of the austere aloneness of meeting God, the transport of prayer, the call to the world beyond worlds, the name beyond names.

9

Christian Salvation

AS I TALKED WITH CHILDREN about their religious thoughts and experiences, about the influence of churchgoing or Sunday school attendance on their lives, I would stop at some point and ask, "How would you describe the heart of your religion, its central message for you and for others?" I'd change the words a bit from person to person, and I'd keep adding essentially repetitive phrases, so that the boy or girl (or the group of youngsters) with whom I was talking would begin to understand what I was seeking. Most children quickly comprehended the intent of my question. Often, as I stumbled along, adding one explanatory phrase after another, they would sit me out in silence, tolerating with equanimity what some of them must have regarded as a grownup's condescension, and then begin their reply. A child might first put my question into his or her words — as if to let me know that I was certainly making myself clear, perhaps clearer than I thought, and to inform me, additionally, that I might try being a bit terser, pithier.

Mary, for instance, was a nine-year-old girl whose Irish Catholic ancestry showed in her classically freckled face, her light brown hair, her pale blue eyes. Not that she reveled in her charming appearance. She had a cousin, Theresa, whose looks she openly envied, a girl whose "black Irish" features (dark hair, brown eyes, a strong chin and prominent nose) Mary was convinced would be more appealing, one day, to boys. The two were close and often went to church and Sunday school together. They also talked frequently about their religion, and so I interviewed them together, because each made the other more attentive to the subject at hand and more voluble. Here is Mary's response to my question about the central message of her religion: "You mean why Jesus came here and why He died?" She stopped to let me digest that. I could tell by the way she took in a larger than normal breath that she would continue with no urging from me. I nodded and smiled to let her know I was impressed by and grateful for her telling précis. She continued, "You see, He was supposed to come, and then He did. It says in the Bible that He'd come, in the Old Testament. So He did, and He tried to be a good teacher, and He was a doctor too — He healed people. But then He was killed. He was 'too good for this world,' the nun says, and we should remember [that phrase]. But He didn't mind dying. He was sad, but He knew He'd live forever, and 'because He died, so will we live forever,' the nun says. That's what our church says, it's what Jesus did for us."

She had given a speech, and she availed herself of the water in a pitcher, put there (in her Sunday school classroom) by the very nun who had encouraged her to memorize certain important phrases and, indeed, tested her on them. She took a long drink, several swallows, then came up for air. She moved the glass away from her; it was still partially full. Meanwhile, Theresa had been watching her closely, listening with obvious care. Once or twice she had glanced at me to see if I was taking in what Mary was rather confidently sending my way. When Mary finished talking and began drinking her water, Theresa looked at the water longingly, I thought, and made a half gesture toward it, only to restrain herself at the last minute. I wondered why. Soon I was given a clue: Theresa started talking, and as she did, I thought to myself that she'd decided to save the water for the end of her own statement. It was brief but earnest: "Jesus felt sorry for us. He knew we were in trouble, so He came here to save us, and He did." Then she filled her glass, drank every drop, filled it again — and then took me and Mary both by surprise: "He was very thirsty when He was on the cross. He was sweating, and I think He may have cried — not because He was scared, but He was in pain. No one could give Him water, though! He was up there on this big cross, and they were all kept away by the soldiers."

We all three now became quite conscious of that water pitcher.

Mary reconsidered, reached for her glass, emptied it. Theresa filled her glass, swallowed its contents in big gulps. I wasn't thirsty but saw the eyes of both girls glance toward the third, unused glass, and instinctively I reached for it, filled it up, began sipping from it. All this took only a few seconds, and by then Mary was ready for me: "What do *you* think?" Her emphasis on the personal pronoun startled me. I thought I heard a nun's voice taking attendance, making sure everyone participates in the class discussion. I felt my feet moving on the floor; I was pulling them in, toward me. I drank some more water, and felt, still, rather blank. Finally I said, "I agree with both of you."

They both seemed pleased enough by those six words, even though I felt rather contemptuous of such a pitiful response. The two of them had said quite a lot, and rather well. I found myself wondering whether their remarks had been less spontaneous than I had initially thought — they were repetitions, perhaps, of the nun's comments. Maybe Mary had memorized a phrase or two; and maybe all I heard was more rote or stale than I wanted to believe. But Mary and Theresa soon taught me otherwise. "I think a lot about Jesus — you know, what He was like," Mary remarked. "I do, too," Theresa joined in. "You do?" I lamely commented, looking first at one, then the other. They seemed, again, far less critical of me than I was of myself as I heard in my own mind the echo of my two words, a worn, reflexic comment uttered the world over by psychiatrists like me in our offices. Mary took the lead: "When I pray to Him, I thank Him for coming here, and I tell Him I look forward a lot to seeing Him, when I get to." Theresa picked up on that angle of thought: "I wonder what He'll say to us! Will He just say, 'Welcome,' or will He talk to us? It's hard to imagine what He'll tell us. I think He'll smile, though. My mom says you should think of Jesus as your best friend, and He came here once to make sure we knew Him, and He'll be glad to see us, and we'll be glad to see Him."

This idea of a welcome-home reception intrigued me; I hadn't at that time, early in my research, heard the beginning of the afterlife described in quite that way before. The girls saw interest on my face and became quite talkative as I asked them for details. I wondered whether they imagined Jesus sitting or standing when they first saw Him. Theresa replied promptly, "I've wondered that — and I was going to ask Sister, but I decided I shouldn't. I asked my [older] brother, and he said no one knows. I asked my dad, and he said the same thing, that you'll only find out when you get there! So I guess that's the answer!" Mary had an opinion: "I think He might be sitting on a chair — a throne. Isn't God supposed to sit on a throne? I think so! I heard it said somewhere — I forgot [where]. Anyway, God has to rest, just like us, don't you think?" Theresa said no: "He's not like us, that's the difference. He's God. We're just us! We'd die and never get to heaven if Jesus hadn't come here — if God hadn't sent Him."

They both were now silent, and I was sent into a reverie. I thought of God distancing Himself from Himself, sending Jesus to us; and I also thought of Jesus standing, then sitting — with Mary and Theresa and me, among others, waiting to see Him. Theresa must have been thinking along roughly the same lines, because she jolted me with these words: "I don't understand how God can be God, and then He's Jesus. I know He wanted to come here and visit, and He wanted to show us that you can be saved, if you follow Him, where He wants you to go. But then He became God again, and I don't know how. Sister said you can't imagine how it happened; it just did. I guess that's the answer. He probably doesn't eat and sleep, the way we do. He might not need a chair. Does he breathe? It's hard to know."

After delivering herself of that, she seemed genuinely perplexed as she sat there. Mary also seemed to be straining to comprehend what is, finally, incomprehensible. She looked down even as Theresa was staring at the floor. I wanted to say something to help us all out, but nothing came to mind. At last Mary broke the silence: "You just have to keep your faith in Him. He'll tell us what's ahead when He wants to — and it's like my mom says: 'Not one day sooner!' "

That last quote, with its worldly humor, relaxed us. First Mary and then Theresa let me know that mystery is a major part of Catholicism. Mary said it this way: "You have to pray, and you can't expect the answers to your questions until you die and go see Him. But don't forget, He came here, and He's the best friend you can ever have." Theresa offered her version of reassurance: "He'll be there, waiting for us. He'll keep us out of trouble."

We went around and around for a half-hour more, both girls

reminding me, in essence, of the gratuitousness of Jesus' voyage earthward. "He didn't have to come here, you know," they both said. The subsequent seriousness of the look on each of their faces made me realize that a gesture of apparent gratitude wasn't quite enough. Mary crossed herself; Theresa lowered her head and also crossed herself. I sat there with no ritual to perform, caught between my admiration for their passionate sincerity and my lingering skepticism. How much of what I'd been hearing did these good young Catholic girls hold true on their own account, and how much was a consequence of obedience to "the nun," to "Sister"? Of course, I reminded myself, all children mouth parental pieties, or ones picked up at school, and so do many of us who think we've got our ideas quite on our own. Still, Mary and Theresa were a bit too sure of what lay ahead of them, or so part of me thought.

They must have noticed my reticence and perhaps a quizzical look on my face. Theresa was bold enough to inquire: "Do you believe in heaven — and Jesus there?" I was quicker than I wanted to be in my retort: "I'd like to." They sized up that wistful rejoinder all too accurately. Mary: "But *do* you?" As I hesitated, Theresa answered for me: "He's not sure." I nodded. It was then that Mary showed me a side of her contemplative life that I had thought was missing: "I know, it's hard to imagine what will happen after you die. I wonder how we get there, to heaven. I wonder where it is. My dad said [she told me she had asked him] you can't see heaven; it's not in the sky — we just think it is. You can't know for sure. My mom and dad say the one thing that we *do* know is that Jesus did come here, and He did His best for us, and He got killed, and they saw Him; He appeared to them — so He'll save us, somehow. But it's not something that you can just sit down and say: this is how He'll do it!"

She had to stop several times as she gave me that lecture. Theresa had kept nodding, and her affirmation clearly meant a lot to Mary. I was touched by Mary's recognition of the impossibility of knowing what she surely wanted very much to know — the practical details, as it were, of how salvation takes place. Yet her impasse did not deter either faith or further speculation, nor a moment or two of thinly disguised doubt: "You have to believe Jesus will be there when you die. If you don't, then there'll be no one. I asked my daddy what would happen if Jesus hadn't come here. He said God would still be up there, but it would be different, because Jesus knows us. Didn't He live here until they crucified Him? He was praying for us all the time He was there, on the cross. I guess that shows He was God. A person — you'd try to stay alive, and you wouldn't be thinking of everyone else."

Theresa gave those thoughts her own thought. She had a reservation, one supported by a memory of a Sunday school lesson: "Yes, but He *did* get upset! I remember when we learned that He was very sad, and He thought He might be in trouble, real trouble, because God had forgotten Him — [we learned] something like that, right?" "Right," said Mary, "but only for a second or two. Then He realized God was watching over Him." They looked at me, and I agreed with a nod: so I had read in the Bible. It was then that Theresa asked me whether I thought "a lot about Jesus." I wondered why she chose that time to ask, and I almost asked her that, but I didn't have it in me to heighten our self-consciousness any further. Anyway, I felt Theresa was simply trying to bring me, out of politeness, further into a conversation she and her cousin had found personally challenging and interesting. I answered, "I do think about Jesus — more and more as I talk with you two and others." They smiled, and soon thereafter our threesome got distracted by a low-flying, noisy plane and the demands of the clock.

In the two years of our talks, every week for almost a year, then every month, I began to realize how strongly the cross shaped their sense of what Christianity meant. These were not morbid or sad girls. They came from reasonably strong families, and as I write this I know a lot about their late adolescence. They are able students and athletes. They are popular. They are headed for good local (New England) colleges. Catholicism is still very much a part of their lives, and they still continue to contemplate the reason Jesus came here, the meaning of His "visit." What an unlikely word for religious introspection — a word used by all of us to describe the casual act of dropping in to see friends or family. Certainly as I read theological books I don't see "visit" used often in describing Jesus' time on earth, His "coming," His brief but dramatic and memorable life. Yet again and again I have heard Christian children speak of his "visit." I asked both Mary and Theresa whether the nuns had used "visit" in describing Jesus' time here, and their answer was no. Their parents? No. I dropped the matter, but not before they wondered why I was asking. I told them that I hadn't often — before then, at least — heard the word used in connection with Jesus' life. They were surprised. What better way to describe those thirty-three years? I agreed.

For many other children, as for those two eager informants, that "visit" lives strongly in the moral and religious imagination as they try to figure out "what church is all about." Most often, as Christian children[1] reflect upon the central thrust of their religion, the word "promise" comes up as well. He came here to visit us, those children keep telling me, and His visit was meant to be a "promise" — of salvation, no less. That "visit" was important, was providential, they take pains to say.

"It was no picnic, His visit here," Theresa told me many months after our early meeting described above. I was always alerted when a child pushed the language a little, as in "picnic." I knew then that the child was probably thinking independently about some aspect of his or her religious inheritance. Theresa, of course, let me know, and not for the first time, how much Jesus suffered, how difficult His brief spell here was. But she almost played with the word "picnic": "He had some good times. He ate with His friends, and they loved each other. They drank wine." What a picnic — bread and wine and love! On the other hand, speaking of "no picnic," she remembered all the "rough times" — the betrayals, the isolation and condemnation at the hands of others, and, invariably mentioned, the final hours on the cross, followed by the end of the visit. Still, if it was a visit that ended in tragedy, it was also a visit that gave the world its "reward," another word children use again and again as they try to describe certain quintessential religious and spiritual elements in their lives. Theresa, now two years into our talks and nearing adolescence, told me, "You know He gave us all this reward, if we want it. It's yours, but we have to ask for it. You should go to church — but just sitting there isn't enough. You have to talk with Him, and He'll listen to you. He's offering you a lot! You go to heaven. But you have to remember all He had to go through so that we could have Him up there, helping us out."

As with Theresa, so with other Catholic and Protestant children. Christianity is a "special religion," a Hungarian boy of twelve told my son, because "it's the only one that God chose." When the boy was asked to expand on that assertion, he gladly obliged: "I don't know about other religions. I only know about ours [Catholicism], but Jesus came here, and I don't think in the other religions God came here to live — and so He knows us, because He was down here, and He'll be looking out for us when we leave here."

I was struck by that proprietary claim to singularity. Accordingly, I asked children in the United States to compare their faith with others. Many told me they knew little of other faiths, but both Jewish and Christian children remarked on the centrality of Jesus' human existence in Christianity. That distinctive kind of divinity registers deeply in children, especially because He is so often presented in church as a child, one who for a long while lived as other children do — in relative obscurity, with a family. Moreover, He was a child who later had an important mission, and for many children, intent even at eight or ten on finding out what the future holds, Christ's life stands as a concrete example. No wonder, then, a mission — the coming of God to earth as an infant, a growing child — becomes regarded as redemptive in a rather heartfelt manner. When children flounder a bit psychologically and morally, Jesus turns into a personal guide: He has been where I am, and so He knows, and He will lead me to an outcome in this life, and in an afterlife, that is "good," that need not be feared. As any parent knows, all children experience, with everyone else, "good" dreams but also nightmares, and they sometimes wonder with apprehension what the world offers down the line. For many Christian children Jesus becomes not so much a revered, inspirational figure, nor God's Son, hence powerful and knowing beyond measure, but a children's Savior: the One who survived childhood and later suffering, and is still very much present.

I am especially indebted to a ten-year-old boy named Charlie, who suggested such a line of thought to me in 1986, when I was talking with him in Sudbury, Massachusetts; it helped me understand what others would tell me later. "My dad is a lawyer,"

Charlie reminded me one day, and I wondered at that moment why he brought up the matter when we were in the midst of a talk about the Episcopal church his mother attended and the Presbyterian church his father used to attend occasionally. With some sidetracking Charlie explained himself, and here I bunch together his comments and omit most of mine: "People forget Jesus had a father as well as a mother, and he was a carpenter. I told my friend Gerry that Jesus' dad was a carpenter, and he said no, God is Jesus' father. We argued. Our minister [Episcopalian] said we're both right: Jesus had two fathers, one in heaven and one here! That's not bad! I know a lot of kids, they don't have any — I mean, their parents have split. 'It's no life,' a friend I know always says.

"I think of Jesus having a dad who was a carpenter because [I had asked] I wonder why God chose that kind of family for Him. He must have had a reason. Right? He didn't do anything without a reason, right? That's how I see it. He must have thought to Himself: Why, I want my Son to be down there with just plain people, nothing fancy. If Jesus had grown up in a plush house and been a spoiled brat — that's the big danger in this town, my folks keep telling me! — He'd have been different. Wouldn't He? Don't you think?"

We stopped there for a while. I confessed that, in fact, I had never really asked myself such a question. The boy kept emphasizing that Jesus was the son of humble parents, that Jesus is the One who wants to "save" us because He has actually experienced the ups and downs of life as we all know it — a theology, one might say, strong on the palpable, the everyday. "They don't tell us [in church and Sunday school] what He was like when He was my age, when He was almost eleven. That would be the year eleven, right? Probably no one heard of Him then. Probably He was in school, and I don't know, He could have been having trouble there. I asked our [Sunday school] teacher one day [a lawyer, like his dad, with a Boston law firm] and he laughed and said, 'Doggonit, Charlie, that's a funny question!' He didn't answer it, and we kept reading from the [Sunday school] book, that explains the Bible, but you know, afterwards we got to talking, my [four] buddies and I, when we were practicing lacrosse, and we decided: if He was a human, like us, He must have gone to school, and He must have liked some subjects and not others. Even the 'brains' don't like every subject the same!"

A long distraction ensued — a discussion of schoolwork and the academic life. I fended off questions as best I could, sometimes feeling uncomfortable, such as when Charlie wanted to know whether I liked "best" the students who got A's. I tried to get us over what then seemed like a barrier. But the boy had his own reasons for the inquiries he was making: "What if Jesus had trouble with something [at school], and people began laughing at him? What if a teacher really didn't like Him, really didn't give Him the time of day, really said these wisecrack remarks about Him, the way they do in school sometimes, you know? He must have felt lousy! That would have been way before He ended up feeling *real* lousy; I mean, when He was on the cross. We don't do that [crucifixion] anymore, but kids really feel left out in school, and you can see them having the worst time, and it can be the teacher's fault, or it can be our fault, kids being no good to other kids."

At a certain point it was Charlie, not I, who wanted to hurry us back to a major thesis: "Our minister told us one day [in a church sermon] that Jesus knew what it is to feel left out, and when he said that, I thought of how you can feel in school — you're alone, and no one gives a damn (that's how my father talks). When He died He knew the score here, and He must remember that — how He felt — while He's in heaven. I want to say '*up* in heaven,' but they tell us in Sunday school that we shouldn't say 'up,' because heaven isn't in the sky. Well, we asked, 'Where is it?' The teacher said its 'away from us here!' We kept asking her, 'Where? Where?' She said, 'Away, away!' Then she got mad, and we shut up! I don't care where He is; I think He remembers."

He stopped then, almost as if he himself had a little trouble remembering something. I waited. He looked at me. Still nothing. I responded, finally, to his intriguing last sentence: "What does He remember, Charlie?" He replied immediately, tersely, "Everything." I was frustrated. Clearly this boy had a lot to say about God's awareness over time — His relationship to His own life, and to ours who follow Him, we who are so distanced from His lived life.

Silence still. Charlie's head was slightly lowered. He was lost in thought, I realized, and I kept my mouth shut. Finally, after five or six long seconds, his head rose and he spoke: "He couldn't forget the way He died. He must remember the way people treated Him. You don't forget, when you're alone. I remember when we moved, and I went to school, and I didn't know anyone at first. Jesus, everyone knew Him — but they didn't like Him, they didn't believe Him, and that's even worse [than what Charlie had temporarily experienced]. So He must still remember. My mom once told me Jesus knows everything because He is God. I was supposed to pray to Him on my birthday! That's better than asking for presents, she said. So He must remember what happened to Him, if He remembers all of our birthdays! (My mom says He does!)"

That last parenthetical remark was made in response to the incredulity on my face as I heard that the Lord "remembers all of our birthdays." With his footnote completed, Charlie was ready to let me carry on my side of our discussion, but I was by now somewhat lost in thought, trying to fathom the mystery of God's memory. Charlie spoke up, suggested this: "I guess we'll only know more when we meet Him." On that note I could smile, nod agreement, speak out with my own memories, not unlike Charlie's, of hearing my mother attribute a kind of universal knowledge to an omniscient and omnipotent deity, even as, at the same time, she read far and deep in science, prodded by her engineer husband. My young friend seemed quite comprehending of what I realized I was saying only as I heard it said — that many of us struggle hard to understand what is, in the end, beyond us. He signaled our rapport with humor: "Maybe God will remember we were trying to figure Him out today, but we just couldn't!"

Perhaps children raised in Christian homes are quick to focus on Jesus as a Savior because they know full well their own vulnerability as boys and girls. I have heard many aspects of Christianity emphasized by their parents — Christ as teacher, as moral and spiritual guide, as healer, as one whose wisdom can help us turn away from various demons. Any number of those parents also stress Christ's beautitudes, His Galilean sayings, His struggle with "the powers that be." For the parents Good Friday was a tragedy and Easter a triumph, but they didn't mobilize that

Easter victory in the direct and personal way their children did. Charlie's mother: "My son talks about Jesus sometimes as if He's working day and night to rescue people!"

In Tennessee my son Bob and I were sitting with three Protestant boys, all twelve, as they discussed their "relationship" with Jesus. I winced a bit at the free use they made of that word — a psychiatric banality for those who, ironically, accept psychology and psychiatry as a secular religion. The boys were all too interested in how Jesus "influences your mind." I wanted no part of this aspect of the research project. My son was angered by my indifference, my unwillingness, as he saw it, to get beyond the psychological palaver, to listen for what those children were really trying to say. The day before, I had heard one "relationship" too many discussed, and I had begged off further meetings. And now here we were again, father and son, my eyes glazed, my mouth shut.

"Jerry, would you tell my dad what you told me last week — about your Jesus versus your parents' Jesus?"

"Yes, Bob, OK."

Jerry looked at Matt and Junior, the more reticent ones: would they speak, too? They somehow perceived his request, responded with ever so subtle nods. Jerry began: "My mom and dad like to think it's all done, so we should have a party! I guess they have more faith than I do! A lot of times, though, they'll warn us that if we don't read the Bible and think of Jesus, we'll be 'lost' — the devil will win out. I believe them! I see the devil doing his work. My grandma says, 'The devil has slippery shoes,' and she's dead right. We've got this 'mean streak' in us, she says, and we take it out on people; we express it. It's Jesus who helps us with that; He wants to be involved in our lives. He needs us — He wants a relationship with us. He wants to save us. But we can't just expect Him to snap His fingers, and that does it, we're saved! You can hear people say, 'Jesus died to save you,' but I don't think He likes hearing Himself talked about like that!

"If you want to think of your life ahead, [think of] not just now but way into the future, then you should be thinking of Jesus as much as your friends. If you've got a good relationship with Him, He'll be there for you, and when the day comes, the

big day, He'll be on your side, and that's all you need. But if
He's not on your side — well, then, forget it! Our minister told
us: people put money in the bank and they buy land, and they
take out insurance policies, and they think they're protecting
themselves. The trouble is, when you go [die], and you're waiting
on the Lord to decide, it's not what you own, it's what you've
been: I mean, have you known Jesus, that's what counts. So you
should think of whether you'll be saved. If you're not [saved],
it's a long time in hell, my pappy [the name he uses for his
grandfather] will tell you. He's close to going, and he's hoping
Jesus will be on his side — but everyone has to worry. You can't
just say, 'All right, He's on my side.' You have to work on how
you're doing with Him, that's what our coach says [he also teaches
Sunday school]."

I was crossing and uncrossing my legs, more than a little offended by a certain bargaining I sensed in all this. My son, alert
to my signals, didn't seem pleased. I noticed *his* signal, a frown.
He turned to Matt and Junior and asked them resolutely and
with obvious interest what they thought. Expecting a rehash, I
reached for a Coca-Cola; that would liven me up and sap away
some excess self-righteousness. I gave myself an inward lecture:
these are decent boys who work hard not only for themselves
but for the community they belong to. They are polite, courteous, warm-spirited.

Matt started talking. He disqualified himself before he said
anything about religion by telling us that he wasn't a "deep
thinker." My son commented, "Deep thinkers can be as phony
as anyone else! They can end up in hell with the best of us."
The three boys loved that brief outbreak of populist anti-intel-
lectual egalitarianism. They smiled broadly — perhaps "defensively." Indeed, I remember thinking that some of their smiles
had been too predictable, even automatic. At any rate, Matt put
an end to this undercurrent of cultural and regional suspicion:
"You have to trust in the Lord. He's all you've got; that's what
I think. I'll be using my slingshot, and I'll go too far — I'll be
having my fun, and some little squirrel gets wiped out, and I
feel the hand, His hand, on mine: Matt, you've got to be more
considerate. My mamma and my daddy will tell me to be 'more
considerate,' and I'll try to oblige. But when the Lord talks to

you, you'd better pay attention. Sure, it's OK to have fun with your slingshot [I had interrupted to ask], but you can cross that boundary, and suddenly you're in trouble, big trouble — because He's watching you (He just does!) and He's keeping track. We know He does — but we want to forget He does! That's how I see it. If you're wanting Him to be there for you, 'to give you the gift of salvation,' like they tell you in church, like they say there, then it's up to you to be deserving of it. He's not up there handing out goodies! No sir, I don't believe He is. He's trying to do right, so the right folks will live forever in His kingdom, and it must be hard, even for Him. I think I'm correct in saying that! I hope I'm not out of bounds! Our coach told us, 'Act as if the Lord is watching over you, and He wants to love you and protect you, but He won't take any of your "small-time stuff"! So be careful, because what you do today can be a step to eternity, and that's the goal, the big touchdown you want.' "

A transcript of a taped conversation, even if it has been sharpened by editing, pointed in the direction of clarity and forcefulness, can't fully convey what a videotaping would offer: in this case, Matt's utterly convincing sincerity, even his passion. His face was alert; his eyes were gazing now at my son, now at me, now at his two friends, with a directness that drew each of us toward him. This twelve-year-old boy from a semirural east Tennessee community was intent on an exercise in self-criticism at odds with the glib, pious cant I had been picking up. Matt was trying, really, to indicate that he perceived in himself a sense of moral jeopardy that ignited his mind's conscience but also his mind's common-sense urge toward survival. Under such circumstances, he was all ears for any counsel and always called upon the example of examples, the life of all lives, for help. This youthful try at psychological and moral immersion was readily apparent on his face, in the timber of his voice, in his awakened body. As I tried to sort out the mix of clichés and deeply felt convictions he uttered, I wanted to filter out many of the words and simply attend with admiration his struggle to look from his twelve years into the great span of future time.

When Matt had stopped, Jerry opened his mouth but quickly closed it. The most voluble of the three had been silenced. I looked at Junior, the least talkative, and concluded that he was as touched as the rest of us. Suddenly, though, Junior signaled us to pay attention to him. Characteristically, he did so nonverbally at first. He reached for the last Coke, awkwardly searched out the bottle opener, made a bit of a spectacle out of opening the bottle by only half succeeding for a second or two, so that foam escaped. He had failed to put the bottle over a glass, and so the floor caught the spill. We were all his audience, though this was not a self-conscious or sly production. Junior could be affectingly awkward and shy in many ways — now he was simply gearing up to have his say.

"I don't know what will happen to me." He abruptly stopped with that, not uttered with the hopelessness of a melancholic or the anguish of an agnostic existentialist. Junior was being matter-of-fact, yet the incongruity between the content of his statement and its manner of delivery made us look at him a little more closely. The boy knew right away what had taken place. He smiled and then started in again, this time rhetorically: "Can you know [what will happen to you], until you die?" Having gained momentum, he spoke confidently right through his short but intense declaration: "You can't." Then came the modest attribution: "Our minister says you can't, and I believe him." Those last three words, uttered gravely, were convincing. I noticed all of a sudden that his eyes seemed glassy — a deep blue that began to suggest two ponds. Was he on the verge of tears? I lost for a second my sense of having a bond with him. I began to feel cool, even annoyed: there was a betrayal at work hereabouts. The phrase "Bible belt" occurred to me, and I found myself thinking of the Bible salesman in Flannery O'Connor's "Good Country People."

When that thought subsided, another one took over: I worried for Junior. What ailed him? Some unhappiness? I was almost ready to break this charged moment; I could feel the words welling up: "Is there something that happened to you, Junior, that you might want to share with us?" Talk about clichés! I glanced at my son; the sight of his complete absorption in Junior's words provided a control I would otherwise not have had.

Junior told us softly why he had blurred up a bit: "I remember my sister when she was dying. She was the oldest. She was but thirteen then — two years ago. She'd been walking on the road, toward home. She went to get some bread and some starch, I think, for Momma, and sugar, too, a small bag. She was minding her business, like you should. She was well off the asphalt. This car came along, and it did the curve, and the man tried to straighten out, but he didn't, they told us afterward, and instead he went straight for our Sally, and he struck her down."

No more words for a while. The boy lowered his head. His lips moved in a silent prayer. His friends lowered their heads, too. In the stillness my son and I exchanged a look. He glanced at each of the boys, then lowered his head. His lips were still, but he wanted to feel close to the children. I sat with my head not really lowered but my eyes cast downward. Part of me wondered how this lull in our discussion would end. Part of me wanted to bow my head, like the others. Part of me vividly remembered childhood: our mother taking us to church, our father sitting outside in the car, reading the Sunday newspapers, waiting for us. When we returned, he smiled that thin, wry smile which, better than any words, reminded us of his attitude toward "mystery shops," a laconic scientist's derisive dismissal. My parents were so happily married, I remembered in the stillness. Try to live with the contradictions or tensions in you, in this room, I thought, even as your parents did.

I noticed Junior's lips stop moving. His eyes suddenly became mobile; they engaged with a shadow a few yards to his left. The shadow seemed to have a life of its own, coming close to Junior, then withdrawing toward the recesses of the room. It was, I realized, a tree's branch outlined by the sun: a dance of light and darkness in our midst. Junior seemed entranced. An intense look eventually gave way to a smile. The others, his friends and my son, had joined with him: all eyes were on the wind's impact on us through its impact on that tree's branch. The wind abated. The mix of shadow and light was stilled. Junior lifted his eyes; they moved from friend to friend and finally engaged with mine, the eyes of someone twice an outsider, from another region and another generation. I tried to hold my eyes in place, return this boy's look. For some reason I simply couldn't. I wondered why he was "staring" and why I couldn't meet his gaze. But such passing ruminations were banished by the reality of his voice: "We pray for Sally, every day, at suppertime. She's with the Lord.

I guess He wanted her bad, real bad. I guess He just couldn't wait. Daddy gets upset even now; he says the Lord must fall asleep a lot, and that's why our Sally was hit, and got killed. Mom doesn't like to hear him talk like that. She says it's doubting Him, that's what it is. She started crying the other day, when he went on and on — saying bad things about the Lord. When he saw her tears, he stopped. But I could tell, he's not a praying man, the way Mom is a praying woman! You know what he says? He says, 'Let them [the ministers in the church] do an honest day's work! Let them stop leeching off the rest of us!'

"When Sally died, Daddy lost his faith. I think he goes to church with us because he wants to do Mom a favor. He wants her to be happy, so he lets her think Sally is with God. Where is Sally? [I had asked him where he thought she is.] That's where she is, with God, I guess. I mean, maybe He did overlook her that day; maybe that's why she got killed. But He must take His people home, after they die like Sally [did]. He can't just let her be there [in the grave], and that's the end of it."

He said much more. For almost an hour we talked, poignantly, of faith and doubt, life's dangers, their meaning — Job's question, and answers to it. Twice Junior reminded us that Christianity was not for him only a weekend ritual practiced (or endured) at the behest of demanding parents. "Without Jesus, Sally would be a big heartache for us until the day we die," Junior said. He amplified: "We still miss her. But we know she's gone to be with Him [Jesus], and that's where you hope you'll go. He was here, and He went back — He died, just like Sally did. It's sooner or later — death. You can't just keep crying for her. You have to think what came out of the accident — that she got to meet the Lord! That's the good side; the bad side is that she's not here with us, and Mom will forget, and set her a plate, even now, and then she'll remember, and she'll take it away, and she cries come each time, but Sally is there, in heaven, and that's where you'd want your sister to be, if she can't be with you! Jesus is the one who will save you, if you deserve it. That's why we're born — to test us, to see if we should go to heaven and be with God and with Jesus and with His friends; or go to hell and be there with the devil and all the people he's got keeping him company! Once I asked how many of us go to heaven and how many of us go to hell, and the minister said you can't put a number to it, and if there is a number, only God knows it. If you're not going to be saved, then it's your fault. Sally did her best to be good, and she prayed to Him, and she must be there with Him. I believe she is! That's what God taught, that He'll look after us, and He's a teacher whose word is good!"

I hadn't before heard Junior remark upon God's teaching capacities. As a matter of fact, most Christian children I'd talked with hadn't emphasized Jesus the teacher so much as Jesus the powerful Son of God, Jesus the healer, Jesus the gatekeeper of sorts, welcoming some, turning away others. I asked Junior about what kind of teacher Jesus was. The boy was at first irritated. Hadn't he just told me? The annoyance on his face was given expression: "His word is good, like I said — that's the best teacher, and Jesus was the best." I looked for more about Jesus' teaching life: "How did Jesus teach? Have you discussed His teaching in [Sunday] school — what He taught?"

Junior did not reply for a few seconds. He looked up at the ceiling, the way so many children do when they are temporarily at a loss for words, and then down at the floor. When he began speaking, I noticed that at first he spoke as if I were way across the room — in a loud voice, directed far off: "He taught everyone to love. He tried to love people; and some of them were glad, and they signed up to be with Him, and others, they didn't trust Him, and they were against Him from the start, and they never stopped being against Him. He tried to be kind to everyone — most folks, I think, except for the real bad ones — but a lot of people didn't want to believe Him. So He was all alone at the end of His life."

Junior stopped at that point. I noted a shift from an initial discussion of Christ's teaching to a description of His final days. I concluded that Junior hadn't really thought much about Jesus as a teacher, that I had more or less pushed him into a consideration of the subject. But I was wrong. Junior resumed, with no prodding from me: "I don't think He taught in school. He taught outside; it [the teaching] was [done] up a hill. A lot of people listened. For a while He had a crowd behind Him. But then there was trouble, and the government cracked down. When He was doing his teaching, He must have made everyone believe in Him; they must have really been on His side then. It was later that He got into trouble."

As Junior talked I thought of Jesus walking in Galilee, throngs attending His words and deeds; and I thought especially of Him offering those hilltop beatitudes. This boy could recite from the fifth chapter of Matthew — one "blessed" after the other. He had even taken the trouble to imagine himself there, project himself back over the centuries to the earliest years of the Common Era, think of himself as living in ancient Galilee: "I'd have been living in a tent, maybe, and I'd be a fisherman or a farmer, I think. There He'd be, and I'd be listening to Him! He must have been a great teacher. People must have stood there, where He was, and listened to every word He said, and they must have remembered every word, too. Maybe some folks didn't listen [I had asked], but I'd hate to be one of them. He was popular then — before He got into trouble. There were crowds, and He was a teacher people loved. They must have known He would save them; they must have known He was special. He probably looked special — no, not the clothes He wore. It was His face, I guess, and what He said, and how He got to you."

The boy himself appeared flushed and animated. While he did his own teaching, my mind wandered. I tried to follow Junior's lead, tried to visualize what it might have looked like almost two thousand years ago as Jesus walked Palestine, stopping here and there to exhort, to explain, to pronounce, to bless and heal, to encourage others to think about what counted most and for which reasons. My mind wandered not only way eastward to the desert villages not far from the Mediterranean, but westward to California, to a dramatic and commanding view of Jesus teaching a crowd of engrossed listeners — a scene that covers the upper part of the entrance wall of Stanford University's Memorial Church. As Junior talked I remembered that church, that scene; and I remembered, too, at Junior's age, standing with my parents, asking them for an interpretation of what we all were seeing, visitors to a great California university. I began to understand why a long-ago experience had suddenly come to mind as I became aware, suddenly, that Junior's most recent words, "and how He got to you," were echoing in my head.

I told Junior of that great mural. He at once seemed to comprehend why I still remembered the mural vividly. "Jesus knew how to teach — you can tell by what the Bible says. People knew He was special, real special, and they waited for Him to tell them things. If a teacher doesn't get your interest, it doesn't make any difference whether he has a good idea or not! No one is listening. Jesus gets to you even now, and He's been gone all those years. You can hear Him talking. You can see Him. He's looking at you, and you don't want Him to leave, ever. He's the one who's going to save you. He's that kind of teacher!"

Those last words brought me back to my childhood California visit — my mother explaining to me, as we both looked at the mural, that Jesus did a very special kind of teaching. This boy, Junior, had been telling me about the Teacher's spiritual charisma, actually the subject of the Stanford mural. For Junior the coincidence — his remarks, my mother's remarks decades before — was itself worth consideration: "He's been the one who has taught us all! If you're a Christian, that means you've put yourself in His classroom, and if you do like the teacher says, then you'll graduate!" The boy stopped to let me know that he was borrowing someone else's imagery — that of his uncle, a high school guidance counselor: "He took us to church when we were visiting him, and he said we should remember that Jesus is our most important teacher, and He's the one who will get us through life, or if we're not on His side, He's the one who will say no, you don't graduate! After he told us that, I thought of Jesus handing you a report card! My mom said it's foolish to think like that — but she said it's true, He does keep track of you, because He has to, it's His job. My cousin [that uncle's daughter] says He's got the biggest computer in the whole universe and no one falls through the cracks!"

The cousin, Jeannie, fifteen, was not planning to be a housewife soon — so she'd told Junior. She wanted to be a computer programmer; she envisioned herself, upon completion of high school in Knoxville, heading up to Chicago for "scientific education." Junior heard the phrase from Jeannie: "Jeannie says a lot of ministers are afraid of science, and she says it's too bad. She says if Jesus returned, He'd buy a computer and use it! He'd fly on a jet plane! He'd drive a car so He could visit a lot of places. If He could only walk, there'd be fewer people to see. He's hoping to save as many as He can, so why not see all the folks He can? With a computer, He'd know more. He'd have everything stored away — all His speeches, and the people who wrote to Him! I can see why Daddy gets upset when Jeannie talks like that — but you wouldn't think God would send His Son here, this year, and expect Him to be at a real disadvantage, would you? That's the way Jeannie answers my dad, and I can see her point!"

I got rather uneasy myself as he talked, but I managed to keep my mouth shut so that Junior could pursue a variant of his salvation thesis. He did so, and weeks later, he and Jeannie (she was there on a visit) both did so. Jeannie, sunny-tempered and lively, looked not much older than Junior. In fact, interrupted by nods from Junior and an occasional question from me, she talked about their similar looks, as well as their beliefs and ideals, in a number of longish monologues: "We look alike — our faces. My mom and his look alike, but mine is shorter, and maybe that's why I'm short for my age and Junior is tall for his! The other day a friend of his said I looked like his younger sister! I like coming here and seeing another branch of our family tree. With a computer we could make a record of our whole family. That's what I mean about computers — they can help you track down anything! If you were trying to decide what will happen to millions of people, like God does, you'd want a computer to help you, wouldn't you?"

She was almost ready to take my answer for granted, but I was just uncomfortable enough with her talk to speak up: "How would a computer help?" As I asked, I was glad I did. Giving voice to what seemed like a simple query released a spirit of anger in me: what nonsense, this way of thinking! Another voice quieted me down, lectured me: Why *not* think that way? Each generation struggles with its own ways to fathom what are, finally, the mysteries of this universe. Jeannie's bold imagination was holding on to her notion of Jesus and His singular existence for dear life: "I can see Him punching His keyboard up there! He must have rooms and rooms of printouts! He must have people helping Him out, don't you think? [I said nothing.] Maybe that's what the disciples do — they help read all the computer sheets!"

She was about to plunge on and elaborate the computer fantasy, which she had clearly found suggestive — but, to my relief,

Junior wanted to point out something, exercise his own critical judgment, set limits: "Jeannie, are you sure those guys are helping Jesus? I don't know if He's really up there with a big computer. Where is 'up there'? They told us in Sunday school not to think of a place, a room, a house, when you think of heaven. I guess we shouldn't think of heaven as a computer. I mean, we can [think along such lines], but we'll never know for sure, will we? Besides, how did He do the choosing before we got computers? Daddy said there weren't any when he was my age. But God has been choosing all His life — and that's forever."

Jeannie did not disagree with her cousin. She told him so in the briefest, bluntest way: "Right!" Abruptly she changed tack, and to my surprise she moved in my ideological direction: "When we die, we'll find out what's 'out there,' and not before! Everyone knows that, but people hate to admit it!"

She stopped and sat still, looking out the windows. Only her right leg, crossed over the left one and moving up and down, showed her agitation. After four or five seconds, she withdrew her gaze from the window, focused it on Junior, then me, then him: "What if God isn't really anyone! What if there's no heaven and no hell, either! No one can prove what He's like. Our minister told us you have to hold on to your faith, because God isn't next door, and you can't go see Him, or call Him up and hear His voice on the phone!"

She was going to continue, but Junior hadn't gone beyond the first inquiring outcry. He lifted his right arm up — another dramatic moment — and made sure that we took notice. "What if God really isn't anyone!" He was repeating her exclamatory question, only moving forward the adverb "really." I expected him to rebut the obvious doubt implied in those words. But he chose to stop with his repetition of her utterance; then he lowered his head as if to ponder the question carefully in his own way, at his own pace. We all do just that, I in my own way: thoughts were rushing through my head, thoughts about God as a person, the Christian view; or God as the elusive "spirit" so many Indian children have mentioned to me; or, finally, God as an "idea," an assertion I heard as a freshman in college. Oh, everything was an "idea" at that heady place! Away from Tennessee for a second or two, I awoke to Junior talking: "If God isn't anyone, then maybe we're not, either. At my [great-]aunt's funeral the minister said 'ashes to ashes,' and I got scared. But if there's no God, that's all there is, ashes. No heaven and no hell. If God is someone, then we're someone, too. He'll make us someone, if we let Him. I hope He will — that's what you pray for: that He'll be something for you, if you've given Him a chance, by being mostly good. You can't be all good, I know."

Jeannie said an "amen" to that last observation, and I found myself joining her out loud — after which we all smiled knowingly, each with, no doubt, a passing thought or two about sinful times. Junior's statement was, however, a rather serious one, as we all recognized. We were getting ready to break up. I was to meet my son and do more interviews in nearby Chattanooga, and Junior and his cousin were to go on a family outing. Junior made one more comment: "You know, I guess the Lord and us, we're all in this together: us hoping to be saved, and Him wanting to save us" — delivered in an offhand manner as we ambled toward the door. All in *what* together? I wondered whether such a question, even if posed and answered with the greatest care, would not ultimately leave us precisely where this child had intended. Why should I ask him to elaborate on what is utterly beyond our knowing. I asked myself as I kept quiet and said my goodbyes. Weeks later, though, Junior's reflective analysis kept coming to mind. So much complex Christian theology worked into such a disarmingly simple, folksy summary! Here was a child who understood not only his own wishes but those of his Lord.

Driving away from that intense meeting, I remembered a seminar of Paul Tillich's back in 1957. I was a psychiatric resident then, but still struggling with religious interests. Tillich had taken the trouble to bring Karl Barth's theology to our attention, with its emphasis on *God's* search. A revered teacher, calling upon a theological colleague, asked us to stop and look beyond ourselves, *way* beyond ourselves, to Another's involvement in this great riddle whose contours, actually, the boy Junior had evoked: "us hoping . . . and Him wanting . . ." That was Junior's contribution to my learning, but also a fine approximation of what so many other children, steeped in various ways and to various degrees in Christianity, have tried to convey as they have given voice to (or drawn, painted) the messages they have learned to carry within.

10

Islamic Surrender

ASIF, OF PAKISTANI BACKGROUND, turning twelve, told me in London that he dreamed of becoming a pilot.[1] That way, he would see the world, not be confined to a city street or two. Often, he said, he heard or saw a plane headed for an airport or leaving for a foreign country; it made him stop in his tracks, look down after looking up, and dream: "I'd like to be flying the plane, and I'd like to get a medal, after I've flown lots of planes for a long time, if I never have an accident."

The boy had heard his parents talk of Pakistan's national airline, and of its strong air force, of their flight by plane to England after the Second World War, their desire to return to Pakistan someday — but their desire, also, to stay in England, where, obviously, the standard of living is so much higher. This kind of conflict was also Asif's: "I'd like to live in my own country, Pakistan; but I like living here. The airplane is the answer! If I became a pilot, I could fly back and forth, back and forth. You smile [I certainly did], but isn't it true? I could live in England one week, and Pakistan the next, if I flew for Air Pakistan."

I smiled again: he knew the name of the airline. We talked more about planes, and he told me he had gone to London's Heathrow airport, seen many planes, dreamed afterward of piloting them. He asked me if I ever wanted to be a pilot. I told him no. He reminded me that I travel a lot on planes. Yes, I said, but that didn't mean I had to *pilot* them! But he objected: "Haven't you worried about the pilots — if they're good?" Of course, I answered, but such a concern didn't make me want to be a pilot. The boy said, "I don't like to surrender to others [who are human] — only to God!"

I was perplexed. I began to feel the psychiatrist stirring in me. I looked a bit more closely at Asif; he seemed relaxed, though, not an anxious or troubled child. It was my turn to speak, and I'd already waited too long. Finally, I stumbled forth with: "Well, Asif, we can't do everything for ourselves. Every day we trust others to do things we don't know how to do."

He listened carefully and quickly got my point: "Yes, but up in the sky, there is Allah, and with Him His messenger to us, Mohammed, and they are the ones I want to obey; and if I was in a plane, I'd be paying all my attention to the pilot — a pity. I'd rather *be* the pilot and think of Allah as I fly the plane!"

I hardly expected this turn to our exchanges. I had known Asif for several weeks, and one of my sons, Danny, had met him a year earlier and explored with him the nature of his religious beliefs. But now we were approaching the boy's sense of Allah in an unusual and unexpected way. I decided to let Asif help me understand him, if he could. "All right, imagine you *are* the pilot — what thoughts would you have about Allah?"

I hoped, with that inquiry, to bury my worry about the logic of Asif's thinking (what has being a pilot really got to do with one's life as a Moslem?) in the interest of letting him explain to me how he did, in fact, connect his fantasies of an occupational future with his religious beliefs and spiritual values, as he was then learning them. He said, "I'd know that I'm nearer to Him than I'd be if I wasn't up there flying! I'd look at the sky; at night, I'd look at the stars. I'd think of Him. He must walk from star to star! We don't see Him. You mustn't think of Him — how He looks! But He's up there, in heaven, and in a plane you'd be nearer [to Him]. I don't know if it would be right — but I'd say my prayers on the plane, and He might hear them better up there. It must be hard for Him, when all of us pray to him [in the mosque]. I asked my father, and he said not to worry, Allah hears every word. But it might help if I was nearer — higher up toward where He is."

I was now ready to ask the boy about the geography of heaven — where he as a Moslem child envisioned that "place" to be. But Asif, who had stopped for a second or so to catch his breath, kept control of our discussion: "He gives us strength. A pilot has to keep awake for a long time if he's going from Pakistan to England, or from England to Pakistan. You have to know how to keep the plane going, but you can put the plane on 'hold' if everything is all right. I saw a movie on television, and everything was explained. I couldn't follow the whole explanation, but I remember the 'automatic pilot' — the plane is operated while the pilot can stop and rest.

"I'd pray — when I could rest I would pray. I'd ask my father and others [of the father's generation] if I could say the *salat* [the Islamic ritual prayer service] in the plane. I'd 'testify'; I'd be high up and I'd say, 'I testify that there is no god but God,' and 'I testify that Mohammed is the messenger of God.' I could say, maybe, 'God is most great,' I could say that. God would hear, I hope."

He was smiling, and his face expressed the hope he had just mentioned. He had already drawn me a picture of the Moslem hell, flames all over, and a few skeletal, black bodies burnt to a crisp in the fiery heat. He remembered that picture, searched for it in a pile on a table, where I'd put his work, now joined to a stack of drawings done by other children, some of whom he knew. When he found the picture, he pulled it out, placed it before me, and pointed to it: "A plane would melt in that fire! In hell, it's so hot that anything could melt — 'Even stone!' my father told me. If you pray to God, you could have Him on your side when you need Him. He could make things get better."

Exactly how might God "make things [in the plane] get better"? I didn't want to sound skeptical to this devoutly Moslem child, so I tried hard to control the tone of my voice as I asked that question — conveying a sincere interest rather than the impatient skepticism of the Westerner. Asif answered at once: "Our God wants us to obey His laws, and if a pilot is praying to Him, then the plane is safer. God knows who will be sent to hell. He could send us there soon, or later. If you pray to Him, you'll be stronger; you will be purer, and you will be a better pilot. If you don't think of Him, and don't pray, you will be weak, and you could make mistakes. Without God, my father tells us, you are already in trouble, even if the plane is all right. No plane goes well if the pilot forgets what he has to do. Pilots can make only one mistake, and that is it! The plane crashes. Don't you see — that a pilot who doesn't have God protecting him will be in trouble, because he's thinking of himself, and not God, and he'll be all by himself when there's trouble? The pilot who believes in God, and prays to Him, will call for everyone on the plane to pray, just as he does, and God will have to hear. He will answer our prayers!"

I was not convinced, as Asif could tell by looking at my face. He was beginning to suspect that I had concluded that he held God to a level of accountability that was preposterous, at least by Western scientific standards. He amplified and enlightened: "God doesn't operate machines; He is not an airplane pilot! But in one [television] program the announcer said that 'the pilot's confidence matters as much as knowledge.' I have memorized that [statement]. I believe it. My father says, 'Not only for pilots' [does that remark hold]! If you have said your prayers — and called to God — He will be there, and He'll answer you. He'll come to you. He'll give you the confidence you need; it's His spirit entering you!"

I suggested that many pilots do a first-rate job of flying without the help of any religion's god. The would-be pilot of the twenty-first century listened politely and attentively. His brow furrowed. He reached for a package of Lifesavers, opened it, and passed over the cherry and orange flavors for a lemon one. He unwrapped it a touch too eagerly and popped it into his mouth, then went to work on it quite strenuously. I began to wonder whether I hadn't been somewhat provocative moments earlier with my offhand secular observation.

After the seconds mounted up, my nervousness began to urge me to speak. Yet I drew a blank, torn between a desire to press my skeptical case and an impulse to apologize. Silence continued until Asif no longer had a Lifesaver in his mouth — what seemed like an exceptionally long time. Finally, quite prepared to explain himself, he said, "I know, it's true, lots of pilots don't pray to Allah, don't pray to anyone. I see pictures of pilots on television, and they are like the teachers in school, or the doctors and nurses in the clinic." He must have noticed a cloud cross my face, so he stopped, and then, correctly assuming the nature of my discontent, addressed it. "It's different being a pilot, I know: you can be doing everything right [in a plane], but there's something that doesn't work, and it's not your fault."

He stopped, looked at me, decided I must need a little more of that kind of analysis, and provided it: "I don't know whether Allah helps us when a machine breaks down — probably not! He could help us fix it; He could make us strong, so we would do the best we could. Beyond that — I don't know. I'm sure He could punish us, even if the plane is good — no problems in the engines; He could make us weak."

He noticed a further reason to pause: I was readying myself to talk. He let me do so. "How might Allah make someone — a pilot — weak?"

"If you ignore Allah or don't obey His rules, you will lose your strength. You will become an enemy of His. He'll attack you. No [I had asked], He won't hit you; I don't mean that. My father says: if you don't obey Allah, you lose His spirit; if you do, then His spirit is in you, inside you, and you'll do the best you can. He wants us to follow Him, then we'll have His help."

I noted some repetition in Asif's declaration, but he was intent on continuing, and I decided only to ask about the kind of "help" Allah might offer. Asif elaborated: "He can breathe His power into you! He can make you feel the world will listen to you, it'll obey you. Sometimes, you can feel everything isn't working. My mother told us of someone who had a car, and nothing [in the car] worked, until the man [the owner] said his prayers, and he kept saying them, and he got up and went to the car, and he could run it, he could laugh at the car and *dare* it to give him more trouble, and it didn't!"

Asif noticed a calm upon my face. I didn't explain to him that prayer can help someone break through a psychological or cognitive constraint. I didn't think my skeptical effort at rapprochement would please him, and anyway, I told myself, the point of our discussion was to hear what *he* made of God, rather than to keep asserting *my* views. Pleased that I seemed relatively unruffled, he continued with a stark picture of Allah's willfulness: "If Allah doesn't like you, He'll punish you. That's hell, where you go. It's hotter there than any fire. It's hotter than the nuclear bomb — I asked my father. [I wondered aloud how "we" could know that, hence this explanation.] There are a lot of people in hell. They belong there because they have not followed Allah; they have disobeyed Him. If you do that, He'll pay you back. He can't have everyone forgetting Him."

Before I even knew I wanted to know, I asked why. He straightened himself in his chair, and when he started talking again, I noticed that his voice was tougher, its pitch elevated. Maybe he was at last beginning to lose patience with my skeptical interruptions. "If you are the Master, you expect people to admit you're the Master. If you let people forget, you'd stop being their Master. Allah is our Master, and we have to respect Him and do what He wants. He has told us in the Koran what we should do; He told us through Mohammed. If we don't listen, He'll remember. He'll check us off."

I began to think this London Pakistani boy had found his own reasons to stop and wonder, every once in a while, about the reality of such an image. Asif sensed my thought exactly: "I don't know how Allah keeps after all of us! I asked my uncle; he is very devout. He said, 'He does!' I wasn't ready to ask any more questions. My father told us when we were little that you don't ask questions of Allah, you learn His rules and you obey them. If you question Him, you are not sure of Him. Always be sure of Him!"

Asif stopped, and I wondered whether he was satisfied with what he had said — whether in some corner of his mind a voice was asking questions. I decided to talk more directly for myself, rather than in response to him. We knew each other well enough. "Asif," I began, "I don't think anyone alive has figured out how God, or Allah, keeps track of us, all four or five billion of us on this planet. But we all wonder about something like that. Maybe I shouldn't say 'we all'; maybe I should say a lot of us do."

I had to go no further. The boy scratched his head, pushed back a lock of hair that habitually fell on his forehead, and seemed ready to start a response to me. But abruptly he sneezed, pulled out a handkerchief, blew his nose, put the handkerchief back in his left pants pocket, and seemed stilled by what had just happened. I waited. So did he. Then Asif started talking: "It's true, you can't ever know how Allah knows everything; but He does. He wouldn't be Allah if He didn't know everything! When

I was small my mother told me Allah is the one who knows everything. She said He can do everything, too. I remember asking her, 'Can He jump from here to there?' — and I pointed to the sun. 'Of course,' Mamma said. I believed her, and I still do, but I don't know how He does that. You have to understand that Allah is not us; He's different, completely different."

I said yes; he said yes, too. I wasn't sure there was anything more to say, and since the hour was late and I was due at another home, I prepared to end our time together. But Asif had more to say: "Do you think Allah will one day come here and visit us?"

I was surprised by that question. I decided to speak my thoughts. "Asif, among Christians it is believed that God has already visited this earth once."

He was not at all surprised. "I know. We in Islam have the greatest respect for Jesus! But He was not Allah — God; He was the one He sent here for a visit. If God, if Allah, came, there would not have been that trouble — the death on the cross. Jesus wasn't God. You could not kill God. Allah would have lifted His right hand, and all who wanted to kill Him would die! He would make everyone believe in Him, and if someone refused, he'd die — that's what would happen if Allah came here."

I had no intention of asking him to describe God's appearance; Moslem children, I reminded myself, are taught not to "represent" Allah in their minds or in drawings or paintings. But Asif added something of great interest: "Allah would wear white robes, and He'd cross the ocean in a few steps. He'd want people to listen to Him, and if they didn't, they'd be in real trouble."

I decided to ignore the boy's description of Allah; nor did I want to contest the great powers he had granted Him. Instead, I picked up on another aspect of what I'd just heard. "Asif, tell me, what do you think the 'people' you just mentioned would hear when they sat or stood somewhere, trying to 'listen' to God?"

"I'm not sure," he replied right away. We were at a momentary dead-end — this child, understandably enough, hadn't given any real thought to a speaking agenda for Allah. But Asif did conjecture to this extent: "Allah would tell the world, everyone, 'God is great, very great.' He'd say that real loud, and if you want Him on your side, you'll say it, too — otherwise He'll make you say it, or He'll send you to the fires [hell] with a snap of his fingers. If you fight Him, you'll lose. If you surrender to Him, you'll win."

I had to go then; I was late. The boy had managed an aphoristic conclusion, and I could tell that he was ready to leave also. Asif's words brought to mind the Biblical moments of my own childhood — Isaiah and Amos and Jeremiah and, finally, Jesus of Nazareth; I thought of their challenges to "the powers that be," their insistence on reversing conventional pieties. Asif told me he'd walk out with me because he was due soon at his uncle's house to babysit a four-year-old cousin. We walked down the street, and I kept hearing the phrase "surrender to Him" in my head. Just as we were to part, Asif wished me well, made sure he remembered the time of my next visit, and smiled broadly. I told him he'd given me, as usual, much to think about — and I mentioned that his last words before we'd left his family's apartment had been especially thought-provoking. He had forgotten them already! I told Asif what had been sticking in my mind — the notion of surrender to God, to Allah, as being desirable. He offered an even bigger smile at that point, and his eyes shone: "Doctor, that is what we believe in Islam: surrender to Allah! If you come with us to our mosque, you'll see us all trying to surrender!"

Rita, ten, was born in England, but like Asif she was of Pakistani background. Their parents knew one another well, and they all worshipped in the same mosque. I had intended to have a drawing and painting session with Rita, but I was still thinking about my previous meeting, with Asif, as she and I began to talk, and I decided to tell her of it. When I finished, she laughed and told me what to say to Asif the next time I saw him: "Let him know that you don't understand our religion! But you know, it is simple — we surrender to Allah. We try to follow Him, as Mohammed said we should. Isn't that what other religions ask, too?"

"Yes," I said, "though I don't hear 'submission' and 'obedience' mentioned by Jewish and Christian children as much as I hear those words used by you and Asif and others here [in England]."

"Oh, I see," Rita responded immediately — but then she stopped, and I wondered whether she would say anything more on the subject. After a few seconds — during which my eyes were noticing the crayons and paper I'd put on a card table standing near her seat — she began a statement for my benefit: "We go to our mosque to tell God we belong to Him. If you don't believe that, then you don't belong to Him! My father says to pray to God — it's to say, 'I'm your servant, so tell me what to do.' God is the one who made us, and He'll be the one to decide where we go. It's heaven or hell, and it's up to Him. He chooses. But we're here choosing, too. 'You choose,' my mother tells me lots of times: 'You choose what to do, and Allah remembers.' I hope I get to see God. But you can never be sure. You have to wait until you die. He can save you from hell whenever He wants, and He can take you into heaven whenever He wants. It's all up to you, and it's all up to God, too. I hope I'm being helpful. A lot of times I think about Mohammed and Allah — and I wish I could always be on their side. But sometimes I'll forget all about them. That means I'm not really good enough. If I was [good enough], I'd pray to them all the time, and do whatever God wants me to do — whatever."

She was a bit sad, troubled, by the end of that presentation, troubled because she had not yet learned how to give her all to Allah. She hadn't used the word "surrender," as Asif had, but she clearly had such a concept in mind at a relatively young age — a yielding of herself to the God she had learned to uphold as all-powerful and important beyond any worldly individual or possession. Already poised and self-possessed, Rita could become anxious and scared as she contemplated the divine power of Islam's God — His capacity for utter rejection on the one hand, for eternal embrace on the other.

Not that Islam as Rita knows it is so different from the Judeo-Christian world other children her age have come to know. The conviction of God's great power is the legendary knowledge of thousands and thousands of children for whom Islam is of little or no significance. But such children as Asif and Rita, and others I talked with in London, in Tunisia, on Israel's West Bank, kept making the point that utter self-abnegation was desirable in relation to that immense power. Rita, later that day, reiterated an injunction she had repeatedly leveled at herself: "When something bad happens, you must accept it as a message from God.

He doesn't want to hurt us, but He has to punish us sometimes. We can't just get our own way! If you can't follow Him and tell Him you accept Him as your master, then you won't be visiting Him in heaven! My father tells us every day — every other day, maybe! — that no spoiled children go to heaven. Who does? [I had asked.] Heaven is where God allows His followers to live, after they die. You start a new life then, and God will be your friend forever, but only if you've been His friend first, here."

I was struck by Rita's use of the word "friend," and I immediately asked her to spell out the nature of that friendship. She drew a blank at first, told me she might have, in fact, made a mistake: "I shouldn't have said we can be a 'friend' of God's; that was wrong, maybe. I mean — God can choose you, He can say, 'You've been loyal, and you've followed the rules of Islam, and so I'll be having you come up here, to be with me.' That's what I should have said! You're just you, but He's the one who rules the whole earth — so it's not a friendship. To me, friends are mostly equal. No one is equal to God! How could anyone be?"

Toward the end of that day's meeting, Rita got to talking about the prophet Mohammed. She had "no idea" what he looked like. She did admit to imagining him riding a horse and wearing flowing white robes. He "probably" was "most familiar" with deserts, she told me, and would be "surprised," she thought, were he to visit late-twentieth-century London and see mosques there, places devoted to him as Allah's great mediator and interpreter. On second thought, though, Mohammed would not be surprised at all: "He must be at God's side always. *They* are friends! I think so! God must be like a father to Mohammed! A father can be a friend sometimes!"

She stopped herself — told me she'd lost her train of thought. She was talking about London, and she had meant to say this: "Our God, He knows everything, and He tells Mohammed all He knows. If they are friends, they talk a lot, and they share secrets like we do! In heaven, people are good, and they can have what they want, mostly. What? Anything. Food, I guess. Nice places to rest." She was not alone among children, no matter their religion, in portraying heaven to me as a place of comfort, contentment, and happiness, though most of them hadn't men-

tioned good food as a heavenly bonus. "You don't get to heaven
by dreaming of going to heaven! You only go to heaven if you've
proven to Allah that you belong there, and it's hard to get there,
because He won't let you in unless He *knows* you're good, and
you believe what He wants you to believe, and you bow to Him,
and if He wants you to do something, you do it, and you don't
complain."

She was very much averse to complainers, this eagerly hard-
working girl who helped her mother, a seamstress, take care of
three younger sisters and a brother. She also worried, as did her
mother and father (a store clerk), about the constant swearing
of many Moslem children. "Swearing will keep you out of
heaven," she let me know several times as we talked about the
future of people after death. "Swearing will get you to hell and
keep you there," she told me emphatically.

By then I knew her well, and trusted myself to say, "Rita, if
that is true, I'll not get to heaven. I'll go to hell."

She looked quite serious as she contemplated my statement.
I wanted to go further; I wanted to tell her I supposed there
were plenty of other reasons I wouldn't make it to heaven —
but I dismissed them as not especially worth confessing. Meanwhile, Rita was contemplating my long-term future with the somber and precise attentiveness I'd come to expect of her: her large,
dark eyes were ever watchful, and the tips of the five left fingers
often touched the tips of the five right ones, as if she was not
likely to let much get by unnoticed. Eventually she addressed
the question of my soul's status: "If you have done a lot of
swearing, you must be in some trouble with Allah. But I haven't
ever heard you swear, so you must not swear too much. If you
fall down once in a while, you can still go to heaven — and if
you beg Allah to smile on you, and promise to do whatever He
wants you to do, then you can increase your chances that He'll
take you [to heaven]. It's up to Him, though. He doesn't like
people who cross Him. He really doesn't."

I noted that expression "cross Him," a phrase I'd heard some
London teachers use: don't cross me! I asked Rita what especially
might "cross" Allah, make Him ill disposed to a person. She was
impressively humble: "I don't dare give you my opinion! It's up
to God. He can overlook some mistakes, but others, He won't.

He knows the good people, who are clean. He knows the bad people. You can't trick Him. People, some people, think they can. They must find out they've failed when they die!"

I wasn't quite ready to let go of the matter: "Yes, Rita, that is when we're told a big separation takes place — heaven and hell. Have you thought about what kind of person will go to heaven, and what kind will go to hell?" She said yes, quickly — but didn't then start talking again for a few seconds. When she did, she essentially asked for more time: "I'd have to think about all this, I guess."

Much silence, to the point that I started talking: "Well, maybe we could discuss this [subject] the next time we meet."

She said yes again. But she had second thoughts. "Maybe I could say this: Allah loves people who are clean, and they pray to Him regularly, and they would follow his orders. If you forget Allah, and don't pray to Him, He'll forget you! If you're doing bad things, you'll be in the worst place, and you'll never get away, because He won't let you. No one can argue with Him!"

I argued with her a little at that point. "Well, Rita, I think some people do argue with Him. They don't follow the teachings they've learned."

"That's true. But they'll be punished."

"Which are the teachings that you think are most important?"

"All of them — that you obey God, obey Allah, all the time, that you do what He wants, all the time. "We're His servants — my uncle and my father always tell us that. You mustn't disagree [with him]. You must be clean, and speak clean, and you must say to Allah, 'I will ask you what is right to do, and good to do, and you, please, give me the answers.' "

I had watched her face and body as she talked. Her eyes were directed not at me but at the ceiling. Her hands were by her sides, both her palms were turned up, and her arms were bent slightly at the elbows — a kind of supplicating posture. Now she had stopped talking, but her mouth was slightly open. I sensed she was thinking of Allah and decided to ask her. "Are you finishing a brief prayer?"

"No, not a prayer. I was trying to remember what my grandfather used to say about Allah — about His wishes. I don't remember much. He died five years ago, so I was small then. But

I know he wanted everyone to be clean, really clean, before we prayed; and he said we should *always* be clean, and that's hard, that's impossible for us [children]. He told us that if we came to Allah clean, and we told Him He is our ruler, and we'll never fight Him, then He'll know we're loyal and we believe in Him. Sometimes people want to believe in Him, but they can't because they are captured. The devil and his angels, they have captured them. There can be wars — and Allah wins if we want Him to [win], and if we've 'earned His desire.' My mother says to us, 'You have to earn Allah's desire for you, or else the devil will win you, and Allah will say: I won't fight for her, I won't.' Why should He fight for someone who doesn't want to be one of His people, and do everything He has told us to do?"

Again I was hearing an emphasis on cleanliness and on obedience, to the point of full submission. Again I was hearing of struggles, military in nature, between Allah on the one hand and the devil and his various lieutenants on the other. I was beginning, also, to see that a rather subtle psychology was being invoked — Rita's life as potentially unworthy of such active intervention on His part. It was as if at a certain moment Allah took the measure of your life, then decided whether to enter into an alliance with you or to walk away and leave you to the devil's power. I suggested this to Rita, and she seemed glad and even relieved — I'd finally begun to comprehend what she had been trying to explain to me. Other Moslem children, I then realized, had made similar efforts.

A few minutes later, as we talked, Rita stopped to summarize. "You can't just go to heaven! Allah has to want you there; He chooses you. But He only chooses you if you've chosen Him! Do you see? [I nodded.] If you pray and He sees that you're one of His servants, and you will give your life to Him, then He'll be on your side. Then the devil and his soldiers won't take you — capture you. But if you say you're a Moslem, and you go to the mosque every once in a while, and you tell people you believe in Allah, but you're not clean, and you drink wine or other alcohol, and you eat the wrong food, and you don't mean what you say in your prayers, then you're not going to have Allah with you. The devil will spot you, and it won't be long before he gets you! Allah won't fight for you when you need Him —

unless you're on His side all the way. Do you have to be perfect? No. No one is, except Allah, I guess. But you have to be trying — to be better and better, cleaner and cleaner, so He will think: I want you, and I'll fight for you. If you surrender to Allah, He'll make sure the devil surrenders to you!" Then she sat up straight and looked me right in the eye. She had learned from hearing herself, I gathered, even as I, sitting through her struggle to give shape to her religious and spiritual assumptions, had learned a lot myself.

As I heard her talk I was reminded of a series of exchanges between my son and two children in Tunisia. Ramzes was nine, Karim thirteen — two sons of quite devout Moslem parents. The boys kept telling my son that a good person should be "polite and clean," should be "kind to people," should use "good language and not swear," should say prayers regularly and "live according to the Koran and the Prophet's words." But they also emphasized that a good person is someone who "doesn't only pray to Allah — it's someone who bows to Him, so He knows you're willing to do anything He wants you to do." They were asked whether they had given thought to what Allah, under such circumstances, would want them to do. One of them, Karim, made very clear that the issue was attitude rather than a list of avowals, rituals, or even deeds: "Allah wants us to be ready to give our lives for Him. He wants us to believe in Him; then He'll rescue us if the devil tries to capture us. You're either with Allah or you're not."

The two boys were glad to spell out the nature of the "evidence" that one is "with Allah." For instance: "A Muslim should eat carefully, chew food well, and not eat too much." But both Ramzes and Karim were quick to insist that such behavior, without a passionate and lifelong commitment to Allah, means very little. Moreover, they, too, used the word "surrender" at a particular moment in a long and quite frank discussion: "Allah wants us to really obey Him; if we pretend, then He'll see right through us — He'll know our tricks! If we surrender to Him, He'll be our protector; He'll watch out for us, and He'll win over anyone who might try to drag us away from Him, like in the middle of the night."

That phrase "in the middle of the night" got my son Bob, a

medical student, rather intrigued. They were sitting in a modest house in Gafsa, a Tunisian town known well by his college roommate, then a Peace Corps volunteer. That young man had assured my son that the town was quite safe and secure for its people, and so, hearing that comment about the night, he wondered whether the boys were referring to objective danger or the subjectivity of nightmares. He asked them to explain, and they gladly did. "When you lie down and sleep," Karim pointed out, "Allah can come to you; He can welcome you or He can warn you! If you are happy in a dream, He has told you something good; if you are upset, and you are scared, and you shout, then the devil is somewhere near, and maybe Allah is warning you, or you've found out yourself that trouble is near. Allah can save you, or you can get caught, and Allah isn't your friend, your master, so it's you against your enemy."

In response to further questions about their dreams, Ramzes stressed Allah's capacity to shape dreams. "He will send us His words; He will tell us what to do. If you wake up and you remember a dream, it could be a message from Allah. He could be telling you something. During the day, you're very busy, and so many people are talking with you. When you're asleep, no one is saying a word to you. But Allah is watching, and He could let you know something important, and you open your eyes, and you have something to think about!"

The discussion of dreams continued, and both boys made clear that they were not saying that *all* dreams were Allah's instrument of communication with us, His frail and vulnerable human servants. Still, they emphasized that Allah is not by any means impassive or unconcerned with respect to us, His worshippers, and that among His possible ways of affecting us, stopping us in our tracks, as it were, intense dreams, harrowing nightmares, are certainly to be considered, their message weighed as quite possibly crucial. Karim said, "Allah watches over us, and He's there [watching] at night, too. When you wake up and you think of Him, it's because He has visited you and told you something."

In London, among the ten Moslem children I got to know rather well, four took pains repeatedly to mention their dreams when we discussed their moments of contact with Allah. Three others mentioned Allah in connection with dreams they had, though less frequently. This response of Moslem children was in my experience quite special and surprising. The Christian and Jewish children I met brought up their dreams much less often than the Moslem boys and girls I interviewed in Israel and England or those whom my son met in Tunisia.

Toward the end of my research for this book, I started reading the transcripts of the many tape-recorded interviews I did with Moslem children, and once more I noticed the frequency of dreams — memories of them, and those memories at least partially religious and spiritual in nature — as a topic. I was reminded, then, of the education I received from a boy named Sajid in London, the thirteen-year-old son of a baker, a man originally from Pakistan. Sajid's mother was also from Pakistan, though she spoke English better and had been better educated before she left Asia for Europe. The oldest of four children, Sajid yearned to get a higher education — to become, perhaps, a lawyer or a businessman. He was interesting and morally introspective as he talked about his future: "I'd like to become successful, so we could move from here. I'd have the money to buy a nice home for myself and another one for my parents! I'd have the money for clothes and the best of food. But I'd have to be careful; I'd have to give half of my money to charity (maybe less than half, but a big amount). If I didn't, I'd never get Allah's permission to come and live in heaven. I'd be sent to a big fire, an oven with a fire that never stops — to hell. Either you give to the poor, to your neighbor, or you risk lots of trouble when you die.

"Even before you die — I know. Last week I was in school and I had figured out the answer to an arithmetic problem, and I was really glad. The teacher told me I could be excused for soccer, because I was doing the best work in class. Later, after soccer, a couple of my friends came to me, and told me they were having trouble with their homework, and would I help them? I said no, they should learn themselves, without help. They said I was being selfish. I thought I was trying to be truthful. I thought maybe they'd do better and better, and I wouldn't be the only one being excused for soccer. Then they'd be better at soccer, too. But maybe I *was* selfish! I told my father, and he

said I should still try to be very good in school, in all that I do;
but I should help my friends, too. You should be generous; you
should give help to others.

"The next day I offered to help my friends. They were glad.
They did better in the class. They thanked me. But that night
I had a dream, and they weren't thanking me! The teacher was
telling me that I wasn't going to heaven — Allah wasn't going
to let me in. A man walking down the street told me I should
read the Koran and remember what the prophet Mohammed
said: I should give to people who need me to give. Then a fire
truck came by, and a siren was going, and the red lights were
going around and around. The fire truck stopped beside me,
and a fireman came out, and he told me I had to go with them,
on the truck, because where I lived, there was a fire. I didn't
want to go on the truck. I was scared. The police came, and a
bobby pulled me to the truck, and the firemen picked me up,
and the truck started going fast, real fast. I was afraid the truck
would crash. When we came to the street where we live, I saw
the fire, and it was in our house and the house next door. My
father was standing on the street, outside our building, and he
was calling my name, but I wasn't there. I was in the truck, and
we didn't get near my father, because the street was blocked with
lots of cars and fire trucks and police wagons. I wanted to get
to my father, but I couldn't, and the fire kept going, and our
truck was hot — the fire was heating up the whole street! That's
when I woke up, and I was hot, and I thought of Allah. I wondered if I'd ever get to see Him: you have to be very good, or
He'll not have you in His house, in heaven!"

I've pulled together this account of his dream from a somewhat
more rambling presentation by Sajid, which was interrupted by
talk of long division, soccer teams, the differences between life
in London and life in the countryside, and a long aside on Margaret Thatcher, whom this boy and many of his friends did not
especially admire. When he asked me if I had dreams like the
one he'd related to me, I told him no, not like that one. His
immediate response: "I guess because you're not a Moslem." Not
knowing how to reply, I said nothing. He thereupon asked me
whether I "understood" his dream. I told him that dreams have
no one meaning — that it is up to us who dream to figure out

what we're trying to "say" in the middle of the night, though someone else, listening, can sometimes help us with a suggestion or two. Sajid by then, correctly, had surmised that I was not readily going to be of help. He gave me his own interpretation: "I think Allah was sending me a warning that I'm in trouble." I asked him why. He did not answer. He looked down at the floor. He looked over at a pile of Lego pieces which one of my sons, Mike, had given to him and his brother. When he talked, finally, the weather was the topic: six days of rain, going on a week of it. He remembered that he'd been to a soccer game eight or nine days ago, and that was the last sunny afternoon London had seen. I felt reluctant to try to steer us back to that dream. Sajid had said all he wanted to say, and the more I considered what he did say, the more I admired his terse analysis of what must have been a rather disturbing nightmare.

Though we never discussed that particular dream again, Sajid did make reference to dreams in general several weeks later when he and I talked about his future life. He was, again, mentioning the life of a barrister, a solicitor (I asked him the difference, and he wasn't sure he knew); he was also thinking about his future life as a Moslem: "I hope I'll be respected by everyone. I hope I'll be the Imam, and give a sermon [in the mosque]. He's someone we look up to. I hope I have a good family, and we all are welcome by Allah when the time comes [for them to die]. And I hope I have no bad dreams!"

I asked, "What do you mean by bad dreams?"

He answered, "Dreams are bad when Allah doesn't want you. He scares you. If He likes you, He won't scare you."

"Has Allah ever scared you?"

"Yes. He warns you. If you're not remembering Him, that's when He can come at night and scare you!"

"Does that happen often?"

"Not to me, so far! I try to obey Him. I try to do everything I should! The Imam told me: if you surrender to Allah, He'll let you sleep and have good dreams; if you don't, you could have a long dream with animals biting you, or some bad accident happens [in the dream], and it's because Allah is not satisfied that you are a good Moslem!"

Sajid was proposing dreams as a measure of one's religious

purity or devotion. In a sense, he was declaring his nightmare to be an instrument of divine direction. A pleasant dream life, he believed, serves as testimony of one's surrender to Islam's principles, duly noted by Allah Himself. Allah is ever demanding and watchful; those who would earn His favor must endure scrutiny at midnight as well as high noon. Sajid and other children of Islam who have talked to me about their dreams do not push the matter too far, do not turn Allah into a "hound of heaven," so to speak, constantly pursuing the Moslem child through dreams. Rather, the point is the child's notion of optimal submission — a surrender under the moon as well as the sun. Sajid's dream told him — reared as he was in a neighborhood utterly unselfconscious psychologically — that Allah's demands are unyielding, are round-the-clock in nature, are as emotionally insistent as they are cognitively detailed. A boy who has learned to abstain from pork, who has learned the fasts of the month Ramadan, who has learned that "Mecca is God's House," that "a Moslem should have a destination when he leaves the house," who always prefaces a meal with "in the name of Allah," and who always ends a meal with "thanks Allah," is also a boy who wakes up with the conviction that Allah has had reason to visit him, upbraid him, or give notice to him about life's eventual outcome.

This nocturnal and unwitting intimacy with God is evidence of a surrender that surpasses the kind put into wordy avowals or even into complex rituals. No wonder one weekend morning Sajid said that he felt "closest" to Allah when he first opened his eyes: "I wake up and I feel Allah has been near me, very near. I almost want to go back to sleep so I can be nearer Him again. But I must not be greedy! Father tells us we should give to others; we should share what we have. The same with Allah: I can't have His attention when there are others who need it too! Once I'm out of bed, I'm doing all my obligations, and Allah is visiting the others who sleep!" This boy once asked his parents whether "heaven is like sleep," and when asked what he meant, explained himself in this way: "You're always with Allah when you're asleep. You've left your life and He's got you in His arms for the hours you're in bed!"

Such a nighttime surrender to Allah's arms, a much sought

and embraced captivity, was not Sajid's alone, as he several times let me know — out of a genuine modesty, but also out of an impressive regard for what he viewed as the truth. On one of our last visits together, for instance, his tendency to be a stickler for what he called "accuracy" became apparent as we talked about his friends in school and the neighborhood and as we discussed what he perceived to be their sense of what Allah wanted from children: "I talk with my cousins, and at school I have three good friends. We try to remember to say our prayers, and we explain to the Christians [some school classmates] what we're doing. They want to know about our religion and we want to know about theirs! I've heard my friends talk about Allah, how they will wake up like me — they're sure He's touched them in the night! They told them [the English, Christian children] that, and they laughed. 'What do you mean, God touched you?' My friend said, 'He just came and made me think of Him, even if I was asleep.' Me too, that's what I said!

"If you pray to Allah, He'll answer you. When I hear the muezzin calling us to prayer, I hear Allah saying He'd like us to come and be with Him. That's what my father tells us all: we go to the mosque so we can have a good close time with Allah; otherwise, we'll be saying our prayers, but not together. When we're all together, and we're all bent on our knees, praying, He knows we are calling to Him, just like the muezzin [is calling], and He is happy. I don't know Christians [the children at his school] well enough to ask them if they think their God keeps His eyes on them like ours does. I should ask them one day! My friends say the [various] religions are different, so you can't be sure what other religions are like, and you should just try hard to do the best you can as a Moslem."

He and his friends had been doing just that, I began to realize. I remember the energy they showed as they prayed, visited the mosque on Friday and Saturday, made an effort to remember rules, rituals, an array of admonitions handed down from generation to generation. I remember, also, what they told me about Allah, about Mohammed, about Mecca, about their own lives as Moslems living in a predominantly Christian England — a collective testimony to their attempts to become members of Islam's worldwide spiritual nation. Once, talking with Sajid about his future as a student, a worker, I hoped to get away from religious matters, for a while at least, but in the course of the long discussion he kept bringing me back to a central point: "I'd like to stay here [in England] — sometimes; other times, I'd like to go to Pakistan. But all the time, I hope I can be the best person Allah would want."

He said that in response to a question about a rather secular interest of mine: "Sajid, which country offers you the best chances for your life?" I knew *my* answer, of course, and I was fairly sure that I knew *his* answer as well: England. But he wasn't going to let me run so confidently down a field of my own making. First he told me, "England is not Pakistan." He explained the obvious: "Here there is a rich country, with good houses and lots of food, and you can make money that only a rich person can make back in Pakistan. You live longer here; you don't get the diseases you could catch back there. It would be foolish to say that I want to go back there with all my heart." A stop in the flow of his speech, and then a poignant resumption: "But part of my heart — yes, I'd like to go back, even if I'd be poorer, and I might die young, very young. You know why? I think Allah must prefer Pakistan to England! There are so many of us [Moslems] there, and here we try to be pleasing to Him, but we are fewer here, and He must notice that. I hope when I make my choice, I'll be thinking of Him, not just me!"

The moralist in me — responding to my own life, needless to say — could only compare that idealism to the crasser materialism some of us somehow reconcile with our religious practices, our intellectual convictions. The research doctor in me kept hearing in my mind the word "pleasing," and wanted to ask this articulate, strong-minded boy to explain what he thought was "pleasing" to Allah, to the God of his Islamic people. "Sajid, please tell me what you think Allah finds 'pleasing.' You just said you and others here in England are trying to be 'pleasing' to Allah, and I was interested in how you do that."

"Well, I've been telling you [all along]." His silence seemed to put an end to that proposed journey. But a look of mild impatience on his part yielded to one of a teacher's forgiving goodwill: "If you want to please Allah, you have to think of Him a lot! Here, in this country, there's much more to think about [than Him], and that's a big difference from Pakistan. My grand-father, his grandfather, they thought of Allah all the time; and Mohammed, His messenger, and what He told us. They lived by Mohammed and the Koran, and they prayed and prayed, and their life, all of it, was a preparation for meeting Allah and Mohammed and the angels, you know, that are in heaven with [the two of] them. My father has told me that a hundred times, a thousand times! Then he points to himself with his finger and to me. 'Look at us,' he says. I know the speech by heart! 'Look at us,' he says, and he says it until he's sure I'm looking at him and at myself, and he's sure of what I see: 'Bellies full of good food, a nice warm apartment with a roof that doesn't leak, the doctors in that [National Health Service] clinic. But where is Allah, *where*?' Father answers the question after asking it! 'Allah is someone we think about, if we're lucky, on the bus coming home.'

"It can't be pleasing to Him, to Allah, that we don't think of Him the way they used to, back in Pakistan. Mohammed must be disappointed in us. Father is sure He is, and so is Allah! That is too bad for us, and it's too bad for them, yes, because Mohammed tried to tell us what to do, what to believe, and Allah wants all of us to remember Mohammed's words, and if we're here, we don't have the time, that's the problem, and I'm sure Allah isn't pleased — that we don't have the time for Him we'd have if we lived someplace else: back home in Pakistan, and other places where they do have the time."

With that comparison he stopped and looked toward the window. Suddenly I heard noises outside I'd not heard before, intent as I was on hearing him speak: the buses his father mentioned to him, the cars, London's urban din. I noticed that the boy, too, was listening to the world outside, even as he had just, in his own way, invoked its powerful, hovering presence in the life of his immediate family. We smiled at each other — a moment of mutual recognition: we both heard the same noise, and, more important, we both could connect what we heard outside to what we both had heard in that room.

The silence continued, and neither of us seemed about to break it. I glanced at my watch, felt reassured: plenty of time. Sajid looked at his hands, scratched his left forearm with his right fingers, then examined them. He must have seen some dirt under one of the fingernails, because he worked hard to get it out with the fingernails of his other hand. I decided the next move was mine, but I had no idea what I would ask or say until I half listened to myself speaking: "Do you think, maybe, Sajid, that your God might well understand the differences between the life of your ancestors in Pakistan, in Asia, and the life of people here in England — and so, not be too upset if you practice your religion differently?"

He understood in a flash exactly what I meant. Such words were themselves part of the Western, big-city clatter — so I realized only when I saw his face, with the faintest beginning of a smile and his large black eyes taking everything in, me and my earnest manner, me and my carefully qualified suggestions, masked as casual questions. He took his time before replying. He moved around the room with his eyes, as if to remind himself that much there once belonged elsewhere (clothes, some luggage, a small rug), proof that worlds can merge as well as forever clash. Finally he handed down his judgment: "I don't know. It's up to Allah. Maybe — you could be right. But He would be losing us, wouldn't He, if He let us get too comfortable in London. I don't think He'd want to do that; I think He wants to hold on to us: He wants us to be with Him, not just think of Him every once in a while. I think that He's like that — that He won't be happy if we walk away and don't give Him much attention. He wants our attention — so He can know us before He has to decide about us when we die."

He spoke quietly, not insistently, not "defensively." He wanted to let me know out of the depths of his being, his soul, how and what he very much felt. His concluding sentence was very affecting indeed — a reminder that some people on this earth still await with great apprehension and desire the final decision that God will be making with respect to them. It is this conviction — God's ultimate hold on them over the span of eternity — that inspires a boy like Sajid to prepare himself for such judgment and to resist the reassurances people like me so good-naturedly offer. Allah is in His heaven, biding His time for only so long.

I had encountered the persistent, unyielding faith of a child who regards his God to be a necessary, compelling guardian and guide, a "ruler." A ruler exerts authority — and certainly Allah must, Allah does, as Moslem children have told me many times, in many ways.[2] For them, Allah the ruler and His messenger Mohammed (who is no weak-kneed, spineless emissary) are both here as well as in heaven. Sajid wondered not only about his future but about that of all Islam: "I hope Allah doesn't let go of us; He could, if we let go of Him." True, he had heard a remark like that from his father's closest friend as they left the mosque a few months earlier. But now the boy speaking was a boy contemplating a distinct (and dreaded) possibility. I concentrated on the words "let go" — as in "let my people go," the American slave's archetypal outcry, the clarion call, too, of blacks in the American South of the 1960s as they struggled for their freedom. Here, in contrast, was a boy worrying that he and others might well be "let go," with disastrous consequences, for eternity. This boy wanted to be tied firmly to his Master, as He is revealed in mosques and in homes, in nearby streets and distant pilgrimages — to experience the Islamic surrender one offers to Him whose verdict is believed to matter more than anything else.

11

Jewish Righteousness

ON HER TENTH BIRTHDAY, I heard Elaine, of Orthodox Jewish background, ask her older brother, Joseph, whether he really intended to go through with his bar mitzvah. (I was sitting with the two of them in their home in Brookline, Massachusetts.) Joseph thought she was being playful with him. Of course he would take part in his bar mitzvah, he told Elaine — such a "foolish question." But Elaine was not kidding around; she was dead serious: "They keep us [girls] separate in shul, and [in our religion] it's the boys who really count." She soon apologized for her remark — she told him she was sorry for not being "respectful." It was a word her father had urged on her for years.

Joseph was inclined to agree with Elaine, and told her so: "I didn't make the rules!" But he went no further, though he knew Elaine wanted him to take a stand of his own. As he sat in silence, occasionally moving his thumb up and down his forefinger, Elaine stared at him steadfastly, even fiercely, a frown on her face. Her look was intended to put him on the spot. He knew that; not once did he let his eyes meet hers. Finally he said more: "Hey, I'll say it again: I didn't make the rules! Anyway, just because we live in America, and its 1986, doesn't mean we have to forget our history. If you're Jewish, you're Jewish, and the rules are the rules; they go way back."

Elaine let up a bit on her scowl, but she kept her eyes intently on him, and he could feel them even though he didn't acknowledge them with a return glance. Indeed, he looked away toward the window, as if hoping that the impasse would end. But Elaine seemed relentless in her determination to keep both of them locked in their tense morning confrontation. Finally Joseph shrugged his shoulders and began to rise from his chair, having given me a look of abject hopelessness. He spoke as he rose: "Elaine, you're right, but I can't do anything that will change things."

Those were fighting words. Elaine rose from her chair and walked toward the door, as if she meant to prevent both of us males from making an easy exit. Then she gave Joseph a piece of her mind: "I know, you are not a rabbi, and you are not even bar mitzvahed yet! But if you were a rabbi, you'd be saying the same thing; and when you *have* been bar mitzvahed you'll say the same thing!"

Joseph dropped his head as he stood accused. He gave me a look, but I was of no help. I wanted to intervene. I wanted to say to Elaine that she was right, and to Joseph that at twelve he was also right not to consider himself a major religious authority — though his sister wanted from him only a bit of moral passion. But how was I to share such an interpretation at that electric moment? Elaine suddenly shifted to a higher gear: "Joseph, you have to make a speech when you're bar mitzvahed, and that's when you could tell everyone what you think — you, Joseph, my brother, not you, the boy who will say whatever they want."

Joseph had been listening carefully, with no apparent response on his face, until he heard the word "they," and then he stiffened. "Who is 'they,' Elaine? Not our parents! You are their daughter, and I am their son, and they wouldn't argue with you, would they? They'd say, 'Yes, Elaine.' I've heard them say yes, when you say this is wrong, and this is wrong, and this is wrong. But what can they do? I mean, Mother and Dad. Are they the ones you meant? Dad is only a lawyer, Mom teaches in a school. What do you want them to do?"

He had straightened out and obviously felt stronger. Elaine looked at him with more warmth now. It was as if their parents had actually entered the room, brought them together. Elaine became tender; her smile broadened; she glowed as she moved a step toward Joseph and said, simply and affectingly, "Oh, Joseph!"

Their mother had told them that Judaism was many things — a traditional religion, but also one that encouraged its adherents to break new ground, speak up when injustice cloaked itself in the conventional.[1] Their mother had also emphasized the prophetic side of Judaism, the voices of Jeremiah and Isaiah and Amos with their righteous determination to stand outside the city gates and condemn those whose privileges were obtained at a cost to many others. The two children seemed ready to bury the hatchet, meet on the common ground of Jewish righteousness. Joseph signaled a rapprochement: "I'll try to say something [upon his bar mitzvah], I will! I don't want to get people upset. Grandpa has a bad heart. He could hear me and get an attack! What if I came out swinging, and he turned real pale, and he got sick right before my eyes? I'd feel terrible. So would you!"

Elaine interrupted: "Yes, I would; I would." I thought she would have a more extended agreement to offer, but she stopped there.

Joseph resumed: "Grandpa used to tell us that you have to be loyal to our people. Maybe they made mistakes a long time ago. Maybe they treated women one way and men the other. I agree with you, Elaine: we should all sit together! But when we go to *shul*, we are returning to our people, that's what Grandpa says, 'returning to all of our ancestors.' In [Hebrew] school, they say the same thing — we must obey our ancestors; otherwise they're forgotten!"

He was not totally convinced, despite the conviction in his voice, and abruptly took another tack. "But our prophets were right — we should shake our fists, plenty of times we should. Our rabbi told us once to 'learn how to shake your fists.' I didn't know what he meant, at first. Weird, I thought!" He was talking to me, mostly. Elaine smiled; she had heard the story before. Joseph continued: "When should we shake our fists? At who[m]? That's what we wanted to know. The rabbi kept repeating, 'Learn to shake your fists.' Like a broken record, I thought! What's his problem? Then he asked *us* what we wanted *him* to explain. He asked us when we should shake our fists. No one answered, so he did. I remember him talking — he told us that to be a Jew is to be fair and honest, and to think of others, not just yourself. To be a Jew is to side with all the people who are in trouble. Jews have had a lot of trouble, and Jews will try to help others in trouble. That's what he said."

It wasn't a new message, Joseph went on to remind me. Here his sister joined in and told me of their parents' concern for the world's hungry, the poor and hurt people the world over, who ought to be constantly on the minds of "all of us," meaning her fellow Jews — the spirit of Passover handed across the generations. Elaine was forthright and vigorous in her presentation, and in case there was any doubt, her brother added examples, repeated her assertions. As I listened I had to remind myself that these were two *children*, he still twelve, she ten. They spoke as if their parents and their rabbi had been personally tutored by Moses himself. ("Love the stranger as you would yourself, for you too were strangers in the land of Egypt.")

I had by then talked with many Jewish children. Not all of them approached this level of righteous reflection. Elaine and Joseph were an especially inward pair of children. Yet their desire to live intimately, even now, with the past of their people, and their interest in the fate of others less lucky than they, were qualities of mind and heart other Jewish children exhibited in various ways. As Joseph once reminded me, "We are the people who gave the world the Ten Commandments, and we must never forget that, and we must always remember them." He had memorized those words in Hebrew school, but he smiled with pride as he spoke, obviously happy to assume that continuing responsibility.

Joseph reflected at some length on "my Judaism," as he called it. "I was told I was a Jew when I was very small. I don't know how old I was, no. [I had asked.] I think it's the first memory I have: My father is sitting at the kitchen table. He is wearing his yarmulke. He is talking to me. I think I have done something wrong. I had kicked our dog. I don't remember doing it but my mom and dad tell me that's what had happened. That's why Dad sat me down and gave his 'big lecture.' Even now, he'll take us to his study sometimes, one by one, and give us one of his 'big lectures.' I used to dread them, but now I like them. That first one — I can hear the words right this minute: 'Joseph, you cannot hurt others, and that includes our dog. We are Jews, and we know what it means to be kicked by others. We try to help others, not hurt them.' Then he kept repeating, 'Help, not hurt.' It's those words that I keep hearing. When? All the time! I'll get angry, and I just want to say something bad to someone, and Dad's voice comes to me, those words! Yes, I forget them sometimes. But a lot of times I'll think: 'Joe, you're a Jew, and that means you don't kick your neighbor, you treat your neighbor the way you'd want to be treated.' That's Dad talking, and it's what a good Jew should be saying every day to himself."

When he'd finished that disquisition — I've omitted my questions and some of his responses to them — he gave me a lecture on the *mitzvah*, the good deed every Jew should strive to do today and tomorrow, a lifelong obligation. "It doesn't have to be something big. It's best that you do it quietly — not in a braggy way! Dad always says that: 'No bragging.' Mom says, 'A *mitzvah* should be between you and God.' Sometimes I wish I could forget her saying that! I want to tell her what I've done — some good deed, my *mitzvah* — but I don't. She'd be happy — she wouldn't lecture me, no. But I lecture myself."

Joseph used the word "lecture" often and with ease. "You see, we have 'the book,' our Bible; it tells us what we should believe, and it tells us how to live. 'I don't want empty knowledge,' Dad always says. His grandfather was a rabbi, and he told Dad, 'A Jew is someone who lives the law.' Dad once told me, 'Don't memorize — remember what you've done that's good, and keep doing it!' But I have to memorize, too. I told him, and he said, 'Sure,' but he was just trying to make a point. He's a lawyer, you know! He lectures in his [law school] course, and he lectures us! His grandpa used to sit him on his knees and tell him about 'the rules' and 'the law' — the Torah and the Talmud. I don't know all of it; Dad says he doesn't — but Dad says it all comes down to being 'a Jew in the eyes of God,' and that means to be a good person during the day, every day — most of the time (you can't be perfect)!"

His parenthetical comment, the stuff of everyday pietistic conversation, was stated with earnest stress — rescued in that way from staleness. Joseph, at twelve, already knew that "excuses are no good," that even if one cannot attain an ideal, it has to be retained as a demanding force in one's life. This boy's perfectionism was very much alive, yet tempered by an earthy psychology. "Excuses are no good," he repeated, and then he added, "But without excuses we'd be lost — we'd have nothing to remember for the next time."

I associate such observations with Jewishness because I have heard comments like them so often from Jewish children. Not that other children, not Jewish, don't hear their parents say similar things. But Joseph had an ear for such remarks, remembered them, and evoked them for others — a religious *and* cultural inheritance embraced and rendered. When a boy of twelve has taken Isaiah to heart, encouraged by his parents and his Hebrew school teachers, and a girl of ten has been taught the story of the Covenant and that of the prophets, with their remarkable urge for spiritual confrontation, an observer need feel no great astonishment at the following exchange.

"Maybe," Joseph said, "you should be glad you're not near us in *shul*; maybe you should celebrate your seats upstairs!"

"Don't be so 'clever,' Joseph," Elaine said.

"I'm not being 'clever'!"

"Well, what do you mean, then?"

"I mean: you and our Isaiah! He'd be *outside* the *shul*, telling us everything we will forget otherwise!"

"You *are* clever! I like it that Isaiah will tell you off! Do you think he'll be there at the bar mitzvah? I hope so!"

"He'll be there! He'll have to be there, because I think Daddy prays to him — not prays, but he mentions Isaiah as much as anyone alive, and more than anyone but God! So Isaiah must hear, and he'll show up!"

"Don't talk like that, Joseph!"

"Why not?"

"You should pray to Isaiah for advice on what to write [for his bar mitzvah speech]."

"No, only to God."

"I guess He hears everything, so He'll decide if you're being a wise guy or not!"

"He will. He'll look at my record!"

"Well, if He misses anything, I'll be sure and tell Him!"

"Stop talking like that!"

"You do all the time!"

"I guess I do. We should leave this subject!"

"I agree."

The notion of God as a moral guide, and — just as important — a demanding judge, is shared by many Jewish children. In Brookline, Massachusetts, I sat with two boys and two girls, each of the boys just eleven, one of the girls eleven and the other twelve. Tony and Al, the boys, were of Reform Jewish background, as was Ilona, the younger girl; Tamar's parents were Jews of the Conservative religious tradition. It was the summer of 1987. I had known these youngsters three years. They had drawn pictures for me to illustrate various Biblical stories, and as younger children they had let me know through those pictures how they connected Jewish religious ideals to their daily lives. Now, a bit older, we all talked about the same matter — in Ilona's words, about "what it means to be a Jew and be living right now, not back then [in the days of the Biblical chronicles]." Ilona mentioned her own struggles: "My dad does a lot of flying; he is a lawyer, and he goes all over the world. He's taken me on trips, and on the plane he points out the cities and the rivers and the farms and the mountains. When you go on a plane, you're nearer to God — because you can see the world, a lot of it, more than you see when you're on land, and you can realize how big the whole universe is, and people, they're not even visible. The cars are moving, and you know that people are in them, driving, but you can't see them.

"That's why you have to stop yourself (once in a while, at least) and say: Are you remembering God, and are you looking at the big picture, the way He does, or are you inside a car, and all you're thinking of is where you want to go, right away (and watch out, anyone else!)? If you do stop yourself, you have to think of what God told us, through Moses, and later, through His wise men, Jeremiah, those people: to be better than you might want to be sometimes, because it's the big picture that counts, and if you forget that, you get lost in going from one place to another, because you don't think of what you should be doing for God, what He's seeing and He's wanting."

She had been struggling with an image, a metaphor, wrenched

out of her father's flying life — struggling to connect the upsurge of moral and philosophical contemplation she experienced with him on airplanes to the everyday life she usually immersed herself in. The others grew impatient with her. "Ilona, you can't look at life as if you're on an airplane all the time, and it [life] is 'down there,' someplace!" said her friend Tamar.

Ilona was unhappy and hurt: "What do you mean, you *can't?*"

Tamar hesitated in the face of Ilona's question and its insistence, by implication, on an alternative moral or religious stand. I noticed Tamar looking at some food I'd brought along, candy and fruit and soft drinks: why not just eat and relax, rather than get into all this "heavy talk"? But the attention Tamar gave to the food and drink (she took an apple and poured herself a Pepsi) was only a prelude to her own plunge into our discussion — as if she had said to herself and us: all right, I'll fuel myself up and get going. She did get going, with a brief but trenchant remark: "If you pull back too much from life, then you're not in it, and that's not living, it's watching other people live."

After a second or two of silence, Tony tried to mediate: "Well, you can do both. You can keep doing what you've got to do — school and sports and vacations and more school! — but you can try to stay out of the rat race just a little, and when you do, when you stop and think, that's the way you stop yourself from being a 'total programmed animal.' My dad says you can become that if you don't watch out. You just take your orders from everyone else, and you do what they're doing, and you're not you anymore — you're what everyone wants you to be. So you do have to stop yourself, every once in a while, and that's what God said to the Jewish people, to us, that we shouldn't just be like everyone else, caught in a rat race. We should be different; we should think of Him. We should ask ourselves what's the right way to live, and we should try to live it, and we should pray to Him, to get His help, or else we'll settle for the rat race."

The children had now been invited to abandon air flights and consider another metaphor, that of conditioned rats scurrying down mazes, and they did so eagerly. Al spoke up, only to undercut all that had preceded him: "I wonder if we should be talking this way! My mom says a good Jew doesn't climb up a

ladder and shout to the world that he's a good Jew! If you're
really going to be a good guy, then you'll remember what you've
learned from your folks and in Hebrew school and the synagogue. You'll try to do your 'good deed for the day.' That's
what my mom says — try once each day to help someone. But
I can't believe God is out there counting! He doesn't want us to
count, either. You just *do!* The more you talk — you can talk all
day and all night — the less time there will be for doing!"

"Doing *what?*"

Ilona fired off that question with heavy emphasis on the second
word. Tony nodded. He opened his mouth but quickly closed
it, as if he realized that any additional comment would weaken
rather than build up Ilona's bold case. Tamar, looking at Ilona,
seemed at least partially persuaded. Her face displayed a hint
of a smile, which was then replaced by a frown. She abruptly
rose, went to the table, took another Diet Pepsi, and brought it
back to her chair. She placed it near one of the chair's legs
without taking even a sip. Al watched her closely. I thought he'd
follow her lead, and his body for a second began to show signs
of impending activity. He uncrossed his legs and began to lift
himself upward, his eyes holding on to the nearby table with its
food and drink — but all at once he let himself slump backward,
and his eyes now returned to his friends, moved from one to
the other, and settled upon his adversary, Ilona, whom he addressed with a question of his own: "What do you think we all
should do?"

He had responded to Ilona in a cleverly suggestive manner
worthy of an experienced philosophical discussant. She sensed
the task his question presented to her, and remained silent.
She looked away; her eyes settled on a door across the room,
the door to a closet. (A lengthening silence awakened self-
consciousness in all of us. I felt an urge to intervene with some
statement that would keep us talking. But what to say? Nothing
fitting came to mind; what *did* come to mind was the thought
that I should leave the young people alone, not patronize them
with a prodding comment.) The children continued to be silent
until Ilona broke the impasse with a question directed at me:
"What do you think?"

I prepared to provide a summary of what Ilona and Tony had

proposed and the opposed reasoning that Tamar and Al had offered, but for some reason I said nothing.

Ilona's response to my lack of response was a mix of the apologetic and the argumentative: "I'm sorry — but it's not fair. You're supposed to be asking us! I'll say what I think: I think a lot of the time we all waste our time doing things we don't enjoy — following orders. I know — I know you'll all say that you've got to follow orders, that there are a lot of things you've just got to do, whether you like it or not, and that's that. 'C'est la vie,' my older sister says. But you don't have to become a *slave!* You can stand up to life! That's what our rabbi told us last week, and I told myself ten times since then: 'Hey, Ilona, stand up to life!' "

"What did he mean? What do you mean?" Tamar had no sooner asked her question than she answered it herself: "There's so much you just have to get through. If you started talking like that in school, the teachers would let you know what they think — wow, would they! They'd say what my parents say when I want to take it easy and they want me to do my chores: 'You have to pitch in and help! This is a family! We all have our jobs to do!' It's the same way when you leave the house — plenty of jobs to do! Sure, if you've got a lot of money, a lot, you can take your time — or you can just loaf, I guess. But most people don't have that option. My dad will tell us, 'Choose your options very carefully, because there aren't that many in life.' " She paused momentarily and resumed with a rhetorical question: "Isn't that right?" No one disagreed; she kept right on: "I wish I could just swim in our neighbor's pool in the summer, and ski in the winter, and then I'd watch TV and eat my favorite foods, spaghetti and ice cream, chocolate chip. That would be great. But I can't, so I do my errands and study."

She seemed ready to tell us more about her responsibilities, but an exasperated Tony interrupted her: "Hey, Tamar, what's your point? What are you telling us — what's new?"

She started to reply, but he wouldn't let her, as they glared at each other like open antagonists, and Tony said: "Hey, everyone's got 'stuff' to do! I hear that all the time: Tony, do your stuff; Tony, you've got stuff to do. Even the maid tells me that! My mother is out there working, and she pays this woman to look after the house and keep her eye on us, and she's telling us about this 'list' our mother gave her — the 'stuff' we've got to 'do'! But that's not the whole story. It's not! I've got time to stop thinking about me, me, me, and try and give someone else a hand — even that maid!"

He was going to make a more elaborate presentation, but he'd surprised himself with that last observation. He stopped and smiled. The others recognized the irony and smiled with him. The tension in the room receded. The children began to unite on the interesting question of their parents' obligations and responsibilities. Tony had managed masterfully to defend the cause of a considered altruism in such a way that the doubters, Tamar and Al, were now amused by the thought of his abandoning his own egoism to lend a hand to a maid whom his idealistic mother employed to keep an eye on the house and its three young occupants, so that she, in turn, could run an ambitious Jewish philanthropic effort.

Rather unexpectedly a war between the generations then began to unfold. The righteousness disputed by four children among themselves turned into a mutual righteousness aimed at — well, "them," the senior authorities on the subject of righteousness. Tamar and Ilona mentioned a rabbi they knew — mentioned his sermons, so urgent in moral intensity, as against the stories they had heard about his personal life. I thought of Salinger's Holden Caulfield when Ilona and Tamar arraigned *their* "phonies" and Tony and Al turned to *theirs*. I was a bit taken aback by the use of the word "phonies" until I realized, as the children talked, that their parents' righteousness, enlisted in the service of moral indignation, had a special vocabulary that these children knew quite well and could use with both delight and vehemence.

Al, for instance, said, "My dad is easygoing most of the time, but sometimes he explodes. He doesn't have a good word for too many people when he's upset. I remember him telling us at breakfast a few weeks ago that the world is full of 'frauds and hypocrites and two-bit phonies'; and then he said God is perfect, but us [human beings], we're not perfect, that's for sure, and a lot of us are 'no-goodniks.' But lots of times he'll say, 'Al, you can weigh in there on the side of good!' That's his slogan. That's what he believes — you try to do good when you can. God put us here to do good."

Al's statement enlisted the enthusiastic support of all four children. Ilona hastened to say that "God wants us to do all we can to make the world just a little better while we're here." Tamar nodded, saying, "That's it, that's what He wants." Tony made more explicit the Jewish imperative: "If you're a Jew, you're here to do God's work. My parents tell me a Jew is someone God has chosen to send here to represent Him and try to improve His world. If you do good things, the world gets better — even if it's only a little better — and that's what God is wishing for, I think."

That last, two-word afterthought was not meant to be an expression of religious doubt so much as a touch of humility: an acknowledgment in a modest, unaffected way of the limitations of our knowledge about the Lord's purposes. In years of work with Jewish children I have encountered such moments over and over again, to the point that I feel it makes up an aspect of the righteousness those children keep espousing, describing, urging upon one another. At its best, this is a righteousness that avoids the fatal deterioration of self-righteousness precisely because it is not accompanied by a professed certainty: I know exactly what the Lord wants, and why He wants it, and anyone in my sight or within the sound of my voice had better take heed. On the contrary, as these four children kept reminding us all, "God doesn't let on all His plans, but He'd like us to show we trust Him, and the best way to do it is by doing some good while we're here."

That comment of Ilona's came a half-hour after Tony's "I think" had sent a handful of children down the road of acknowledged uncertainty as an aspect of religious passion. I was impressed by the energy these young people displayed. Taking God's secrets for granted and even upholding His secrecy as a defining quality of Jewish righteousness, they talked about doing good deeds gladly and without sure knowledge of what the Lord has in store for them or for the world. Indeed, Ilona's words bring to mind the Biblical figures of Abraham and Isaac as embodiments of the struggle to know a God who will not be known, even as He exerts such power in the lives of those who seek to do His will.

When Ilona spoke of God's "plans," Tamar promptly reminded her that some of His plans *are* known: "It's true, we don't know all He's planning, but He did tell the Jews a long time ago what He thought was most important. He gave us the Commandments. He was letting us know His plans that way. Our rabbi says God chose the Jews to be the ones He'd talk with, and He did, He talked with them [in the Bible], and after a while they knew what He was thinking. Maybe they didn't know *all* He was thinking. I agree, there's probably a lot He's been thinking that we don't know — a whole lot! But He did give us plenty to think about — and you know, He could have decided that there's no point in overdoing something, and it's best to start with what's the most important things, and see if they [the Jewish people] can handle that, and then if they can, He could always tell us more, or He could find another Moses, and give him some new commandments for us. But first let's show Him that we can follow the ones He's already given us, and we haven't gotten an all-A record, so why should He give us new homework when there's the old homework to do and it's not finished!"

With that speculation she had thrown a new log on the fire. At what point in history, if ever, will the Jews (or any other people) prove themselves worthy of receiving additional revelations from God? There, in that room, two boys and two girls, Jewish and American and alive today, unselfconsciously wondered aloud about God's ultimate relationship to them. "He'll be coming," Tony said — but not in an evangelical tone, and not with a messianic fervor. The natural, matter-of-fact assertion made an impression on the others; they followed suit. "I guess so," said Tamar. But Ilona shrewdly asked, "Why, *why*, should He bother with us any more than He already has? He's given us enough guidance! It's our fault if we still have troubles!"

Then came another of our long pauses, but during this one both of the previous coalitions became sundered. Tony soon took issue with Ilona: "Everyone's to blame, sure — but you could include God, too: He's the one who made us!" Ilona was surprised both by the argument itself and by Tony's defection: "All right, Tony, I agree; but you can't blame God [for the world's evil]. That's terrible! What do you think the rabbi would say?"

"I don't know," Tony answered. That seemed to be that. He looked down toward his sneakers, leaned over, untied the loosened knot of one of the shoelaces, made a new and very tight knot, and then sat up and looked toward the window. No one had spoken, and I noticed Ilona stirring — ready, I thought, to say something. But Tony looked back at his friends and addressed them rather poignantly, his voice raised to a pitch higher than usual: "I know what the rabbi *should* say; he should say that we're all in this together, and that God isn't out to blame us and make us feel bad, and we shouldn't be feeling sorry for ourselves and saying it's His fault — and the thing to do is stop trying to figure it all out, and just be good! Actions speak louder than words: both my grandmothers tell me that once a month or so!"

Next to him sat Al, who seemed as moved as everyone else by the declaration of principles — but with one reservation. "When you said the rabbi 'should' say what you said — is that [the] right [thing for a rabbi to do]? We've just moved, and we go to a different synagogue. The rabbis — the old one and the new one — are different, way different, 'like day and night,' my folks say. The one [we went to] before told us God 'must be fed up with us,' because of all the wars and the poverty and the nuclear bombs we've built. The one [we go to] now says it's getting better, everything, and we should keep trying to change the world, because if you try hard, you'll succeed. 'It's all in the Bible,' my dad says — if you're an optimist, that's in the Bible, and if you're a pessimist, that's in the Bible — so it's not right when the rabbi says you 'should' do something."

"Hey, that's what rabbis are *for*, to say 'should,' " Tony shot back. A second's hesitation, a glance at his friends and me, then an elaboration: "If there's no one telling you what you should do, there's no Jewish religion. There's no *any* religion, I'd say! Isn't that what religion is all about? I think so — to tell you how to behave. God made a Covenant with our people, that's what we learned the other day in Hebrew school. Moses was given the Ten Commandments, and that's the biggest time in our history, when that happened. Just because we can't get all A's, make a perfect record, doesn't mean we shouldn't keep trying."

The use, once more, of "shouldn't" struck sensitive ears in the room. Tamar took her turn: " 'Shouldn't,' 'shouldn't,' you're right. 'A Jew obeys the laws, the Commandments,' that's what my grandmother tells us every hour, sometimes twice an hour! But my [older] sister is studying religion [in a high school course] and she says that you can be religious and talk out of both sides of your face. She says Jews, even the most religious Jews, can be as big a bunch of hypocrites as anyone else. So we need our rabbis to keep us as honest as we can be."

"Sure we do," Tony acknowledged, but his face displayed the sardonic cast of his mind. We all thought he'd continue, maybe give us a splendid jeremiad, but instead he slumped on his chair, stretched out his legs, crossed them at the ankles, folded his arms into one another, and capped off his body's message with a brief burst of whistling. We all laughed, and we all got his point; and, strangely, his cessation of the argument won him whatever converts he might otherwise have failed to make. He could see the smiles on his neighbors' faces, but he dared test everyone with an almost military challenge: "All with me say aye!" In a couple of seconds he had three hands in the air. He changed his smile into a big belly laugh, said thanks, and then decided to get quite serious: "I like going to Hebrew school. But I don't want any rabbi breathing down my back. A good rabbi — just like anyone else! — is a guy who doesn't come spying on you and running after you. He leaves you alone. He prays for you, but he isn't counting up your right steps and your wrong steps. OK, OK, he's a *rabbi!* But he should be a rabbi in his life, and that'll be the way for us to line up behind him!"

His slightly cynical and colloquial language did not mask his sincerity, even his moral passion. The flush on his face slowly disappeared as he straightened up, uncrossed his legs, separated his arms. The others, after a fashion, did with him what he said others might do with the right kind of rabbi: they "lined up after him" — pulled themselves up, straightened themselves out, uncrossed their various limbs. When Ilona reached for her school bag, long since neglected, the others started searching the floor for their possessions. As we departed Ilona smiled broadly at me and said, "Heavy!" I heard in her tone a bit of exasperation, a bit of weariness, but also a bit of unaffected pride at this foursome's vigorous introspection. Two nods and grunts and one "yes" made a chorus to that "Heavy!" and moments later the street had dispersed us.

*

In Jerusalem, during the summer of 1987, with my son Bob and a former student of mine, now a colleague, Bruce Diker, I sat with the three children of a family once American, now fervently, patriotically Israeli. The thirteen-year-old boy, Joshua, bar mitzvahed only weeks before, gave us a short lecture, while his two younger brothers, eleven and nine, Isaac and Aaron, sat and listened carefully: "Our parents made *aliyah* [immigrated to Israel] when I was two. I have no memory of the States. (I was born in Albany, in the state of New York.) I have two uncles and an aunt on my father's side, and an aunt on my mother's side. I have two grandfathers alive; both my grandmothers have died. Only my one [maternal] aunt has come here to visit us. Our American relatives think we made a mistake. Our parents were not from religious families. They were from nonreligious families! Our parents were 'hippies' when they were younger! They had no Jewish life — no education in our religion. My father did not even have his bar mitzvah when he was my age! He was an atheist! He was in all the political movements — against the [Vietnam] war and against the separation of the Negroes in the Southern states. He was an idealist, but he was not a Jew! His father was born in Lithuania, I think, or Poland — I'm not sure. He [the grandfather] was brought to America when young. He started out being a religious Jew, but he gave it [the religion] up and became a member of the Democratic Party. The same with his mother; she was from Russia, I know. She was in favor of socialism, my father says. As for my mother's family, they were very much like my father's people. They came from Russia, all of them, but my mother was born in Brooklyn — also in the state of New York, just like Albany is.

"My parents —" He stopped, looked at his younger brothers and a bit self-consciously changed the pronoun, emphasizing it: "*Our* parents met because they both went to a college in Schenectady. I don't know its name. [Union College, I later learned.] Then they married, and I was born, and it was after that, not long after, that they met some friends who were Zionists, and they were Jewish, too." He noticed me paying close attention to that expressed distinction and writing a word or two down on a pad of paper. His already didactic, slightly formal English (his "second language" to Hebrew) then became more formal. I heard a long lecture on the history of Zionism — I interrupted it now and then — parts of which emphasized the political and religious tensions he knew interested me: "A lot of the Zionists weren't Jews; I mean, they weren't believers in Judaism. They were Jews who wanted a country, a nation, for themselves. My dad says he never would have come here to be an Israeli only. He came here because he became a Jew, a real Jew. My mother wasn't so sure, but she went along with him. Now she's stronger, even, than he is! They say they don't want to turn their clock back; they don't want to see the States again. If the relatives want to come here, good; but if they don't want to, then it's too bad for them."

I suspect he saw in my eyes a glint of sadness, even irritation, at his seeming indifference to his blood kin. He pulled back a bit — mindful, I suddenly realized, that I too was an American. "We are facing plenty of troubles here, and we have to keep our eyes on why we are here," he continued. "We say our prayers four times a day. We pray to the God who gave us our Covenant with Him. We are here because this is where He came to us and gave Moses His Commandments. This is where He wants us to be. That's why we can't keep going back and forth to other countries, to the States; we're here to be near God and be part of His people."

At one of our meetings Joshua took a back seat while his younger brothers talked with me. Isaac told me he wanted to be a rabbi "someday"; Aaron wanted "to teach," but he wasn't sure what or where. We got to talking about those two professions and about the work people do in the course of their lives. Eventually Isaac told me this: "If I become a rabbi, I'll read the Torah, I'll know it by heart. I'll become 'learned in God's truth' — my father says that. [I had asked about the origin of the expression.] I'll try to live a holy life: I'll obey the laws of our religion, and I'll try to get others to.

"In school we talk about the future. If only Israel would become the land of Moses. Yes, the prophets, too. They are important, I agree. [I had suggested so.] But first it was the Covenant; later came the prophets, to teach our people when they fell from the truth. You see, the Jews were given the truth by God. He chose us to teach; we are His students! We've failed sometimes. Our rabbi says: We all fail — but tomorrow we have to start in again, and ask God to keep inspiring us, so we will learn better and better what He wants of us.

"He has so much to tell us: We could spend every day for centuries and not know all of His wisdom. We're sent here by Him to prove we can learn His knowledge — what's right, and what the truth is, and what He thinks we should do, and all the things that are wrong. A rabbi tries to learn from God so that he can get others to learn, and that's the best you can do, to listen to God and read the Talmud and think about it."

His brother Aaron was contemplating another direction for himself: "I'd like to be a teacher, like my favorite teacher, Mr. Benethon. He was going to be a rabbi, but he became a teacher instead. He reads to us from the Bible [Moses, David, Isaiah]. He tells us stories about our ancestors. He tells us we should be strong like them — and the only way [to become so strong] is to believe that God wants you to learn from Him. You see, if you do that, then you'll live a really good life, and you'll be smart — that means you'll know what He means, what He said to us. [I'd asked for a bit of elaboration on the word 'smart.']

"If you keep thinking of God, then you'll be headed to His truth. Mr. Benethon has told us that even when we study arithmetic or spelling we are learning from God. He [God] wants us to know all we can. Why? [My question, repeated by him.] So we can show Him we're paying attention to His word. You see, it's His gift to us, that's how he [Mr. Benethon] says we should think of the world here. It's a place we should explore, and we should explore what He told us — when Moses heard Him, and others.

"Once you know your religion, you know how to live the way you should live, and you'll be a good person. You'll live according to the rules; and then others will respect you and look up to you. That's important — if others respect you. Mr. Benethon says if your neighbors 'hold you up as wise and good,' then you're the biggest success in the world. My father agrees. He says it's not what you own, it's who you are; and who you are depends on what you've learned, and if you remember it all. If you forget, then you haven't really learned. Also, you've got to know what's important. Not every subject is the same [in importance].

You have to know how to spell, but it's the Jewish religion that's the most important subject. I don't think I'll be that smart — to teach it. But I could teach, maybe, Hebrew; I'm good at languages. You can't learn from God without knowing Hebrew — it's the best way to understand what our religion teaches. [I had questioned him on his use of "can't."] It's true, there are other things to do when you grow up, but if you grow up and you forget God and your people — what we're supposed to be, what God wants us to be — then you're in big trouble, Daddy will tell us."

I was quite intrigued by Aaron's phrase "what we're supposed to be," which he expanded, upon my prodding questions, to "what God wants us to be." Already, at nine, a very learned boy, Aaron had obviously became a favorite of his elementary school teacher, Mr. Benethon. The more we talked, the more I began to understand the depth and intensity of Aaron's yearning for a life that would let him be connected to God in the way that a student relates to a teacher. When he suggested teaching as a possible career for himself (so he explained to me during a late-afternoon visit to a nearby market, where he was doing some errands for his mother), "the reason was this: to be a good Jew." I couldn't quite fathom his logic, and told him so. He happily amplified: "If a Jew stops asking what a good Jew is, he's not going to be a very good Jew much longer!" Still surprised by the terse elegance of his initial formulation, I asked him whether he'd ever heard others make such a remark or whether it was all his: "Yes, it is mine, but I've heard my father say much the same thing, and Mr. Benethon, too." I liked the way he dodged my inquiry — and the way he disarmingly tried to teach me something: that one can learn from others, and do so with originality, with an eager mind that takes in experience and lays proper claim to it.

I began to see, conversing with Aaron, that the Jewish tradition of Biblical study as a central passion was not to be confused with that of academic inquiry, even the kind that is quite determined and zealous. For Aaron, a Jew contemplating the Talmud is a Jew living in accordance with God's wishes, hence a righteous Jew. No wonder Aaron asked one day as we sat in his family's living room, "What would I be like if I lived in the States?" I didn't know what to say — nor was I sure why, suddenly, he had posed that question to me. But when I asked him to answer his own question, he made it quite clear that he had other fish to fry than those I'd suspected: "I'd be trying to get a good job in a business. I'd be trying to be president of the United States!" I wasn't able to let him continue; I laughed, then asked him if he had any moral objection to his fellow Israeli citizens who wanted to do well as businessmen or even become the nation's prime minister. His answer was revealing and right to the point of his family's life: "No, I don't want to tell anyone what to do, even my own brother — only myself."

I had nothing to say. I felt a good deal of respect for a child whose ethical life enabled him to make such a remark. Moments in my life came to mind — times when I'd lacked the reflective restraint, the personal humility, that this boy showed. I wanted to speak my admiration, but somehow my words, in their multitude, seemed inadequate. I settled for a "thank you," and Aaron returned a nod. Silence held us, interrupted by the street noise of other children playing their games. I wondered whether to wind up and leave, or stay and ask more questions.

Aaron must have sensed our situation. He scratched his right leg (he was wearing shorts) and told me he'd been bitten the day before. He pulled together the crayons he'd used earlier in the day to draw pictures for me. I began making my final preparations for a departure — inserting the drawings under the clip of my clipboard, having written the date on the back of each drawing, and then putting the clipboard in my red knapsack. He got up; I did too. As I said goodbye and tried to arrange a time for our next visit, he looked at that knapsack, which I was holding in my right hand, and looked, next, at a menorah on top of a chest in the living room where we had sat and worked, a large, decorative candlestick with many branches. His eyes held to that direction for a few moments; I thought of the Friday night religious celebrations in this home, in other homes like it, the candles lit, the parents and children in prayer and family communion. Finally Aaron looked toward me and said, "I hope I'll learn and I'll remember the Halakah." This parting acknowledgment of the importance of Jewish law in his future life impressed me, made me want to suggest that we sit down again

and continue our conversation. But it was late for both Aaron
and me.

A few seconds later I was walking away from the house, Aaron's self-effacing words still sounding in my head. An exceptional righteousness, I kept thinking to myself — a righteousness
directed inward; a righteousness denied the thrill of conquest
or pride in proclamation. A boy whose parents might have stayed
in America and embraced a secular world's various pieties was
now trying hard to learn how to live up to a religion's ideals and
cautioning himself against the temptation to advise others about
what does or does not matter.

When I returned to Massachusetts and met with a group of
Jewish children who had recently visited Israel with their parents,
Conservative and Reform Jews, I described Aaron, and especially
the moment when he renounced the right to lean upon others
morally in favor of a candid, even self-critical look at himself.
This group of eight children, all about Aaron's age, give or take
a year or two, had been brought together by a rabbi friend of
mine. I had never met the three boys and five girls before and
had a hard time fitting each of them to a name on the list of
names I'd been given. Anyway, names didn't seem to matter on
that early September afternoon of 1987. Israel was on our minds,
and Judaism, too, and its central tenets. I heard much discussion
of the nation we had just visited — a good deal of affection for
it, some misgivings about it, some stern criticism of it. I heard
"Jewish values," as one eleven-year-old girl called them, celebrated. I also heard, surprisingly, one boy, ten, turn not only
against Israel's Arab neighbors but on the Christian world at
large: "You go to Israel, and you see that the Jews there have to
wake up every morning and say to themselves, 'Who's going to
throw us a curve ball today?' It's terrible — and it goes to show
you: the Jews are always in danger. The Arabs want to get rid
of Israel, and the Christians, a lot of them, from all over, don't
care."

Another boy spoke right up. "You are not being fair. The
Arab countries *are* Israel's enemies; I agree. But why do you
bring in the Christians, too? We've got lots of friends, the Jews
do! This country is Israel's friend!"

"Well, sometimes," the first boy said.

"A lot of the time," the second boy replied. "You're being unfair to America," he added.

"The only way Israel will survive is by being strong," the first boy retorted. Then, apparently aware that he had just side-stepped the controversy he had started a few moments earlier, he offered this: "Anyway, people don't like the Jews, they don't."

"What do you mean, what are you saying?" With those words the second boy obviously spoke for everyone in the room. Nods and murmurs of approval greeted his question.

"They don't!" the boy repeated defiantly. Then he launched into an explanation: "Look, the Jews told the world there is only one God, because He spoke to us and told us [that]. Do you think all those other people liked hearing what the Jews said, way back then? When Jesus came, he was a Jew and He said He was there to bring a message from God — I think that's what He said. Pretty soon you had the Christian religion; it's based on what a Jew said a long time ago. If you're a Christian, you're worshipping a Jew. Jesus told people to be good — just the way our Jewish [moral] leaders did, Isaiah and the others. But did people, most people, pay attention? Just read your history books! They worship Jesus, but they don't follow His ideas! So they must be mad at Him, don't you think? That's why I say: the Jews — they make everyone nervous, and people don't like them, because we're the ones God chose to talk with, and He told us how we should live."

He stopped because the others were champing at the bit to object, clarify, amend, refute, and, in the case of one girl, en-thusiastically applaud. The liveliness of this discussion took me by surprise. Not all the children knew all the others, yet they talked freely, almost urgently, with one another — perhaps be-cause they shared an important common experience: a first trip to Israel. They were stirred to vigorous reflection and no small amount of anxiety by the first boy's description of the Jews (and Jesus with them, He who was of them) as a moral agent uniquely approached by God. "Ridiculous," one girl said in response. "The Jews aren't the only people who have given the world something. You can get so into yourself, you forget all the other people out there!" Another girl both agreed and disagreed: "Sure, there are people in Africa and Asia who don't owe anything to Jews or Christians, nothing; they have their own religions. But he [the first boy] was talking about America and Europe, the countries where there are Christians and Jews, and maybe the Arabs, too. He was just saying that with the three religions — there was us, first, and God spoke to us and told us how you should behave, and then came the other two religions, and the others have resented us, because that's what we are, the religion of the Commandments. You always want to take shots at people who tell you what you should do!"

General amusement and apprehension greeted the statement made — quite delightfully — by the third boy in the room, who had kept silent until this moment: "Parents beware!" There was much laughter and more than the usual amount of leg movement as the children let his rather charged remark settle in their minds. Then came further talk of the special Jewish religious destiny and the vulnerability that went with it. As they talked I was remembering Israel — remembering, as these children did, the sights and sounds of a land whose history is so much a part of the ethical, spiritual, and intellectual life of many millions. All at once, the boy who had started us down a series of exchanges that lasted over an hour asked for a truce: "We'll never solve all of this! Maybe the best thing is to mind your own backyard and let others mind theirs! If only people would just leave Israel alone!" The others agreed with him, more or less. A girl warned that Israel couldn't be simply "left alone" — that is a fate no country can expect. Another girl seconded the "backyard" assertion, saying that "too many times we want to point our fingers at others, and meanwhile we're messing up ourselves." Her way of putting the matter hit home. Everyone in the room said yes or indicated assent by smiling or nodding.

It was then that Aaron came back to my mind, forcefully, vividly. His memorable words kept sounding in my head, and I saw him as I heard him, the round face, the freckles under his brown eyes, the brown hair covering part of his forehead, the thin, sturdy body of a boy at once athletic and contemplative, even scholarly. In the midst of a silence I heard my own voice sending forth more words than it had hitherto done — Aaron's message, not directed at me, his listener, but at himself: "I don't want to tell anyone what to do, even my own brother — only myself."

The children sat still, said nothing. Aaron's words held their own temporary sway over us until a girl who had said very little all afternoon decided to state an objection: "You have to let others know what to do, because they see what you're doing, don't they? Even if you don't *say* anything, they see, and if they don't agree, well, they won't like you!" No one else spoke for ten or so seconds, at which point I did: "True, but there's a difference between setting an example and *telling* people." I could hear, in the sound of my voice, a certain annoyance. I wondered why. Wasn't the girl's point as thoughtful as Aaron's? Still, Aaron's humility struck me as admirable, and eventually this girl's psychological wisdom (once I'd let it stand on its own, not as a rebuttal to Aaron) also seemed valuable.

Both these children, from such different backgrounds, albeit both Jewish, had in common a zeal for righteousness. I thought about their zeal later that day as, the meeting over, I sat with my notes, tapes, memories. A righteousness lived out certainly speaks to others — but with attendant dangers: the envy, shame, guilt, and rage of many of those others, as well as the admiration and applause of a few. Yet righteousness can certainly get out of bounds, a major danger for any of us, whether we've been told we have a special body of truth to protect or simply left to our own moral resources. Aaron's admonition was not meant, I suspect, to fly in the face of the psychological reality of righteousness-by-example, aptly summoned by the young girl; nor was Aaron forsaking his future responsibilities as a son of Abraham, Isaac, Moses, Isaiah, Amos, and others. Indeed, it was an important part of his Judaism which spoke on that day in Jerusalem; his remarks, like "the Proverbs of Solomon the son of David, King of Israel" or like "the words of the preacher, the son of David, King of Jerusalem" (Ecclesiastes), granted full leeway to the danger of "vanity," the constant temptations to self-importance and self-aggrandizement that go with righteousness.

One does not reproach oneself, usually, with respect to a danger that does not really threaten — that is something the boy Aaron surely knew in his bones as he tried to find his place in a powerful tradition of religiously sanctioned righteousness while worrying about the personal hazards of the tradition. So with other children whose Jewish faith has stimulated them to sift the just and the worthwhile from the fake and the phony, from the outright wrong or evil: they, too, have not always avoided finger-pointing even as they have not stopped wondering what is fair, what is wicked. Listening to them, at times I've heard Biblical cadences joining the everyday slang of America's (or Israel's) late-twentieth-century streets — evidence of a continuity of righteousness, thousands of years old, constantly nourished in family after family, synagogue after synagogue: covenantal and prophetic Judaism become an ethical endowment of one child after another.

Sometimes, though, I have felt these conversations getting too abstract. However vigorously argued, they seem curiously at a remove from the glorious heart of Judaism, from its emphasis not only on moral exposition and analysis but on the sacrament of the family's lived life, one in which metaphors are not only spoken but connected to the everyday rhythms of existence, as in Job, as in the Psalms and the Proverbs, as in Ecclesiastes and the Song of Solomon and Lamentations and Habakkuk. Every once in a while, as some of the children I knew argued with one another and with me, I saw that Judaism, no less than Christianity, could be turned into yet another contemporary "subject," to be connected to other "subjects," to be aligned with this or that viewpoint, to be fought over and claimed. At such moments I've often thought of Leah, ten years old when I came to know her in the initial stages of this research, who died of acute leukemia in Boston's Children's Hospital toward the end of the summer of 1986. Leah was a quiet girl when I met her, tall for her age, of light complexion and delightful auburn hair. Every once in a while, though, amid intense discussions of religion, she yawned openly, then apologized; it was her way, actually, of expressing her sense that we were all getting lost in talk and more talk. (Her yawns made me want to follow suit — and so I'd engage in the work of stifling.) One spring day, during Passover, she suggested that we all shut up, go get "Cokes and Pepsis and ginger ale" and some matzoh, and, as she put it so pointedly, "just *be* Jews." She was overruled, so on we went with the exchanges over the difference between Conservative and Reform Judaism.

A year later Leah fell sick. She seemed to have the flu. She was weak, chronically tired, short of breath. She felt dizzy at the slightest exertion. A visit to the doctor did not turn out to be reassuring. He wanted tests and more tests. In no time he was suggesting hospitalization, and soon he was calling in various consultants to help arrive at a diagnosis. From a school friend of hers I learned the terrible diagnosis: an acute leukemia, of a kind not so responsive to chemotherapy as other leukemias of childhood. The girl who brought the news did so in tears, and when I met the group of five children (in Brookline, Massachusetts) who had been talking with me and Leah, our shared sadness was obvious. It was then that I heard God questioned as I never had before by children explicitly "religious" in their background, education, stated beliefs. "*How* can God let such a thing happen?" "Why — why does He permit this?" "*What*, tell me, what has she done to deserve this?" "Where is He, where is God?" "When you see a girl like her get sick like that, you want to scream and scream, because God must not know — He couldn't know and just sit back and do nothing!"

I waited for the Old Testament to be called in — those stories with all the mystery of pain, suffering, and hardship, all the challenges to faith, all the questions men and women have put to God. But these decent and thoughtful children did not at first call upon the Bible, either for solace or in indignation. After they had expressed their raw emotions, they peppered me with medical questions, ones that I felt unable to answer. I promised further information at a later date — whereupon one member of the group, a girlfriend of Leah's, remembered her in all her recent health, and connected such a memory to Job: "I heard our rabbi once read from the book of Job — when he saw himself healthy, the time before he got sick." But immediately she wanted to know — why not? — if there was some drug that would "reverse all the leukemia." Maybe, I finally said.

I started visiting Leah at the Children's Hospital. I had trained there; I knew her doctors and nurses well. They began to be quite fond of her and her parents, no rare event in hospitals, but not an everyday one, either. They began to tell me of her "remarkable faith," of the religious life that unfolded daily in Leah's hospital room. Her mother brought the Bible, read from it — the Psalms especially, one after the other. Leah loved hearing her mother and father and older sister read those psalms; loved reading them aloud to her family; loved a "book of psalms" that was given to her and kept it at her bedside; and loved the matzoh her mother brought, the taste of wine her father offered. Yes, Leah loved the 23rd Psalm especially, but she loved others, too — the 40th, the 42nd, the 92nd, the 96th. She wanted to offer an emphatic salute to God, it seemed, an unquestioning and undemanding one. She wanted Him addressed with reverence and affection and trust rather than from the vantage point of the vulnerable or enraged beggar. She was inclined to impute righteousness to God rather than demand it for herself. Hers was not the impiety of Job — not even his nostalgia for the good times of yore: "Oh that I were as in months past, as in the days when God preserved me; when His candle shined upon my head, and when by his light I walked through darkness." Once, during a visit, she told me this: "It's been hard for us [the Jewish people]; we've had troubles, lots of them. We'll keep going, though, and we'll remember our God, and we won't forget all the troubles, and we won't forget that God has His eyes on us, and He listens to us; and if you read the Bible, He's there, talking to us, and like my daddy says, and my mom, 'He touches you mightily.'"

Through all the disfigurement and pain of chemotherapy — a modern agony — Leah recited sentences from the ancient psalms, said her prayers to God, listened attentively to her parents as they upheld His name, His eternal goodness. Watching their child slowly die, modern medical science notwithstanding, Leah's parents continued a steadfast, prayerful vigil. This family brought a living Jewish ceremonial tradition to a hospital bed. They spoke of the only hope they knew, God's ultimate wisdom. Leah's family remembered not only its own better days but those of its people — God's call to them, God's gift of intimacy with them, God's deliverance of them. "Leah is part of Israel," her father once said. He must have seen the sad doubt in my eyes — at which he closed his and spoke a prayer in Hebrew. I found out later, from Leah's sister, that his prayer celebrated the historic vulnerability and suffering of the Jewish people at God's hands — part of the Jews' destiny but also a major reason for their longstanding concern for the poor, for those who suffer.

I remember my last visit to Leah. She was not far from death. Her body had withered; she was jaundiced, dehydrated, sweaty, feverish. At her bedside was her father's Bible. Nearby, her mother sewed and sang a song the girl's grandmother (now dead) had loved, had taught Leah years earlier: "Three o'clock in the morning; we danced the whole night through." It was a romantic ballad from the 1920s and somehow meant a lot to Leah, for whom it was a pitch-black, melancholy three o'clock, with only a handful of sunrises left. Her eyes shone, however, and she listened carefully, her mind and soul bravely alert. I saw in Leah a child intensely attached to a family's religious and spiritual life, its prayers and food and ceremonies, its spoken acknowledgment of the Lord, its remembrance of His words, of what He and His people had experienced together in the past and were still, in that hospital room, in our time, undergoing together. "I'd like to go to that 'high rock,'" Leah told her dad just before she slipped into a final coma — and from then until her death, her heartbroken but proud and strong father could be heard by nurses and doctors and ward helpers and visitors and family members saying in Hebrew the 61st Psalm: "Hear my cry, O God; attend unto my prayer. From the end of the earth will I cry unto thee, when my heart is overwhelmed: lead me to the rock that is higher than I." The rock for Leah, for her family, was a Judaism that would not break or yield, even at the death of a young girl.

⁂ ⁂ ⁂

12

Secular Soul-Searching

AS A MEDICAL STUDENT I heard Reinhold Niebuhr deliver a memorable sermon on "moral reflection." He had invaded Harvard, one of the precincts of Boston Unitarianism, to attack some of the shibboleths and icons of America's mid-twentieth-century secular bourgeoisie — for instance, a self-important, messianic faith in psychology and political reform as the harbingers of a coming utopia. A master ironist, Niebuhr walked a tightrope for the half-hour or so of his sermon in Harvard's Memorial Church. He himself had, by then, become very much a venerated figure among many who may have had their doubts about Christianity and Judaism but were quite willing to admire a minister who was properly "intellectual." In his sermon, however, he reminded us that Jesus did not spend his time learning to become a theologian or leading thinker but was, rather, an itinerant moralist and storyteller, even as the Hebrew prophets carefully, and with righteous indignation, distanced themselves from the institutions of their time and place. Standing in an influential institution of our time, Niebuhr asked us when we ought to stand apart, live (as he put it) "outside the city's gates."[1]

He was trying to strip himself of some of the authority vested in him by his listeners — while at the same time earning their respect for his bold, even sardonic message. He was, of course, a stunning preacher. His electricity gripped us; the charisma in him poured forth, engulfed us. He was also unsettling to both the believers and the skeptics in his audience as he wondered aloud what hidden sources of pride and idolatry were at work among the liberal, agnostic intelligentsia.

Not that he was any great friend, in that speech or elsewhere, to those who espoused the established religious faiths. He had a keen eye and ear for religious hypocrisy and smugness, and at times, as he railed against them, he sounded like H. L. Mencken or the Sinclair Lewis of *Elmer Gantry*. He took aim, also, at not only the easily targeted fundamentalists of rural and small-town America, but the self-satisfied cadres who professed a "modern" polish in their religious doctrine and practice. For such men and women he invoked the fiery radicalism, the insistent eccentricity, of the Hebrew prophets and of Jesus of Nazareth — individuals cherished in our time, but in their day dismissed by religious authority as outsiders, as wrongheaded, as violators rather than custodians of a religious tradition.

All of the above was meant to serve as prelude to what, we slowly realized, was his main point — the distinction between the religious and the spiritual. The religious tradition, he reminded us, can successfully stifle a good deal of valuable and suggestive spiritual introspection. He was, of course, working St. Paul's territory — the difference between the letter and the spirit. In the Jewish tradition any number of mystics have chosen to emphasize their own private and inward manner of faith rather than the conventional and ritual kind. But Dr. Niebuhr pushed the matter rather hard, wondering out loud whether spirituality doesn't best renew itself in the most surprising ways, at the hands of those who may not lay claim to any interest in religious or spiritual speculation.

I have remembered that sermon often as I have worked with boys and girls who go rarely or never to church, to synagogue; who may not in any way consider themselves religious; indeed, who shun such a word as utterly inapplicable to themselves; and yet who ask all sorts of interesting, even stirring questions about the nature of this life, and who can be heard sweating over and playing with ideas that are clearly spiritual in nature — wondering about the meaning of life, expressing their own sense of what truly matters. Often I've met these children by accident. I did not intend, at the outset, to work with boys and girls whose parents were avowed agnostics or atheists, or who themselves denied explicit religious involvement. But then, at the outset, I had a somewhat restricted sense of this research project — limiting it to the religious life of children. Soon, however, I was talking with a wide range of boys and girls in schools all over this country, as well as abroad; and I began to see that even many youngsters brought up in a strict religious tradition were generous in their estimates of the spiritual life of certain classmates who claimed no particular faith.[2]

In a town near Boston, in a private school that attracted both white and black students, both Catholic and Protestant children, and a substantial number of Jewish ones, I listened to Gary, just thirteen (the son of a churchgoing, Episcopalian businessman and a mother who is Catholic and a college professor), talk about his own religion and that of his classmates: "My parents have joint custody of me! One week I go with Mom to her church; the next week I go with Dad to his. I'm a Catholic, I guess, but I like our Episcopal church, too. My parents visit each other's churches! We make it work! Lots of kids at school don't have my problems — they don't have any religion to worry about. Sometimes I wish I was one of them. I know that most of the time we're all happy in our family, but there will be bad days, and 'when you're looking for a fight,' Dad says, 'you find something to fight over' — so it'll be religion sometimes, and it's then that I say: for crying out loud, let's remember what Jesus said about love, and not hate each other over whose church is better!

"You take the kids whose folks aren't into any religion; we have lots of them in our school, and they're no different than anyone, and some of them — I talk with them about what they believe — are really great, because they ask a lot of questions about life, and they want to stop and talk about things, about what's right and wrong, and what you should believe, and after I'll talk with them, I'll say to myself, hey, maybe if you have no religion, you end up being more religious. You know what I mean?"

An irony worthy of Niebuhr, I thought and nodded with an enthusiasm growing out of statements made by several of his classmates as well, all eighth-graders. Gary had two younger sisters and "sat" for them often when their parents went out. He would sometimes talk with his sisters about "serious things." "Carrie [nine] and Molly [eleven] aren't deep thinkers, but they have good friends, and they hear them talk, and they talk to each other a lot. Carrie says she's tired of going back and forth to those two churches, just to please Mom and Dad. Molly says she wishes, sometimes, 'religion wasn't invented,' so there'd be less for our mom and dad to fight about! Molly's best friend doesn't believe in anything, Molly says — no God, no way! She [the friend] believes that the world just happened, and it'll die one of these days, when the sun just gives out, and that'll be that. Our science teacher, I think he agrees with her! He doesn't quite say it — he *almost* says it! I mean, he tells us what the 'theories' are. When a kid said his parents 'believe' the same thing, the teacher smiled. That was when Eric [a friend of his] spoke up in class; he said that science is science, but where does God fit in, and the teacher said that's up to each of us, and it's not a 'subject' in school, what you believe. But he was telling us what *he* believes!

"I talk sometimes with Carrie and Molly about God and what the science teacher says, and they talk with their friends, and some of them will even say that it would be a relief to be growing up in a home where you don't say prayers and go back and forth the way we do from one church to another. Like one of my friends, Eric, says, we're all 'churched out' in our family! When my sisters and I talk, the best times we have are thinking about being grown up, and being just ourselves and not *Catholics* or *Protestants!* Some kids will say to me: 'I think for *myself*. I think about God and all that stuff, real deep stuff, and no one's dictating to me, no priest, no minister, and no rabbi. It's just me and my thoughts.' That's great!"

Later, Gary suggested I talk with his friend Eric. A twelve-year-old, tall for his age and lanky, Eric was bright, well-spoken, forthright. He was "amused" that Gary had brought us together: "I'm not into religion, and he [Gary] really is. It's because his parents are always going to church, and they go to different ones, and if you go there [to their home] they'll say grace, and I never know what to do. Sometimes the father will even read from the Bible . . . on Sundays, mostly, before dinner. That's not the way my parents are! They think for themselves, and they want us kids to think for ourselves! My dad [an engineer] laughs at religion a lot. He says, 'Millions have slaughtered millions in the name of religion!' If you think about it, he's right! That's what we've been learning in school, in our history class. People should think about that — what's been done in the past by all those churches. It tells you something about human nature, my dad says.

"My mom's a teacher; she teaches math. She reads a lot — history and biographies. She says people turn to religion because they want answers, and that's all right, that's okay, but then they go that step further: they want to tell everyone else that they either believe 'our' answers or they'll be in real trouble. That's the whole story of religion, my parents will show you from their reading: each religion says it's the right one and all the others are wrong, and they won't stop there; they'll go after the other religions, and pretty soon you have big fights, and lots of people die, and that's supposed to be good, because some religion has 'won,' and everyone is believing in it! No way, I say!"

He had become more excited than he'd realized, and now he sat silently, trying to regain the kind of "cool" he and many of his friends tried so hard to present to one another. He stared at the floor, then scratched his head. That gesture seemed to energize him again. He asked, "What do you think?" I was, as I often am, quite surprised by the suddenness of this question. I had expected a continuation of his vigorous argument, or maybe some second thoughts. Instead, I was supposed to say something — and not just utter a conversational piety. I hesitated longer than I ought to have, for I wanted to hear more from Eric, not hear myself drone on. Sadly, I wasn't thinking of Eric, what *he* wanted. He, understanding my pause, came at me head-on: "I'd really like to hear what you'd say."

I nodded and then told him my nod was substantive: "Eric, it would be hard for anyone to disagree with you — and I sure don't." I stopped. I could have reiterated his thesis, but he had spoken with force and economy. He reminded me, actually, of what as a boy I had often heard my father say, much to my mother's anxiety, even displeasure: she the deeply religious person, happily married to a scientist-skeptic with no small knowledge of history's unsettling lessons. As I sat with Eric, I could feel some of my dad's blunt factuality stirring within; and I could also feel my mother's apprehension and shame, often covered by the sudden (and intimidating) appearance of melancholy. "The sadness of it all," she would say — and who could really disagree? It was a way, I later realized, for her to pull us all together! So, suddenly, in that "conference room" of a school, decades later, I heard myself repeating a familiar observation: "It's very sad, isn't it?"

But Eric wasn't simply going to assent. He did say yes, but he quickly took issue with that comment: "It's sad, yes, but you can't just let it drop there; you have to remember that the same terrible stuff is going on right now. That's why I'm doubtful about organized religion. I'm not talking about whether it's true or not, what the religions tell you; we could discuss that — 'It's a separate issue,' my dad would say. I'm talking about what happens when these religions become 'big deals.' You get fanatics, lots of them. You get people who won't give the next guy the time of day, unless he goes along, swallows the line."

I was made uneasy by that last phrase, perhaps because it so relentlessly, even precisely, describes what happens with many of us: an initial righteousness becomes self-righteousness, supported on a large scale by the institutionalization of a faith or a creed. Eric sensed, I believe, my combination of agreement and surprise. Rather impressively (and I was touched by his thoughtfulness) he pulled back a little, discreetly, using abstract, impersonal language: "Maybe it's a little harsh to go after everyone! I know lots of people who go to church a lot, and they're nice people, and they don't go around trying to make me or anyone else do their thing. There's a minister whose son is a friend of mine — and he's a real nice guy." He stopped, just when I was quite sure he had much more to add. I didn't feel, this time, that he expected me to talk. He seemed to be coming up for air, engaging in a bit of self-examination. Finally he resumed: "I was getting to be like the people I was knocking!" Now he was dead silent for a good reason: he wanted his own words to sink in, stay with him, never mind me.

Now I felt impelled to speak. "Eric, you're hitting upon something we're all tempted with — the way we criticize others and exempt ourselves from the criticism. You're sure right about the religions — how they've become the inspiration for wars and persecution and murder. But people have found other reasons to attack other people — for the ideas they have, for the way they look, for what they do to make a living, for where they live; it goes on and on."

I felt I was getting into a speech. But I'd said quite enough, and I shut up. Eric replied with one word: "Right!" He also smiled, as did I — it was not only an acknowledgment of agreement, but a moment of shared confession. Eric stretched his legs, decided to take off his sweater. I sat still, trying to figure out whether I should follow his lead and doff my own sweater. No, it was still a bit chilly in that room, governed by the restrained heating habits of a school with a remnant of Puritanism in it. I decided to try to change the subject.

The boy didn't need my lead, however. "Religion doesn't mean much to me — going to church; but I sure can stop and wonder about things."

I felt, suddenly, a surge of interest. "What things?"

Eric wasn't shy with words. "You look at the sky, and you wonder what's up there, except what we see, the sun and the moon and the stars. Anything else? Who knows? Not me! Most of the time, I'm just going from minute to minute; I'm trying to get from here to there — all the chores my folks give me, and my own hassles I've got to get through. It's when something unexpected happens that I stop myself and ask what's going on: what's it all about?"

"Do you find any answers then?"

"No, not really. Only more questions!"

"Could you give me an example?"

"Sure. I'll be asking myself what's the cause of this or something else — like we do in science class when we study gravity or atoms and molecules and fission and fusion, that kind of stuff. Then I'll wonder how all that got going. Is there a God? Did He get it all going? Are there other people somewhere in the universe? I guess you just wonder about that kind of thing — and a lot of the time I stop myself and 'get back to the basics,' like my dad says you've got to do, and leave the 'dreaming' to others. But when there was this accident right near us, and the driver got killed, and we saw her being taken from the car — they had to cut her out, she was 'glued in,' a cop said — you had to stop and ask why that happened to her. And it wasn't her fault. A drunk guy crossed over the white line and smashed into her, just like *that!*"

Eric snapped his fingers to emphasize his point, and to remind both of us how utterly arbitrary this life is. The snap somehow registered more persuasively with me than what he had said. Not that I expected startling and original reflections, but I had already enjoyed and been instructively confronted by the boy's polemics, and now he was saying what we all say, even most religious people — or so I thought for a second or two until he reminded me otherwise: "You should have heard our next-door neighbor; she kept telling my mom it was 'God's will,' that accident. She said, 'God will take her [the victim] to heaven.' Can you believe that? Lots of people would say the same thing — millions, my folks say. Wild! How can people think that way? Did God tell that guy [the drunken driver responsible for the accident] to do what he did? Was God punishing someone? I can't buy that, all that!"

He stopped — for an interesting reason, I soon found out. He had heard the sound of his own voice. He was chastened by his lack of cool, reminded of an earlier moment in our discussion — and I was again quite impressed. He didn't say anything; I didn't either. A faint smile on his face told me everything, and a faint smile on mine declared my awareness and agreement. "I'll tell you, Eric, every day there's a new temptation!"

He laughed, answered: "You bet. I don't want to sound like a real crackpot, ranting and raving about all the neighbors who rant and rave! Dad says the world is 'full of ranting and raving,' and the only people who don't rant and rave are him and me, and sometimes, he says, I do a little ranting and raving myself! See what I mean?"

"I sure do."

"Do teachers fall into the same trap?"

"Yes."

"In colleges, too?"

"Yes, definitely."

He picked up on the emphasis I'd just put on "definitely," with another smile. "I remember Dad talking about his college days once. He said there were professors who were in love with their own lectures; they just talked and talked, and no one can argue with them and get away with it, because all they want is to hear themselves talk!"

He looked at me quizzically. I felt myself squirming. I looked at him — to gauge his intent, I realized, and decided he was not being an accuser, though I couldn't be so sure of myself in that regard at that moment. I wanted to get us back on my sense of the right track: "Eric, do you think that people change the way they look at the world as they get older?"

After I asked the question I worried. I had in mind the greater interest in moral and spiritual introspection that one encounters in some people as they get older, but a moment's reflection of my own made me think I'd presented my young friend with a query that seemed to come out of nowhere and be headed no-where. But I was wrong. He answered me right away and at some length: "My grandfather should answer you. He's a great guy, and he takes me to lunch every couple of weeks. He talks about 'old age'; he says he never stopped and thought about 'life' until he was sixty-five and he retired. Then he started read-ing a lot — books on politics and history — and he took long walks, because the doctor said he needs the exercise, and he joined a book club, a discussion club, [held] in his town library. My dad knows his dad, and he [Eric's father] says, 'The old guy is different, he's much calmer and thinks about things more.' That's my dad's reading on the situation!

"When you get older you're nearer to death, so you must think about that. Besides, it's natural at the end of a game to take time out and try to figure out what you did right and what you did wrong." He stopped there and looked down at his legs, which he moved forward and back, away from the chair, back to it. He seemed lost in a reverie. Abruptly he resumed: "I guess that's what you do even at my age. I'll be riding my bike, and one minute I'm looking at the people and the houses, and I'm won-dering how much time I've got, before I have to do something else; and the next minute I'm all into myself, and I'm thinking the kind of stuff — I guess it's what philosophers think. I'm thinking that I'm here, now, but one day I'll be gone. That's far off, I hope, but it could be tomorrow. Look what happened to my cousin, Ned. All he was doing — he was crossing the street, and that truck went wild, and he got killed, and that lady, too, in that accident [which he had mentioned earlier], and she had two little kids, and they lost their mother.

"I had dreams about Ned for a while. He'd be standing on the sidewalk and telling me not to cross there, where he got hit; or he'd be on this roller coaster going up and down, and he was alone in one of the [roller coaster] cars, and I wanted to be there with him, but I couldn't. Then the coaster stops, and he gets out, and he's walking away from us, and there's a big field there, beyond the coaster, and Ned is still alone, and I call out: I say, 'Ned, Ned,' but he doesn't hear me, and he keeps walking, and that's when I turn around, and I walk toward the roller coaster — I guess I'm hoping to get on it, and that's when I wake up."

Eric seems quite perplexed by that recurrent dream. (The roller coaster is not an unusual image, I have noticed — rather, it seems to be a common way for children to symbolize life's up-and-down journey.) He told me that he now had the dream only rarely, but that after Ned's death "almost every night" that dream or a "scarier one" took place. When I asked him about the "scarier one," he was brief in his description: "It was the same dream, only the roller coaster goes crazy, faster and faster, and then it crashes, and I don't know what happens to Ned, because I see the coaster — all the cars — go off the track, and then I wake up."

As we talked he decided to call that "scarier" version of the dream a "nightmare." He is glad he hasn't had one of those "for a long time" — meaning "six or eight months." [Ned died a year before our conversation.] He also decided to advance an interpretation of his dream: "I guess Ned's accident, his death, got to me. He was five years older than me, and I really looked up to him. Everything he did — I'd say to myself: you'll be doing that soon! Then, all of a sudden, I'm coming in the house from school, and my mom is there, in the kitchen, and she says I should sit down, and she has something to tell me. I can still see her face; it told me there was bad news. She sat down, and then she told me. She started crying, then I did. At first, I think I was crying because she was. Every time Mom cries, no matter what the reason is, I'll get tears in my eyes, too. It was later, in the night, that it really sunk in: Ned was gone. I'd never see him again! I was lying on my bed, on my back. When I really do some 'thinking' at night, I'll lie there with my arms behind my head, like an extra pillow, and just look up at the ceiling and think! That's what I did, for a long time: I just stared, and I thought.

"I was conscious of my whole body. I made my toes move, and my hands; I bent my legs and I lifted my arms — strange! I said to myself, 'You're Eric, and you're alive! Ned is gone — there's no more Ned. You're still here, but there will be a time when you're gone, too.' Then I remembered some of the family pictures Mom and Dad used to show us — a guy, and this woman, and three or four other people sitting in chairs, all dressed up. They'd tell us who those people were; they'd give us their names. They'd tell us how they're related to us. I forget more of what they told us. I can remember the picture of my great-grandfather, though. He had a mustache. He's sitting in a chair. His children are standing around him, three or four, I think. He has his hands on his knees. He's staring right at the camera. He's glaring, actually! He looks a little scary! I wouldn't want to mess with him! He was tall, Dad said, and he had big muscles. He owned a store, a hardware store, and he did carpentry. You know what else I remember from that picture? He's wearing a bow tie. I've asked my dad a couple of times why it is that in all the pictures of him [the great-grandfather] he always is wearing that same bow tie."

I wondered aloud, of course, what answer Eric's father had provided to that question. Eric had the answer, but he had also realized, upon hearing it from his father, that the question tapped into a family's past, a nation's past, more deeply than was intended: "Dad told me they were poor, back then, and they lost the store, and that was probably the only tie he had, and he got sick, and he died young. The story is that he was heartbroken, once he lost his store, and he sunk into a bad mood, and then he caught the flu or something, and he never got better. My father is always telling us how lucky we are — that we've got so much, compared to our ancestors, and we should be darn grateful, and if we're not, then that's a big sin."

He stopped himself with that last word. He was silent. When

he continued to be silent, I asked him what he was thinking. He replied, "Nothing."

I took the initiative. "Eric, what's a sin?"

He answered, "When you do something wrong."

I persisted. "Is it a religious word — sin?"

"Yes," he said — then changed his mind and amplified: "It's [a word] used by ministers to scare you, but it can be used just to say you're doing something real bad. My mom will say: 'It's a *sin*, the way people waste food, and they won't care about the hungry, *two* sins!' Sometimes when Dad talks about his family, he'll say they weren't 'churchgoing,' but they believed in sin — and so they tried to be good people. He's not sure they believed in God!

"I guess I don't, either. When Ned got killed, and I was doing a lot of thinking, I'd ask myself if I believed in God. You wonder, sometimes. A lady [a neighbor] said, 'God took him.' My mother told us that. Mom said she wished there *was* a God and He took Ned; then there'd be some 'sense' to it, what happened, but there isn't any, just an accident, a guy who wasn't even drunk, he was just in a rush and he lost control and *bang*, he killed someone! That's what I thought about as I was in bed, lying and thinking. That's life! My mother, my dad, they both say to us, 'That's life.' I was telling myself the same thing in the night — and the next thing, it's morning, and you've got to get up and get going, because 'that's life,' too!"

An afternoon's memoir; a segment of an American family's life turned into a boy's introspective effort to figure out human destiny. Eric's dream — occasionally terror-struck and agitated — had its own story to tell, as I sensed Eric knew while describing it. To be sure, his imagery was not unique or magically suggestive; but he managed (with a certain economy of symbols, and with some narrative power) to say rather a lot about that final moment of aloneness each of us experiences as we walk into territory that has been explored by all who have preceded us, yet is, also, completely unknown this side of heaven and hell. At one point I was poised to comment on Eric's dream, but I couldn't quite bring myself to do so, and I think I know why: no comment was necessary. He himself had fitted a middle-of-the-night story into a broader aspect of a life whose events had spawned what for him was not only a nightmare but a burst of existentialist rumination. It is as if he were telling himself, while asleep, what his parents were telling him, *and* themselves, at the breakfast table. Life is each person's to receive as a gift (from where or whom nobody knows for sure), to seize, to contemplate, and, ultimately, to feel ebbing away. Such knowledge, such awareness, can sometimes be awesome. Eric had his own way of acknowledging that mix of awe, curiosity, frustration, apprehension: "Even now I'll think of Ned — I'll see him, in my mind — and I'll tense up, tense up real bad. He's gone, so I'm tensing up for myself, I guess." I was moved by that concluding remark of his. It *was* a concluding remark, for he decisively ended our meeting, telling me about an impending athletic commitment he had. It was just as well, given such a luminous moment.

A terrible accident or other tragedy is not, of course, a prerequisite for intense, penetrating rumination. As mentioned earlier, I have taught in an elementary school near Harvard, attended by a diverse group of children — some from academic families, but most of working-class background. Alice, ten when I got to know her, was a girl whose parents were an automobile mechanic and a part-time salesclerk. She is a middle child, with an older sister, fourteen, and a younger brother, eight. In 1988, in the fourth grade, she was a most conscientious student, though not without a sense of humor and, more generally, a sense of fun. She responded with spirit and intelligence to the class I taught — again, a sort of art history class meant to help the children think about the various ways artists have represented reality, and to encourage them to discuss their reactions to the paintings or drawings that they viewed as slides each week. As those boys and girls looked at the work of Rembrandt and El Greco, van Gogh and Gauguin, Picasso and Henry Moore and Edward Hopper and Käthe Kollwitz, they singled out elements of the artwork that connected with their own lives.

We met that year on Thursdays, in the late morning, and the children often nibbled on fruit, nuts, or candy as they looked at a particular picture and talked about what they saw. I well remember the day I showed them Picasso's *Les Saltimbanques*. The

children, noticing the attenuated human forms the artist presented, immediately became a bit self-conscious. "I want to share
my food with them," Alice observed. Then she turned inquisi-
tive: "Why do people get like that? [Are they] on diets?"

Her neighbor, whose name I kept forgetting, perhaps because
she was constantly disrupting the class, shouted her response to
Alice's question: "Those are strange people. They may not be
on a diet; they could just be real kooks!"

Alice frowned then. Later that day, when she and I were sitting
alone in the classroom (school was over, and I was interviewing
her), she remembered that moment: "It wasn't nice, to call those
people 'kooks.' My mommy says she sees 'every different kind
of person' when she sells, and you have to be tolerant, or pretty
soon you're calling everyone a bad name! Maybe some people
would think I'm kooky or *she* [her classmate] is kooky. You should
be careful of what you say about people. The other day, a boy
asked me what is my religion. I said, 'None.' He said, 'What,
none!' Then I said, 'Yes, that's right!' You would have thought
I'd just gone and shot someone dead! He said, 'If you don't
believe in God, you're going straight to hell, and you'll stay there
forever.' 'Well, so what!' That's what I said!"

She stopped — reliving, perhaps, the drama of that moment.
I wanted to hear more, hear about the further give-and-take of
the encounter, but I could see that she was still troubled by what
she had experienced, and I decided to leave her the initiative.
She stopped recounting that confrontation, shifting instead to a
more personal, though abstract, line. "I wasn't going to tell him
about my ideas. He's not the only one who thinks about God!
Just because you don't go to church and don't believe what they
tell you [there] doesn't mean you don't think about God, and
about how you should be good, and what are the really big things
in life, and the things that don't make any difference. I can sit
and look out the window, and I'll watch it snow; and I believe
in God then. So does my mommy; she says each snowflake is
different from every other snowflake that ever was and ever will
be, and that shows you there's something out there that makes
our world so special."

Clearly not satisfied with what she had just announced, she
held up both her hands for a close inspection of the fingernails.

She spotted some dirt under two of the nails on her left hand and started working to clean them. I sat watching, irritated by her self-absorption at just the time when I was hearing a meditation that interested me. As I was thinking of questions to ask her, she resumed: "It's hard to know how to take care of other people! My mother knows how to figure out other people. She sells: men's shirts, and sometimes, in the women's department, dresses — she can do both. She sees a lot of people, and she can tell in advance what they're like, a lot of them. She says she can see them coming. Some want you to cut prices on your own, even if there's no sale. Some are nice, and some are terrible; they're rude. Mommy says, 'God made them all'; she says the trouble is, if He made them all, then what's the reason, because a lot of them aren't so nice, and He's nice, so why did He do it?"

With that long sentence, she stopped and looked again at her nails. They were clean, and she moved her eyes toward the floor. I asked my obvious question: "Do you have any idea why He might have done it — God?"

"No, I don't."

No more for a while, and I scurried for more questions. I asked them and got little back. Alice had finished for the day, I concluded, at least with respect to the subject I was trying to explore, so we bantered for a few minutes and then began to take leave of each other. We walked to the door together, then down the hall and down the steps, where she would join some of her friends for the final "study period." As we walked we chatted, but at one point Alice stopped and said, "Look, the sky is blue, and there aren't any clouds!" We were both looking out a hall window, and it was indeed a beauty of a day, sunny and cool, a good breeze about; a bracing autumn feel had even entered the building. I smiled and said nothing. Alice seemed uninterested in conversation, despite her remark, which I interpreted as meant for herself rather than me. We continued down the stairs, reached the bottom, and prepared to say goodbye. As we did so, she said, "Next time, if you want, we can talk about churches. I don't understand why people go to them, but if you do, I'd like to know."

I was surprised, a bit perplexed, and quite awakened by her

statement. I replied, "I'll remember, and we can begin next week where we've just left off."

That is what happened — I recapitulated, word for word, Alice's almost plaintive request. I told her I could surely manage to put forth a few explanations as to why people go to church, what they hope to find there, but the whole point of my work, I reminded Alice, was to hear young people like her talk about such matters. Did she, then, have anything to say? Yes, but she worried about something: "I might be saying the wrong thing. I remember — it was last year — I saw the people next door coming home from church, and I looked out the window after they'd left and I tried to ask God if they were right and we were wrong, because we never go. But how can you talk with God? He doesn't talk to us! Daddy says some people hear His voice, but they are hearing things! That's what he thinks. I tried to be serious, though. I said, 'All right, God, please, I'm young, and I'd like to know, so give us a signal, me and my mommy and daddy.' I knew He wouldn't — and He didn't. Later, when I went to the park, I thought there might not be a God, but somehow we have this park and the flowers are out, and how did all of this begin, that's what I'd like to know!"

I told her that most of us are as interested as she is in exactly that — how this world, with all its lovely sights and sounds, ever got going in the first place. She was a bit relieved to hear my essentially innocuous restatement of what she'd said; apparently I had at least reassured her that she was not alone in her speculations and her self-directed (or God-directed) inquiries. She pursued our discussion further: "Just because you don't go to church doesn't mean you don't think about God. I don't know where God is, but if He's somewhere, He'll be noticing all the people, not just the ones who go down the street to the church — I hope. He might not be anyplace, or He might be hiding someplace, and no one will find Him, until He decides to show up.

"Sometimes, at night, I'll see shadows outside, and I think there might be someone there, but maybe it isn't anyone, or that could be God, or some angel, in the shadow. My aunt [her mother's sister] said a dog can be nicer than people, because the dog is loyal and trusts you, and maybe if God came here, He wouldn't be a person, He could come as a nice dog!"

She stopped there, then right away retracted her assertion: she was being "silly." Her crusty, politically populist, free-thinking father had also once proposed such an idea — that God might be found in nature, in animals such as dogs, who seem "purer" than people in certain respects, or so he argued, and so Alice now conjectured. But her heart wasn't in that thesis, even as she knew her father was merely tossing around ideas in a manner meant to express, basically, an amused skepticism. Alice, however, was serious that day as she tried to describe her spiritual life. "I try to think what's right," she told me earnestly, and then, with an almost Augustinian candor, she turned to the other side of herself: "Sometimes I forget, though, and I'm not very good. I say the wrong thing, or I just do something, and later I know I've been bad. I'll look up at the stars, and I'll wonder if there is someone up there who can see right through you, and He knows what you're up to, all the time He does! Before you accuse anyone, you should think of yourself, my granny said, and she's right. She doesn't go to church, either. Mommy said she [the grandmother] liked to sew on Sundays and cook, but she did listen to the ministers preaching on Sunday [on the radio]. She'd laugh at them plenty of times!"

This distanced, wry skepticism with regard to organized religion on the part of a grandparent had already become a child's intellectual and spiritual inheritance. Alice knew of her grandmother's mocking response to radio evangelists, knew of her parents' amusement or annoyance when certain television ministers appeared on the TV screen, and was already prepared to think twice, upon watching a crowd coming out of a church: "I wonder whether it does them any good, going to that [Catholic] church. My daddy could be wrong; maybe if you go to church, you have got God's help, and you're better. But there are all these different churches — so many. Kids in my class — they fight over which religion is the best. I'll hear them, and I'll be walking home by myself, and I'll still hear them [in her head], and I'll think: now, God, what do *you* think? My mommy isn't as against religion as Daddy, but she says I should pray to God that all the people who want to 'own' Him, and fight over Him — that they stop, and then the world will be a better place. It'll be a more Christian world then! That's what I'll be thinking, and then I see a nice old lady who lives near us going to church, and it's real hard for her to get there, but she does, and she'll be so happy for the rest of her day when she comes out, so that's good."

I'd tried, on several occasions, to learn more about Alice's own spiritual life — disregarding the anticlericalism she had heard so strenuously argued at home and had already included in her moral sensibility. She was poignant and powerfully affecting when she abandoned the sarcasm (lively and astringent though it was) that her mother and father had used when surveying the neighborhood religious scene — when she, instead, looked inward, and looked ahead, as well, to future years: "The moon moving through the clouds — that's really something! I know, I know — it's the clouds moving; the moon is just there. But it looks the other way around to me! I'll see that [picture] in my eye; I'll think of the clouds, and the moon trying to get through them; or I'll think of the moon as someone beautiful, and we want to see her, but the clouds won't let us get by. Then you wonder if there's a God, and He's telling you, 'Look what is up here, and say thank you, and don't forget the moon and the stars while you're in a traffic jam someplace!' "

She apologized after uttering that statement — it wasn't especially coherent or convincing; yet she also felt it had told a lot about her struggles. She continued: "I'll never be the kind of person everyone likes. I know it. I'm not popular in school. I guess I say the wrong things sometimes. 'You can be like night and day,' Mommy tells me — because one minute I'm OK, but the next, I just want to go to my room and sit and look out the window. That's why I like the night; you can be alone, and it's quiet! My friends want to get tan; I'd rather watch the moon and the clouds. To tell you something — I'm kind of disappointed when there's only the moon in the sky! I like it better when there are clouds, and they're going by fast, and the moon slips in and out, it keeps doing that. I feel like I'm hypnotized, watching! It's then I think of God, and I think to myself: What are you going to do when you get older? My granny says, 'What do you want to be?' I don't know. If I had a choice [I'd asked], I'd be a teacher, maybe — or I'd work in the Science Museum. It's my favorite [of the museums she's visited]. I like looking at the stars, and I like seeing the rabbits and snakes and chickens. I like seeing the Charles River, and the boats. It's all part of the world, and I like looking at the people who come there [the Science Museum]: they're part of the world! I don't know who made us all, but it's nice to be here!"

As she talked, I suddenly, for the first time in a long while, and thanks to her, thought of that Boston Science Museum, of all the parents and children who walk through it daily — men and women, boys and girls, an exhibit of sorts, a procession, an aspect of the world on display. Such a broad view of things was an aspect of Alice's inward-looking mind. Although she had obtained from her parents a jaundiced view of institutional religion, even as countless millions of children in country after country obtain from their parents an unblinking devotion to what is preached in churches, mosques, or synagogues, she was no budding ideological agnostic or atheist. Rather, she was attempting to find her own values and ideals, and attempting to connect herself to the universe. Her grandmother, as a matter of fact — a blunt, utterly unpretentious woman who had put in years of factory work before she retired — was the one who described Alice's spiritual life in a most satisfactory way: "She has a real spirit to her — and she is a 'deep' girl. She looks honestly at herself, and that's rare. When I was a girl, they'd talk of 'soul-searching time,' a time to be as straight and open with yourself as you can be, and a time to figure out what you believe and where you stand. Alice is a soul-searcher!"

Others, too, are drawn to soul-searching, even though religion is no great part of their lives. Alice was not the only child in the elementary school class I taught who came from an essentially agnostic family. Two of her classmates, a boy of twelve named Norman and a girl of eleven named Sylvia, were from academic families; Norman's father taught chemistry, Sylvia's father, philosophy of science. Those two youngsters were relatively indifferent to religion — not the case, clearly, with Alice — but they were not loath to speculate on the reasons for various natural phenomena, even the possible explanations that are not strictly verifiable or "scientific." As I sat with the two of them sometimes, after class, I often marveled at their interest in and their devotion to the natural world. Their response to van Gogh's paintings was one he would have appreciated. The restlessness, the anxious upheaval, the urgent energy of his fields, skies, trees, rivers, were meant to be, collectively, a very spiritual statement: the surging transcendence of those canvases attests to the painter's sense of the divinity of all we see and hear, of the planet and beyond it the inscrutable, waiting universe, in which the entire course of history (past, present, future) becomes a mere moment, and in which, too, the most solid of places, the greatest sprawl of space, of distance, becomes a mere pinpoint. Mind-boggling ironies and paradoxes are not beyond the contemplation of children reared under no religious aegis yet encouraged at home and school to search soulfully for some view of things, or "some way," as Norman put it, "of figuring out what's going on all over the place."

Once Norman and Sylvia and I were discussing the van Gogh painting *Wheat Field and Cypress Trees,* in an enjoyable, edifying colloquy. Norman was especially effusive. (I remember thinking to myself that the artist would surely have been pleased to hear what his work could still provoke a century later.) "You look at that painting," Norman said, looking at Sylvia, "and you see an explosion — it's what is happening in the world, but *you* don't see it; van Gogh does. My dad says the guy [van Gogh] was one of the greatest. You're not supposed to expect a photograph. You know what? I was sitting and reading [at home], and it was windy, real windy out, and the wind was probably going for an hour, but I didn't notice it; but then I did, and I got up and I looked out. The wind was whistling, and you could see the trees bending. I watched the trees, and I couldn't stop, and I thought: they're dancing, that's what, they're excited. The leaves — the wind went through them. You could hear it, and the grass was bending, and some branches went in one direction, and others in the other. It made me stop and think about the world. I was looking out there and I felt different — I mean, someday I'll be gone, but the trees will be there, and the wind, and the grass. I have a friend who thinks the wind is God talking. That's what he says. I sure don't believe that. I don't know if there's a God. I don't think there is any real evidence [that He exists]. But you listen to the wind and the trees, and you stop yourself, and you realize you're part of it all. You know what I mean?"

His friend Sylvia had been listening intently and signaling yes with nods. She was much interested in art and had dreams of becoming an artist, though she would always add that she might end up with a career in business because her parents were in serious debt — a younger brother, Joey, had congenital cystic fibrosis, entailing substantial medical expenses. "When there's a storm, I always stop and listen. If there was a God, He'd be saying something! I don't think there is one, though. I've tried to pray; I've asked why my little brother was born with that disease; why he suffers so much, why he won't live a normal life; why he'll probably die when he's young, the doctors say. That's not fair; that's not justice — for a boy to be sick, always, with colds, and his lungs don't work right. When we took Joey to the hospital the other day, he seemed brave. He said whatever happens will be all right with him. I wasn't happy at all! I saw a priest come and pray for the kids, and I wanted him to come over to our room and explain why it's so unfair, what happens, and why, if people pray to God, He doesn't answer their prayers a lot of the time. My brother has seen such misery in his life — he's been in the hospital so many times, and each time he comes back with terrible stories: you just can't imagine how bad it can be for some people! Does God know about all this? — I'd like to know!"

She was taken aback by her own anger. She stopped, lowered her head, and then, in a dramatic gesture, raised it about as high as her neck would allow. A second or two later she was looking directly at Norman and me, and her blue eyes glistened. Her right hand moved toward them, wiped them. She addressed Norman: "I agree — maybe there's something out there that made us, and there's an explanation for why the world is like it is. My parents say it's all by chance — that things just happen. The teachers tell you they can explain a lot of what's happening, and we know a physicist, and he's an expert; he'll tell you how everything works — the trouble is, I can't always understand him, even when he's trying to be nice and explain things to *me*, not his college students! When we drive by a cemetery, and I see those stones, I think of my brother, and I just start crying sometimes. Maybe someday there will be a cure for cystic fibrosis. Maybe they'll be able to prevent it before you're born. But it's us — we're the ones who will make the world better that way. I don't see where God enters into the picture! I'll walk and I'll ask why I'm here and why I'm healthy and my brother isn't. Every day I'll ask — and I don't come up with answers. None. 'Look at how beautiful the ocean and the sand is,' my brother says. 'We should be so happy today.' That's what he'll say when we go to the beach. I'll say to myself: if he can be sick, and be like that, talk like that, you should be like him, Sylvia, you really should be. But a lot of the time I'm asking all these questions about things (about why this and why that) and I don't get any answers, and I begin to think that it's always going to be like that, and unless you're willing to kid yourself — like people do, a lot of them, my mom and dad say — then you just have to settle for what you've got, and expect no miracles. That's how I see it."

I saw Norman's face respond to the end of Sylvia's penultimate sentence, and as soon as she had stopped speaking, he began: "I agree. I think about things, too, just the way you do. At night, a lot, I'll be looking out the window, and it's real quiet, and you can sit and wonder if there are people like you up on other planets or stars; and you can wonder whether there is a God watching you — or maybe there are several gods, or lots of them, or angels, I don't know, but I think about it, about how it's not fair, like you said, that you and I are healthy, and others, your brother, aren't. Sure, we've got to 'settle for what you've got'; you're right — though the world's different now than it was for our parents when they were our age. Isn't that right? My folks say that all the time.

"You've got to change the world, not just 'settle for what you've got.' Maybe, if there's a God out there, that's the one thing He's given us, that we can change things. There are scientists; there are doctors; there's the space program; there's exploration in the oceans. I don't know about God, whether He exists; but we're here, you and me and your brother, even if he's sick a lot, and we can do something before we leave. I mean, if your brother was an artist, like van Gogh, he could paint, even with the cystic fibrosis, and we'd appreciate him, like we do van Gogh. Even if he's not an artist, he can be what he is, he can be your brother, and he's influencing you (isn't he?), just the way van Gogh does, influences us. It's complicated, all this, I know. But you have to find something to believe in; you can't just say it's all nothing out there. Like your own brother says, there's beauty, there's the ocean and the waves and the sand and the seashells, and there's people, your parents, my folks, our friends: all that, and that's a *lot* to 'settle for.'"

He was surprised, I thought, by his own coherence in articulating his point of view, and especially by the way he rounded out his presentation with a rhetorical flourish that nicely echoed his opening comment. He seemed to trust the flow of his thinking. "I guess I said what I wanted to say," he added — and then: "I really did." He wasn't boasting. In a way, he was (with humility) marveling at his own personal authority. His effort to think about life's meaning, to look inside himself, to utter certain deeply felt truths, were things both he and Sylvia (and the rest of us) could regard with some satisfaction and maybe even awe.

In a memorable occasion of symmetry (one I only appreciated days later as I listened to the tape and then read the transcript), Sylvia responded to Norman's declaration of commitment to this world, if not his faith in an overall meaning with respect to everyday life: "I didn't say there's nothing out there; I know there is a lot to live for. I love my family, and I love my friends. I love it when we go to a new place on a trip, and I can see new people, and you can stand there — like up in Vermont or New Hampshire — and look at all the land, for miles (if you're up a mountain), and the trees, and you're nearer the clouds. Once I was on top of Mt. Washington with my dad, and I said, 'You know, this must be the view God has of us.' He liked that. He laughed. He said, 'Right, Sylvia.' Then he told me he hopes there *is* a God. He asked me, 'Sylvia, do you believe in God?' I didn't know what to say." She stopped — and of course we both wanted to know her answer, and she knew we did, and so she told us: "I said, 'Daddy, I don't know.' I said, 'Sometimes.' He said, 'That's a good answer: sometimes.' But sometimes I don't, and that's the truth. I'm not being 'negative.' A minister told my mother she's 'negative' when she says Christmas and Easter are big fakes now — they are holidays designed for the stores, and people just buy and buy. If you know that's true, you just have to say it. That's being positive, not negative!"

Norman liked that and said so. The two of them fell silent.

They had exhausted their respective lines of argument, and themselves as well. They both smiled, a message from each to the other that they were not any the less friendly for their energetic, intimate, at times strained discussion. As I sat there, I wondered whether the very intensity and candor, even at times passion, of their exchanges weren't something each would agree to uphold as worth a lot, deserving respect and esteem, even veneration. Norman and Sylvia were not about to say that to each other; nor had they articulated the obvious regard and affection they felt for one another. But what I couldn't stop remembering, afterward, was not only some of their words and ideas but the looks each gave to the other: the acknowledgment and appreciation that a friend tenders a friend.

To be sure, those two young people had learned at home a kind of doubtfulness that accounted for their own second thoughts and qualms about the received religious tradition. Many "religious" children I spoke with had second thoughts, too, of course. Much of their soul-searching partook less of religious reflection than of an individual's struggle to make some persisting sense of life. Indeed, many of these children proclaimed to me their conventional faith one day, and the next, emphasized the difficulties they had in holding on to that faith through thick and thin. One of my students in the Cambridge art history class, a devoutly Catholic girl, asked me after a class in which I'd shown a slide of a medieval *Angelo Musicante* (a musician angel), "whether those angels always were good Catholics." At first I answered that I couldn't be sure. I explained that the artist (Fra Angelico) was a "brother," who took his vows seriously, I assumed, and who perhaps wanted to express an order of faith, of devotion, which we would call "angelic" in nature. I didn't like what I heard myself saying — it was evasive, academic talk, evidence in this instance of my own hedging. Talk straight to this child, I said to myself; shrug your shoulders, say "I dunno"; shake your head, say "It beats me," a phrase William Carlos Williams used to use. But this girl, only ten years old and a relative stranger to me (I didn't even know her name yet), was quite unintimidated by — or perhaps uncomprehending of — my short speech. "I say my prayers at night," she said, "but afterwards, sometimes, I'll lie there and think, and I wonder about how I came to be the one who's here, and why I was born me and not someone else — all that, and I know lots of people have those thoughts, they just do."

Yes, I certainly do, I thought as I smiled and nodded and reassured her and thanked her for her willingness to be so frank about and generous with her personal life. She had let me know that her pious moments were followed by other moments — that, like Pascal, she knew the bedrock perplexity and aloneness that make both faith and reason quake before them. Pascal's dilemma is the dilemma of many of the children I have met, who seek faith with all their heart, all their might, yet also know much of honest self-confrontation, of twentieth-century secular soul-searching, during which, as with Pascal centuries ago, "nature confutes the skeptics, and reason confutes the dogmatists."

So it goes: with respect to faith and doubt, belief and unbelief, we are all "on the edge," as Reinhold Niebuhr told us in a seminar of his I took long ago as a medical student. He used that expression convincingly. We rather guessed his own hesitations, reversals, and lapses. He would take us aside amid the solemnity of a place called Union Theological Seminary in order to converse, to acknowledge, to ponder, to vacillate, to confess.[3]

"I don't know where the soul is," the ten-year-old girl said to me at the outset of a conversation, "but it's in me, I'm sure — I feel it." She was telling me, as a matter of course, that she had heard of a soul, had wondered about it (where? of what nature?), and had launched her investigation. The result was a sense over time that within her "it" was there to call upon, to address. Other children, more adventurous and even more secular and sophisticated, have been known to ask themselves, ask teachers, and often ask me wherein "this soul," as one boy put it, "differs from the mind." A few children, truly and highly secular, have even asked me about the unconscious — whether *it* might be where the soul is, or what the soul is. Yes, I say; probably, I say; to some extent, I say; I say, I'm not sure, or I'm not so sure. As for them, the nature of their question sometimes reveals their conviction: "Isn't the soul the unconscious?" But some who ask are truly unsure, while others are wise in their philosophical directness. One girl of thirteen cautioned me, "It's not important, where you think the soul is; it's what you're looking for with it, that's important." I wanted to know what *she* was "looking for with it," and she had no trouble giving me an answer: "I guess for some clues about what this life is all about." Then she laughed with a kind of self-assurance that not all American children her age possess. She had helped me consider an interesting possibility: that at least one small part of the unconscious is not Freud's "seething cauldron" after all, but rather, as Isaiah would have it, an alert "watchman," asking and being asked, "what of the night?"

The Child as Pilgrim

ALL DURING MY PEDIATRIC RESIDENCY in the late 1950s, children were being called "healthy" or "unhealthy." We young physicians-in-training had charts, graphs, lists, a host of memorized numbers or "indices" to call upon — and we used them in the constant decisions and judgments we had to make. We emphasized other words for the sake of variety — a "normal" child, a "well-baby clinic"; or a "sick" child, an "ill" child, a child with "a disease." When I switched to child psychiatry, the same polarities governed our daily practice. One boy had "serious problems"; another boy was in "serious trouble"; a girl required "prolonged treatment," while the next girl had, we all knew, "major emotional difficulties." On the other hand, a supervisor would remind us, rather rarely, it seemed, that some people are "basically intact, psychologically," and even appear to be not only "sane" but of "solid psychological make-up." After days, even weeks, of hearing about the various forms of "insanity" or the "serious character disorders," I'd always perk up when a child was given even the grudging designation of an "adequate personality." When the attending physician or guest lecturer went a step further and made mention of "mental health" or, more quaintly, "good mental hygiene," we were both interested and perplexed. I remember, in fact, the time a fellow resident dared to ask a supervisor exactly what "mental health" actually is. "Good question," he replied — but then this shrewd diagnostician, usually a talkative teacher, turned unusually reticent. He described the concept of "mental health" through repeated emphasis on what was absent, what was *not* to be found by an astute psychiatric observer: no "psychosis," no "character disorder," no "serious acting out," no evidence of an impairing "neurosis." We all by then, of course, had come to know that everyone has a neurosis, large or small.

By the time I had finished my work in child psychiatry and begun psychoanalytic training, I was fairly savvy about all those labels. I'd even learned, with the help of an older child psychoanalyst, Marian Putnam (so wise, so blessed with common sense and a sense of humor), to go easy with those labels, even to use plain, ordinary "lay language" when thinking about and "working up" the children I would be treating. She once said as I sat in her Cambridge study, "Since we've all got our problems, it's what we do with them that distinguishes us." I was impressed — but, reluctant to surrender pathology at one swoop, I countered with refutation as well as acceptance: "Yes, but some 'problems' are much worse than others," the plaintive cry of someone who was just finishing a five-year stint of struggling with those "problems" and was beginning to feel like an expert. Dr. Putnam replied, "True, but some people are also much better able to deal with their problems, however severe, than others; and some people whose problems don't seem all that serious nevertheless get quite undone by them — and you and I wonder why that happens."

I recall, even now, my anxiety. If some were troubled badly, yes, but had the knack of living with those troubles, and if others impressed us — or, at the least, impressed *her!* — as not so deeply disturbed, though they hadn't figured out ways to come to terms with what ailed them, what, then, should I think or do? I began to feel the ground under me giving way; I fell silent, unable to ask those two questions aloud. Dr. Putnam read my face with the canniness of someone who had sat through many a spell with silent, confused, alarmed children and adults, not to mention a psychiatric and psychoanalytic trainee. "Maybe, at a certain moment, it's best to think differently about the people we see. Maybe we shouldn't be emphasizing so strongly what 'problems' they have, but how they get through their lives — with a reasonable kind of psychological success or with obvious personal failure."

She was, I understood, restating her message, but she was pushing it a bit further, too. Her first sentence was a general one — the advisability of changing one's point of view and, with it, one's language. In her second sentence she was reminding me, by implication, that doctors, child psychiatrists, are sometimes blind to some aspects of what children present to us, even as we are alert to others. We are not obliged to try knowing all things or being all things to our patients. Nevertheless, it is in our own best interest that we not succumb to an occupational hazard, the psychiatric version of synecdoche: confusing the whole lives of children with the aspect of those lives to which we are privy.

By the early 1960s many of us in child psychiatry and psychoanalysis were eager to follow Dr. Putnam's advice. We emphasized the ego defenses, as Anna Freud had started suggesting we do way back in the late 1930s. Rather than endlessly concentrate on pathology, on instincts and drives, on eruptions of looniness from the unconscious, we looked closely at how people came to terms with the lusts and rages that inhabit everyone. However, we kept on separating the good from the bad, the favored from the criticized, even the saved from the condemned. Some patients had "immature" defenses, whereas others relied upon the "mature" kind. When we liked a person, we talked of "ego-syntonic" defenses; when we felt otherwise, we grimly diagnosed "primitive" defenses. I began to notice that class was a bigger determinant than we cared to admit. I well remember the agreeable psychological adjectives we applied to alcoholics who, though not very nice to their families, were rich and well educated; and I well remember the negative labels pinned on those alcoholics, some of them quite amiable, who were poor or from working-class families. To be blunt, though we had changed our angle of vision, our adjectives were still sorting people out morally as well as psychiatrically.

Such distinctions really came to my mind in a painful way one day when I attended a psychiatric conference at the Children's Hospital in Boston and heard a child discussed whose parents were well known in Boston's social and intellectual world. The boy was exceedingly troubled. We all knew he would need a long hospitalization. We discussed the child at great length, worried over his future, made our recommendations. We also, I noted, bent over backward to be nice to this family — not only in person but in the way we talked. Though honest and thorough both with ourselves and with the family, we were also trying to put the best possible light on things, and our language was, I noticed, rather tactful. We would even choose lay euphemisms (among ourselves) to spare the child and his family some of the grim clinical words we usually attributed to children with a similar diagnosis and prognosis. He was, one of us pronounced, in a "sad situation"; another added that it was a "troubling picture." How kind and sensitive, I thought — and how civil, too.

That morning we also discussed our second "case," also a boy, a year older than the one we'd just been holding up to compassionate scrutiny. This boy came from a rather impoverished family and neighborhood. His parents had not gone to college. The father was a furniture mover; the mother took care of a large Irish-American brood. (She was born in Galway and had come to America at sixteen.) This boy, like the first, was quite troubled, and we thought he, too, might well need extended hospitalization. But we were not nearly so shy with him or his parents. We used one clinical expression after another. Absent were the delicacy of language, the hedged remarks and guarded comments, the evasion in a pleasing vernacular, the discreet or diplomatic circumlocutions. We thought of these two boys, and talked of them, differently. Their "charts," the write-ups of their "case histories," were also quite different in terms of tone, of phrasing. The subjectivity of doctors, our social values and our personal experiences, decisively influenced the way we responded to those two children.

If the observer's personal life determines how he or she regards a child, the observer's intellectual interests are also of considerable consequence. A pediatrician looks at weight and height charts, at x-rays and laboratory reports, at "positives" and "negatives" found on physical examination — and says a child is "normal" or has some suspicious "lesion" or "process at work," or indeed is "sick" because in the throes of a "disease." A psychiatrist listens to emotional "problems," whether declared by the child or, quite often, by the parents or schoolteachers, and makes an "evaluation," writes a diagnosis, then a recommendation for therapy. But both those doctors would gladly admit that there is more to any child than the state of his or her physical health, the nature of the child's emotional condition. There is, for instance, his or her cognitive and intellectual life. How lively is the child's interest in reading, writing, arithmetic? How responsive is the child to the things of this world, to sights and sounds, to the messages brought outside the schoolroom by radio and television and movies, and, inside it, to the instruction offered by teachers, athletic coaches? Or the learning offered by scout leaders, members of the clergy, friends and relatives?

A child can be sick in body or troubled in mind and still do quite well in school. A child can be healthy in body and reasonably solid emotionally and do poorly in school. Plenty of children who are vulnerable physically and emotionally find ways to excel in school — at athletics, with hobbies and extracurricular activities. Words such as "bright" and "talented" and "skilled" and "outgoing" ought to remind us to regard the child as a member of a community or as a potential worker, to mention roles not always considered important by some of us who work with boys and girls in well-to-do American suburbs. In Latin America and Africa, millions of children are already at work by the time they are nine or ten. "He is the best of my children," a mother in a Rio de Janeiro *favela* once told me. The son she was boasting of was an accomplished entrepreneur at eight: he had organized a group of children who washed cars and shined shoes in the city's affluent Copacabana district. The boy's ingenuity, his shrewdness, his initiative, his ability to organize and lead others, made for his "excellence" in the eyes of his mother and also in the eyes of the nuns who tried to work with the poorest of the poor in that neighborhood. This boy had not done well in the few years of schooling he had with those nuns, and I can, alas, vouch for his severe pediatric and psychiatric difficulties. Still, he was an outstanding success story in his community, and I must admit that it took me a long time to see his achievements for what they were. Moreover, his moral life was of considerable interest. He was anxious to share the money he earned with others — his mother, his brothers and sisters, his friends, even those nuns, to whom he gave a substantial sum each week.

To know that boy was to be reminded of yet another way of looking at children — distinguishing those who are considerate, good in their behavior, from those who are callous, mean-spirited, self-absorbed. Are the boys or girls who are in the best health, who are fairly sound emotionally, who do well in school — are they necessarily the most decent and kind and thoughtful toward others? No teacher I've met in the past three decades wants to claim that a pediatrician's report or a battery of psycho-diagnostic tests or an IQ test will tell much about the character of children, about their everyday moral life.

More and more these days we pay heed to the special problems of children with disabilities, and to the special problems of children who have experienced the terrible stresses of war, of forced migration from their nation, of homelessness, of racial or religious persecution. None of these ways of thinking about children need be exclusive, of course. The child's "house has many mansions" — including a spiritual life that grows, changes, responds constantly to the other lives that, in their sum, make up the individual we call by a name and know by a story that is all his, all hers.

Over the years, I've asked children to tell me who they are — by saying whatever words they wish to say, or drawing whatever picture will enable them to forsake words for a visual statement. I am interested, obviously, in which of the analytic constructs, which of the theoretical paradigms, these children themselves have chosen to regard as congenial, inviting, suggestive. To my constant surprise, the variety of responses is enormous. Even when I am in a particular neighborhood — and therefore the national, regional, social, and racial characteristics are the same for child after child — I find astonishing differences in the choices made by children as they prepare to present themselves through one perspective or another.

One day in a fifth-grade classroom of a Lawrence, Massachusetts, elementary school — with a mix of white, black, and Hispanic children from working-class families — I noted many angles of self-analysis at work as child after child responded to the following question: "Tell me, as best you can, who you are — what about you matters most, what makes you the person you are." I would then qualify: "If you don't want to emphasize any one thing, any one quality or trait or characteristic, then include others, but try to single out one for special mention or consideration."

The children were not as perplexed by that request as I thought they might be. Some asked for further explanation, but most sat and thought about themselves, then swung into action with a pencil or pen, writing, or with crayons and paints, depicting themselves alone or in some situation that made their point. One boy told me about himself very pointedly: "I'm just me. I'm a good athlete. I'd like to be one when I'm older. A professional. I haven't decided, baseball or football. I like both." Right across the aisle another boy wrote: "It depends. Some days I take care of our dog more than anyone. I'm his best friend. On the next day I could be lazy. I'd like to be a doctor that cures animals. I forgot the name [of that kind of doctor]. But I think I'll work like Dad on cars. I don't know."

Nearby a girl sat longer than the others with her eyes fastened on the ceiling. I wondered whether she'd write or draw anything. Suddenly, as the others were finishing their efforts, she began hers: "I'm the one who's writing this! I'm the one at home who can make our Gramps laugh. He's old, and he doesn't laugh much. I don't tickle him. I just tell him jokes. My mom said without me Gramps would be sad." When she had finished, she turned the paper over, the only child to do so. I said nothing, but when she took the paper in her hand and began crumpling it, I became concerned. I caught her eye, motioned with my head for her to come to the front of the room. She obliged readily. She brought her wrinkled piece of paper with her, and I asked her if I might read it. She did not hand the paper to me, so I leaned over and read what she had to say about herself. "This is quite good," I told her. Her face was blank. I added, "It's very moving." She looked at me directly, then told me this, a bit despondently: "I don't know what else to say about myself." I answered, "You've said a lot, a whole lot." She was still holding the paper in her hand, not quite knowing what to do with it. I hadn't collected the papers of the other students and had to decide whether to ask for hers or let her throw away what she'd written, if she wished. I told her I'd love to keep her paper — show it to my wife and sons. Her face now displayed a full smile, but she was still apologetic, even self-critical: "OK, but maybe I should do another one, too, because in this one I'm boasting, and you shouldn't do that, the nuns tell you." Yes, I told her, she could do another one — but I wanted to keep this one. I also wanted to talk with her more about those nuns and their philosophy, but this was a full and busy class.

Back at her seat the girl seemed not at a loss for words, I noticed, as she worked on her second statement. Others were coming up to me to hand me their words and in a few instances their drawings, and were then beginning to whisper softly but noticeably; yet the girl didn't seem at all disturbed. By the time she finished she was the last one in the class to hand in her paper — and only upon doing so did she seem to realize that by straggling she had earned the obvious displeasure of some of her classmates, who were anxious to get going on our next assignment. I sat there at the teacher's desk holding a stack of papers, reading hers, the one most recently handed to me: "I'm like I am now, but I could change when I grow up. You never know who you'll be until you get to that age when you're all grown. But God must know all the time."

I was taken by that last sentence; I smiled and then looked up at her. There she was, watching my face and responding to it with a full smile of her own. I asked the students if I could read aloud their answers, keeping the authors anonymous. They enthusiastically endorsed the idea with many yeses, a ruler or two slapped on the desk, and, best of all, a sudden, welcome stillness in that room — such a contrast with the mix of bodily restlessness and whispering that make up a low-level background noise many teachers learn to accept as normal, until a hush descends and a taste of true quiet can be enjoyed.

As I read the statements, the room filled with applause or snickers or groans or, mostly, a combination of all these. Sometimes the identity of the author became apparent with a blush, a head bent, a smile, a frown. Sometimes the author was wonderfully adept at concealing his or her identity. But the children all seemed quite excited by this exercise. (Because of their enthusiasm, it was an exercise I would repeat many times in various classrooms in Lawrence and other cities.)

That day, several statements earned the ultimate award from the students: they all held their tongues, their faces registering surprise or strong interest or sometimes befuddlement. One girl attracted a good deal of attention with this: "It matters to me that I do one good deed every day. I try to. Then I feel better. If I keep it up, maybe I'll go to heaven." Another girl had a quite different approach: "I'm already a good cook. I have lots of menus I can do. My mother says I do better than her. I might get a job in a restaurant, or I could go get a job in some office. I don't know which." A girl who sat beside her shunned such ambitions: "I'll be a pilot, maybe, or fly in space. I'll get a computer. I don't want to sit at home and mend clothes. My mother hates it. She says I should be the one to show what I can do. Then, I won't be poor, if I do."

The class clapped after I read that one, the only time. These boys and girls lived close to poverty, lived in a city once full of mills that employed thousands of newly arrived immigrants at low wages. Now the city was struggling with unemployment, even as new immigrants from Puerto Rico and the Caribbean islands attempted to catch hold of the fabled American ladder. In their self-presentations, some children made reference to that aspect of the city of Lawrence's life, of their own lives. One boy remarked: "I'd like to be the one who owns a good car. I'd like to live in a nice house. I may be a lawyer. I doubt it. I'll go into the service. I get good grades, so I might be a lawyer. Who knows?"

I was touched by that second mention of law, that rhetorical question, and my voice must have shown it. The children heard the emotion and responded without first raising their hands: "You *can* be one, you *can* be a lawyer!" They didn't know whom they were addressing — but I began to understand that they were addressing themselves, though I fear it took me longer than it should have. The look on one boy's face at last made me see.

I remember how impressed many of us were by another rallying cry, this by a girl: "I'm here. I could have been born there, on the island [Puerto Rico]. I'm staying in school. My sisters ask why. I'm the youngest. I'm the one who will graduate. I'll try to get a good job." Some children were more original or idiosyncratic in the way they defined themselves. A red-headed girl, the only one in the class, described herself in this fashion: "I'm the one with red hair. I have a birthmark. Everyone knows me for that. I have learned how to swim. I swim very fast. I am tall, and my legs help my swimming a lot. I'd like to be a champion, but I don't know. I'll try, and I have a good chance, the teacher says. If I become a good swimmer, I could be on TV. That would be a big day!" For that comment she got a few encouraging cries of support.

One boy's contribution was truly different: "I don't know what to say. I was put here by God, and I hope to stay until He says OK, enough, come back. Then, I'll not be here any more. By the end I hope I'll find out why I was sent down, and not plenty of others. There must be a lot waiting. God decides." This autobiographical paper produced silence and elicited looks of curiosity, even apprehension. The children looked around, but the author was being quite impassive, laying no claim to authorship or notoriety. A boy raised his hand to ask the only question: "What does God decide?" I was in a bit of a bind: I wasn't going to ask the child who wrote the statement to explain himself or herself (all the papers had been unsigned); nor did I think it was my right to do an *explication de texte*.

In a dramatic move, the only one of its kind during our long time together, the boy who had written those words raised his hand and spoke: "I can tell you; I was trying to say that it's up to God — He decides who's born. He puts us here, and then He's the one who says we should go back and be with Him." The result was absolute silence. Someone outside the school gunned a car. A nearby church's bell announced the eleventh hour of the morning. Several children raced down the hall outside, laughing and scuffling — but still the quiet held. As I prepared to read another paper, a hand went up — that of a Puerto Rican girl who was bright but didn't usually say much. "Well, how *does* He decide? How can He possibly keep track of everyone? I asked our priest, and he said all kids want to know, and you just have to have faith, and if you don't, then you're in trouble, and besides you'll never know, because that's God's secret. He can do things and we think they are impossible, but He does them, anyway. But I still can't see how God can keep His eyes on everyone, and my uncle says it's all a lot of nonsense."

The class broke wide open. Hands shot up. Mercifully, the children started speaking to one another without waiting for me to call on them — which I dislike having to do, because it dampens enthusiasm. "Your uncle shouldn't talk like that," said the boy whose paper had caused the uproar.

"Why not?"

Then others were speaking thick and fast: "We'll never know about God, until we die."

"True, but we know *something*: He did come here once!"

"Yes, but that was a long time ago. What has He been doing since he died and left?"

"If you go to church, He'll be there. You can go and get Communion."

"Right, but I still don't see how anyone, even God, keeps all those records on everyone."

"No, no, there aren't records! He just *does!* You can't explain it. God isn't a person like us."

"He *was* one! Isn't that so?"

"Yes, but just for a while. Then He went back to being God."

"I know, I know — but I still can't understand this business of God 'choosing' people. Isn't that what we're talking about?"

"Yes, but we'll never get the answer. You just have to have faith; that is what the priest would say."

"Do you think the priests know the answer?"

"No more than we do! They just know that no one does, other than God."

"I believe in God, but it's hard to know whether you're doing the right thing, what God wants, or the wrong thing."

"That's where the priests come in."

"And ministers; I'm not Catholic!"

"But how can you say the priests can tell you (or the ministers) what's right to do and wrong — if only God knows? Who says the priests are right, or some minister?"

"Well, they pray a lot more than you and I do. Isn't that true?"

"How do you know how much they pray? Just because you're a priest doesn't mean you're praying more than someone who isn't a priest but he just prays a lot!"

"Most people don't have time to pray. They have to work all day, and they come home tired."

"Those priests, they don't work as hard as my dad. He says a lot of the priests, they've got it pretty easy!"

"You have to have the priests and the ministers!"

"Why? Why can't anyone just try being good, and pray to God? If you keep doing that, you'll get there — to heaven!"

"I agree!"

"So do I!"

"I do, too — but our priest is nice, and he helped my mother when she lost the baby just before it was supposed to be born. They operated, and the baby was 'gone'; he'd died. It was a boy. The priest really helped us out."

"I know a priest, and he drinks all the time, and you can see: he has a red face. Daddy says he starts with the wine, from Communion, and by night, he's into vodka."

"How do you know — how does your father know?"

"He knows! We know! You don't think priests are any different than the rest of us, do you, or ministers?"

"They *are* different; they spend their lives trying to get closer and closer to God. That's what they do with their lives!"

"*So,* good for them — but that's what we're all supposed to do! Isn't that right?"

"Right, but do you do it? Do most people?"

"Wait a minute, a lot of people *do* — they try to find out what God wants, and then they do it!"

"What do you mean? Who?"

"My mother. My father. My grandparents. My sister — lots of people."

"They're all in your family! How about other families?"

"Hey, come on! I know my family the best, so I'm mentioning them. How about your family?"

"Don't be a wise guy! I'll match my folks to yours! My mother starts the day with her rosary! She's in there pitching, I'll tell you! My dad comes home and he's white as a sheet. He's been up from early morning — when it's dark — and he can barely take a shower, he's so tired. He says prayers for us when we sit down to have supper. Every night he says, 'Please God, look at us, and smile, and help us be as good as possible.' I know it by heart."

"Why are we fighting now? We should stop!"

"We're not fighting! We're talking! We're discussing what he said [pointing at the boy who had said, "God decides"]; at least we started because of him — I think."

"It doesn't make any difference who started it; we're just talking about God and church and all. What's wrong with that?"

"No one said it's wrong! Let's just take it easy! Soon the bell will ring."

"I still say, everyone here can try to be good and God will notice — whether you go to church or not. It's up to you, whether you go."

"OK, OK. The time I'm closest with God, I'm in church. You can have it your way, though."

"Do you think God likes what we're saying here?"

"How do you know?"

"I didn't say I know! I just asked!"

"No one knows, right? Only He knows, right?"

"Right! But you can try to find out what He wants. That's why you pray!"

"I agree. I see my grandfather, he's way in his sixties or seventies, praying, and it's nice. I pray, too."

"We all should! I hope I remember to, when I'm as old as your grandfather. I might forget!"

"Not if you make a habit of it. That's the way, make a habit."

"Each person prays the way he's learned. My mom says: pray when you feel you want to, then it's genuine. She doesn't force us to pray just because it's bedtime or we're eating."

"I agree with her. She's right."

"That's what *you* think! Other people have *their* opinions!"

"Let's not argue over when you should pray! Let's pray that we keep praying for the rest of our lives. Isn't that what you should do?"

"I agree."

"I do, too."

"It's just as important to pray to God as it is to be smart in school, right?"

At this point the class suddenly fell silent. All eyes turned toward the teacher's desk, where I was. I realized how closely they were listening, and I wondered not so much how to answer but whether I could be brief and somehow not block further discussion. I'd been enchanted, and I hated to be the one to ring the curtain down through some ponderous judgment. I said, "Yes, I agree."

I expected the lively, even heated exchanges to resume right away, but the silence continued. No one's hand in the air. No one's voice. Are they tired? I wondered — and they had good reason to be. Let's call it quits, I thought, though we had some time left. I had planned to ask the class to do some more drawing or painting, maybe of a Biblical scene they found memorable. Perhaps that — yes, I'd suggest to the children that they pick up their crayons or paints and use them. But I found myself thinking about the great run we'd had, and I felt that somehow we'd gotten sidetracked at a time when many of the children still had more to say. We'd stumbled into this gloriously edifying moment; had we said goodbye to it? Just as I was glancing up to make yet another suggestion about what to do, one of the children, a girl who had said rather little until then, spoke up: "We should do this more often. You think a lot when you're listening, and then you say what you're thinking, and you don't forget what you've heard — when it's this kind of talk."

"Right," said the girl sitting beside her. "I'll hear my mother and my grandma and grandpa talk like this some times, especially when they've had lots of trouble. They try to figure out what they should do. They get upset, then they calm down. You have these bad times, and you learn what to do. You think about God — how He had his bad times, too; my grandpa reminds us of them. He says you should keep thinking of them. You march through life, he says. It's a long time you march — if you're lucky. My sister, she died and she was only four, four and a half."

She took a long time saying those words. She hesitated between the sentences, and she had a slight stammer. I had on other occasions seen some of her classmates snicker behind her back, and I was worried they'd do so now. Two or three were tempted at first, but by the time she was quoting her grandfather, telling us about the march we make through life, she had the room quite still. When she mentioned the death of her sister, the children looked at her with great concern. Some faces tightened up, and the girl beside her wiped her eyes.

We were all, again, quiet. The idea of life as a "march" captured my imagination. I wanted to explore the image with the children. Would they be agreeable? Should we take a break? I was about to do so — suggest we meet after lunch — when the girl who had begun to tear up decided to speak. She looked at her neighbor and said, "If you die when you're only a young kid, then you'll go to heaven. So your sister is there, up there. It's when you get older that you can lose out!"

Nods of agreement, a few smiles, a couple of "yuhs" — both from boys, I noticed, one of whom addressed the question of age and its hazards: "Sure, you get older and you can get in trouble, big trouble. Look at all the kids from the high school who get arrested. There's drugs; there's gangs. You can end up in jail if you don't watch your step. My dad, he'd like to move us out of this city, to some place that's nicer, but where's the dough? You need big bucks to live in Andover."

"Do you think — where did you get the idea that if you move out of here to some fancy town, that'll get you to heaven? Crazy! The priest tells us every week that Jesus loved the poor. My mama says there has to be some advantage to being poor!"

"He's right, she's right!"

"Come on, come on: I wasn't saying Andover is a ticket to heaven. I was just saying that you get into more trouble here than you do in Andover. There's more trouble here, so you get into more trouble; it's that simple."

"If you don't want to get into trouble, you won't. It's up to you. You can get into trouble in Andover, too, if you want to. Besides, the town is full of snobs. Who wants to live where snobs live?"

"I do!"

"Well, go move there!"

"I would — we would, if we could. We don't have the money."

"I'd never leave where we live, our street. If you're thinking of heaven, I'll tell you something: Andover won't help. You've got a better chance right here in Lawrence: that's what I think."

"I'm not thinking heaven; I'm thinking of my life — when I grow up. Who wants to live here, if you can do better! We came here [from Puerto Rico] to do better, and you mean now that we're here we're not supposed to do better?"

"Hey, no one's telling people they shouldn't do better! Someone said it makes a difference whether you're good or you're bad when you get older. Right? Someone said if you get into trouble, then you won't get into heaven. Right? Then someone said the way to stay out of trouble is to move away from it. Right? So what's the big deal? They don't want people like us in Andover. Everyone knows that! If we moved in, they'd move out! That's how it is."

"Maybe we're on the wrong track — we're really off base. Jesus got into a *lot* of trouble! In Sunday school they're always telling us He got into trouble. The priest spelled this word, 'outcast,' on the blackboard, and he made us memorize it. He tested us on it. You think there are lots of outcasts in Andover? Big shots, not outcasts! Let's all stay here! We can get to heaven if we try hard. We can go to church and ask God to let us in. We can stay away from gangs in Lawrence. There's no law that says you have to join a gang!"

"No law, but plenty of guns and knives, and they use them!"

"Come on, look at my folks and yours; they weren't in gangs — ever. My papa, he's been working all his life. He has two jobs. He slaves away, and he says he's glad to do it, so we can eat and have a roof over us. He'll get to heaven! I hope I can be as good as him. That'd be great!"

General applause, and I joined in. We stared at each other. I thought we were at an end. Still half an hour before lunch, I noticed, looking furtively at my watch. The school clocks weren't working — hadn't for a month. Suddenly the girl who had talked about "marching through life" said, "That's right; we should try to be as good as our parents, as good as the best person we know. God will help us if we try. He's sent us here, and we've got a good chance to get to see Him in heaven, if we're good in our life."

"I agree, but look at all the trouble around. My father was robbed the other day; he lost his whole week's paycheck. You can be good and people just take advantage of you."

"I know," she answered, "you're right. But you can fight back. You can be as strong as possible. You can remember that God will help you at the end."

"That's true, but what about *now*? I know people, they pray and they go to church a lot, and they're still in bad shape. People still take advantage of them." She fell silent. She nodded her head and looked sad, downcast.

A boy across the room came out fighting: "Life is a big boxing match and wrestling match. You can have the worst luck. But you mustn't give up. My uncle had polio. He's in a wheelchair for life. But does he give up? No. He doesn't feel sorry for himself, either. He doesn't need Andover. Andover needs him! He tries to be useful. He gets around. He's good with kids. They've got him working, and he'll give his shirt to you, if you need something from him and he has it. You talk about 'marching through life.' He can't walk but he's 'marching.' He says God has been good to him! My mom says, 'Can you imagine it — your uncle saying that!' You see it's all in what you decide to do with yourself."

"I agree, a hundred percent!"

"I agree — but you can decide to do lots with yourself and not get anywhere, and it's because you get bum breaks or people are unfair to you."

"Yes, but if you know you've done your best, then you'll be all right."

"I'm not sure you'll be all right! What if you can't pay your bills? What if you don't have money for food or rent, enough money?"

"That's right! I think religion falls down sometimes — I mean, the priest gets his food and he lives in the house near the church, but the people who go there on Sunday, it can be real tough on them. The priest shouldn't give us too many lectures, my dad says!"

"Our priest is nice. He'd give us anything. He's a real nice guy. He told us in [Sunday] school, 'Think of God and He'll think of you, all through your life.' I hope God does think of us while we're thinking of Him! The priest says you mustn't expect God to get you out of every mess you get into, but He'll be your friend at the end when it really counts!"

"Lots of people could use some favors right now; that's the truth! My dad lost his job. What should he do? Pray? He's trying to find another one — but so far, no luck!"

"You're right, we need help now, not only when we're dying!"

"I agree, but that's not what God does! We're here, and we're kind of on our own, I think. That's what they tell you in church, don't they?"

"Well, they do; but they're always telling you to pray to God, and He'll help you. It doesn't make sense — there's one opinion, and there's the other. How do you get the right answer?"

The girl who had us marching through life spoke again: "You don't get a right answer! You try to be good; you try to be good as long as you live — and then God will welcome you. I think that's right. I think you have to wait, and in the end He'll be on your side, so long as you've been good."

"But what if you're in real trouble! It's not so easy to be good if you're hungry! If you're rich, it's easier to be good!"

"Hey, that's not true! A lot of rich people, they're crooks! They don't care about anyone but themselves. Anyway, she wasn't saying it's good to be poor! She was only saying: if you try and be good, God won't forget you, and He was poor Himself, remember that!"

No hands raised. None of the spontaneous exclamations that had dominated the classroom during this intense time. Some children, of course, would never speak at all unless called upon, and I had been trying to negotiate on their behalf while also letting the less inhibited children speak out. The urgency of the vocal students had carried us along for over an hour. As I sat there, watching my tape recorder's small red light, writing a few words on a piece of paper as reminders of the magic that I'd heard in that clasroom, the outpouring of ideas and sentiments and deeply felt attitudes confronting one another, I found myself, finally, looking at those children in a new light, one they had provided, actually, as young pilgrims just setting out on a journey, getting ready to "march through life." Here they were, after all that, sitting quietly and remembering that "He was poor Himself." They weren't fidgety. They weren't whispering furtively. They weren't arranging and rearranging things on their desks. They weren't moving around. No yawns. No impatient stares at the slow-moving, inaccurate clock. No glances at the dirty windows, which offer such inviting alternatives to children who feel inadequate, irritated, misunderstood. No hands raised with the endless diversionary requests boys and girls have learned to throw at their teachers. (Can I go to the bathroom? Can I sharpen my pencil? Can I get some paper for my desk?) No sullen faces — no eyes glaring out of frustration and anger, none of the resentment that follows the experience of classroom put-downs at the hands of grown teachers.

I corrected myself. I was, perhaps, romanticizing this eerie lull. The children were spent and tired. I had no need to embellish, to exaggerate, to attribute anything to anything. I watched them a bit more warily. *There,* a girl had dropped her pencil and was leaning down to find it, pick it up. *There,* another girl was brushing off dust, real or imaginary, from her dress. *There,* a boy had yet again violated school regulations, taken a stick of gum out of his pants pocket and put it into his mouth. Now he squeezed the densely crumpled gumpaper in his right hand and self-consciously chewed the gum slowly enough not to be caught. (I am not his teacher, I thought; I'll never report him. Even if I were his teacher, I'd not wage such a struggle with him. Or would I, if I had the day-to-day responsibility for the class? It's easy for me, an outsider, to be so kindhearted to the students, so condescending to the teachers, in this school where I'm a guest.) *There,* too, was the girl who, more than anyone, started us off — and now she was looking at her shoes, wiping off with her right hand some dirt from one of them, then inspecting her fingernails: no saintly gift to us sinners from on high, but just one more child struggling to make a go of life.

I began to think of announcing the after-lunch agenda for the twenty-seven boys and girls who had been earnest and good enough to put up with me once a week for many months — and today, since nine-thirty. But the girl who had become our prophet spoke instead: "What do you think — do you think God heard us talk here this morning?" I was stunned by the question. She had a slight smile on her face. I felt uncertain about her intent with the question, and I thought of blaming her for trying to put me on the spot — as if she couldn't have asked the question with no animus at all, after all our frank exchanges. I had to say something. "I hope so." "Me, too," she replied. The children, in a general murmur of assent, echoed her exact words or said "Yup" or "Uh huh." The morning came to an end as I spoke of the smell of spaghetti sauce from the cafeteria.

That evening and during the days that followed, my wife and I mulled over what had happened on that one morning. By afternoon the children were altogether different. They'd eaten, and for that reason were a bit slow. They also had no more to say, wanting instead to draw pictures. Their pictures were no different from others they'd been doing — with the same levels of artistic ability and of devotion or commitment to the task at hand, the same sorts of subject matter. Nor did my wife and I, for all our contemplation, have much to conclude — other than to reflect on a metaphor given us by the young girl. (I did at last learn to remember her name: Ginny — a nickname for someone who didn't like the name Virginia. "I'll never call a kid I have *that!*" she had said.)

They are marching through life, they are pilgrims,[1] my wife kept insisting — travelers on a road with some spiritual purpose in mind. But what proof did we have? The children certainly hadn't called themselves, or thought of themselves as, pilgrims in any way we could see. For a time we had our doubts: Jane defended her designation, while I insisted we were pressing something on a group of children for our own reasons, or out of our own convictions. No, she said — and pointed to certain passages in the transcript, which she had underlined with a yellow marker. Without Ginny, I argued, we'd have no case at all for our notion of childhood as part of a pilgrimage. No, she insisted: "All of you got caught up in that discussion because you'd all had some personal moment in your life that connected with what you were hearing in class from each other." We decided to try to explore the notion of pilgrimage further with the young students of that class, using Ginny's phrase about "marching through life," and starting with her.

For Ginny, we soon learned, the choice of the word "march" was perfectly natural. Her grandfather had been a career army man, and her father had followed suit, only to be badly injured in an automobile accident while on duty. The family got by on his retirement and disability benefits. Her mother had rheumatic heart disease and could not work. Ginny had four sisters; she was the second youngest child. I'll quote one crucial moment in a conversation I had with her at her home, when we talked of that memorable schoolroom morning: "Maybe I used the word 'march' because I was thinking of my dad; he used to march his men when he was in the army. I don't think God is a sergeant, though!" I loved that, and we both laughed. Then Ginny got serious, and what follows is drawn from an hour of back-and-forth talk: "I try to talk with God, when I say my prayers. I don't know if He's listening. He must be watching us, every one of us — that's His job! My dad says he wishes he could run like he used to, but he can't. Sometimes he'll tell me to run for him, so I run harder and faster; then I win [in school events]. Each day, you have to 'settle your accounts,' Mommy tells us. I try to, when I'm going to bed. That's when I say my prayers.

"You never know what could happen to you. Look at Dad; one day he was in the best shape, and the next day a lot of his bones were broken, and he lost the use of his legs, except for standing, and he can go very slow for a little bit, and then he has to go back to the wheelchair. Mommy stopped going to church then, she told us; she was real sore at God! She went back after I was born! She says my [younger] sister and I, we made up for all the pain!

"They give us report cards, and I do pretty good. I wish I could do better. A lot of the times, I get lost in my thoughts. I'm either way behind myself, remembering something that happened last year or the year before, or I'm way ahead of myself, sitting there and dreaming of what I'll be like when I'm thirty or forty — I mean, the man I'll marry and my kids, like that. I once asked our priest if God can see way in advance what'll be happening to us. The priest said he didn't know, but he thought God just lets it all happen, and I guess he's right. If I was God, though, I'd try and peek! I'd like to know what'll be going on next year or later! Something real good could happen — or something real bad. Maybe, if you behave and do what you should, you'll be rewarded. I hope so.

"I'd like to meet a man who is good-looking, and he's got a job, and most of all he's a nice person, and he'll be a good husband to me, and a father, a good father. [I had asked her what kind of man she hoped to marry, because she repeatedly referred to such daydreaming.] I'd like us to be happy together. We'd like the same movies and food. We'd be good to our kids. We'd teach them to be good to others. When you're going to meet God, He must want to know about your kids, don't you think? Our daddy says he thinks he'll 'make heaven,' because us girls, not one has given them grief, so far. 'You never can tell,' he says to us, but I told him last week, 'Dad, I'll do what you said, I'll walk the straight and narrow!' He laughed, and said I'm one of his 'best troopers ever'!

"I sure hope I live up to what he thinks of me! You try to be good, because it's good to be good; but when your dad and mommy are sick, you try harder, maybe! Sometimes I'm afraid I might get sick, too. My cousin [she is sixteen] told me everyone gets sick, then they die. I know. I told her: I know! But you can live to be a hundred if you're lucky. Maybe you're lonely, then, because everyone you know has gone. Maybe you wonder why God doesn't want you. He's taken everyone else and left you here, all alone! I hope He doesn't put us through the third degree! My dad can do that — he'll question you until you don't know 'if yes is yes or yes is no,' like Mommy says! If God did the same thing, I'd get all mixed up! I forget what happened last week sometimes!

"If I knew my own children were all right, and I had nice grandchildren, and my husband was happy, I'd be happy, and then God would probably decide we all could go and be in heaven with Him. Then we'd be happy for as long as there's time. We'd be marching in step with Him, wouldn't we!"

Unquestionably the former drill sergeant had made a strong impact on his daughter. Yet she was not only her father's daughter but a child of some religious sensibility with her own moral imagination, with a willingness and an ability to call herself to account. She was centered on the here and now, as ten-year-old children tend to be, but she was no stranger to the past, hers and her family's; nor did she hesitate to look far ahead, in the thoroughly conventional, even trite ways of her social and cultural world — but also in the ways of a Piers Plowman or a John Bunyan, or any number of awakened voyagers. She was not an especially religious girl. To be sure, she went to church with her parents almost every week, and she said her prayers regularly; but she was already a rock music fan and a movie buff, one whose tastes were surely not the same as those of the priests and nuns in her parish. It is hardly an original observation that young children wonder about the life they will lead, and form ideas about how that life should go. This girl simply made her predictions more explicit than most because she had, in her language, a military penchant for marches, for taking steps, for arriving at goals.

Ginny reminded my wife and me of the age-old preoccupation of the spiritual wanderer or wayfarer, yet she was an ordinary child whose pilgrimage consisted of the days and nights that a working-class Lawrence, Massachusetts, neighborhood had already imposed as her personal fate — a set of circumstances she herself acknowledged. "When Dad gets upset, he hits the side of his wheelchair. Once he cut himself. We were scared. I asked him if I could help, and he shouted *no* with all his might! I left and went and visited my cousin. My grandma was there. She said, 'Lord, you only live once!' She said, 'Your father, he forgets that. He thinks he's in bad shape, but he's alive, and he's got a wonderful family. You have to talk with God and get some sense into your head!' That's a lot that she said. I can hear her saying it, and I'll say it to myself on a real 'down' day, when all my friends are away and Dad isn't doing too good and Mommy is crying. That's the time to remember you're only here once, and it could be a lot worse!

"They show on TV terrible pictures, on the news. It makes you wonder, Dad keeps saying to us, 'How can these things happen?' He says it — what I just said: 'It makes you wonder.' He means that there's so much trouble, and God must be seeing it, and He doesn't stop it. A priest came to visit us, and we gave him coffee, and the pumpkin pie my mommy made, a piece of that, and Dad told him he wasn't afraid to go to hell after he died, because it's hell now, what the world is like. My mommy argues with him: there's plenty of good in the neighborhood — the people we know, and the guy who runs the grocery store, he'll give you stuff for free sometimes, just to show you he knows you're a good customer. Dad said he'd rather starve than go to a big supermarket, where you don't know people. I hope when I'm older and I have a family of my own, I'll be lucky, and live in a good home, and we'll all look out for each other. Not everyone on our street does, but a lot are the best people you'd ever want to meet. You feel God has been looking out for us, and that's why we look out for each other. I guess He doesn't choose streets; they'd tell us in [Sunday] school it's not what God would do. But there are people who pray to Him, and then you have people who don't, and He must know that, and maybe He'll remember and help us out. I hope He'll be keeping His eye on me and my family all through my life."

As I listened to Ginny during that school year, I thought of a woman I first met in the 1950s, when she was well past the middle point of her life and, like Ginny, hoping to meet the Lord at some indeterminate moment in the future — Dorothy Day, a twentieth-century pilgrim if ever there was one. She called herself that. "Yes, I use the word 'pilgrimage' often — I think it describes the way life unfolds for a lot of us. I hope I'm not flattering us here" — at the Catholic Worker hospitality house, St. Joseph's in New York City, where we were sitting: a soup kitchen for the poor and the homeless — "when I use that word! It's people here, or anywhere, thinking about what life means, searching for God, searching for the answers to the riddles that come to mind as we ask our why's and how's. To me a pilgrim is someone who thinks ahead, who wonders what's coming — and I mean spiritually. We are on a journey through the years — a pilgrim is — and we are trying to find out what our destination is, what awaits us when the bus or the train pulls in. (I don't fly!)

"No, I don't think spiritual questions have to be asked in a religious language. No, I don't think my own 'pilgrimage' began when I converted to the Catholic Church. I think my 'pilgrimage' began when I was a child, when I was seven or eight. You ask why then — well, I have a memory and to me it's the start of my life, my spiritual journey. I'm sitting with my mother, and she's telling me about some trouble in the world, about children like me who don't have enough food — they're dying. I'm eating a doughnut, I think. I ask my mother why other children don't have doughnuts and I do. She says it's the way the world is, something like that. I don't remember her words, but I can still see her face; it's the face of someone who is sad, and resigned, and perhaps she was embarrassed for the sake of all of us human beings, that we keep letting such terrible injustices remain. (I'm putting words and ideas into her mouth now!) Anyway, I remember her face — she was troubled. Maybe she was trying to decide what to tell her bothersome daughter! Most of all, I remember trying to understand what it meant — me eating a doughnut, and lots of children with no food at all. Finally I must have decided to solve the world's problem of hunger on my own, because I asked my mother if she'd take my doughnut and send it to some child whose stomach was empty. I don't remember my words, I just remember holding the doughnut up and hoping she'd take it and give it to someone, some child. I also remember her saying no, she couldn't do that, because the children she'd been telling me about didn't live nearby. I didn't eat that doughnut! I put it down on the kitchen table, and I can still see my mother's face: she didn't know what to say or do! She was puzzled, and so was I! I must have taken that moment to heart, because years later my mother told me that I kept asking her whether there wasn't *someone* who needed my morning doughnut more than I — someone we could find and feed with a doughnut or two! I asked her if *God* knew someone nearby, or if *He* could help us with our modest doughnut plan — to give the hungry some of our abundance! I don't remember asking her that, asking her how we might enlist God in this effort; but she says I kept talking about God and Jesus and feeding the hungry with doughnuts, until she told me, please, to stop!

"What I *do* remember is being a little older, maybe ten or eleven, and walking with my father past some beggars on the street, and asking him if we could go and buy something for them — some doughnuts! He said no, we were in a hurry. I can see us right now in my mind, so clear! And I can feel my sadness and my disappointment. I remember, after that, walking by myself and wondering about the world, wondering why some people had so much and some people had so little, and wondering what *God* thought about such matters. I even remember asking my mother that question. She said she was sure God didn't like it, that there was injustice in the world. I must have bothered her with my questions (the innocent questions of a little girl), because I can also remember her telling me — after one question too many about what *God* thought — that she had no idea what He thought! It was then that I'd ask Him myself in those prayers I'd say sometimes when I was in bed and wide awake. I'd ask Him to tell us, to show us, what He thought, so we could do what He wanted us to do. Of course, I didn't know — no one had explained it to me — that God had already come here and told us what He thought and how we should live and what the right things were for us to do!

"By the time I was, I think, eleven, twelve, I was having talks with myself. I was wondering about what my life would be like. I was trying to figure out who God was, and what He wanted, and what I'd be when I grew up, and whether I should go to college, and what I'd do with my education. I dreamed of the man I'd meet who would be my husband, and I'd look at the map, and wonder what city I'd live in, or *we'd* live in. I'd imagine myself talking with God, or one of His saints — St. Francis — and mostly I'd be asking them questions. They weren't *religious* questions. We were Episcopalians, and we went to church now and then, and my mother had God on her mind in her own way. But we weren't given any special Christian education; it was just me, reading books in the library all by myself, learning about how St. Francis lived, and thinking of Jesus, and thinking about books, and thinking about my own life, what it would be like — *dreaming*, I guess you'd say. If it wasn't a silly pun, I'd say day-dreaming! I was a child with spiritual worries or concerns — and don't we all have them, I hope, and they start earlier than we think. My daughter Tamar: I remember her spiritual questions when she was eight or nine — they reminded me of mine!"

Dorothy Day resisted the attempts others made to see her life as something quite special — a preparation for sainthood. She wanted no part of such claims and was at pains, over the years of discussions I had with her, to show how much of what she did with her life was at the behest of others — Peter Maurin, of course, who helped her found the Catholic Worker movement, and the many friends she made during her long life. I once asked her if she thought others had experienced some of the childhood spiritual experiences she described — had, like her, found their spirituality in childhood, as in the message that Wordsworth gives us in the "Ode on Intimations of Immortality": ". . . Those first affections, / Those shadowy recollections, / Which, be they what they may, / Are yet the fountain light of all our day." Here is what she said to me on the afternoon of April 20, 1971, as she sipped tea and thought about a life then drawing to its close: "In many ways I feel I'm the same person now that I was when I was a girl of nine, maybe, or ten, or eleven. You look surprised! I thought you folks [psychiatrists] believe we're 'made,' once and for all, in childhood, so why the shock?" She paused only because I insisted I wasn't "surprised," only "interested." (She clearly didn't believe me.) "Jesus kept on telling us we should try to be like children — be more open to life, curious about it, trusting of it; and be less cynical and skeptical and full of ourselves, as we so often are when we get older. I'm not romanticizing childhood, no. [I had mentioned that often we do.] I can recall my 'bad behavior' when I was ten (that's what my parents called it), when I got stubborn or sullen or difficult to deal with. But I also remember all the *wondering* I did, all the questions I had about life and God and the purpose of things, and even now, when I'm praying, or trying to keep my spiritual side going, and before I know it, I'm a little girl. Some of the things I asked then — asked my parents, my friends, and a lot of the time myself — I'm still asking myself now, forty or fifty or sixty years later!

"I don't think it's been any different with my daughter, or with the many children I've known during my life; they all want to know why they are here, and what's ahead as they get older — heaven, hell, nothing at all, or as Tamar once said to me, 'Mother, will it be the cemetery, and that's the end?' A natural question. I'd call it her spiritual side expressing itself — and we, as parents, should take notice!"

That was what Ginny had been trying to encourage us to do in class, I realized, finally, one day as Jane and I and our sons, Bob, Danny, and Mike, sat and talked about all the children we'd met over the years we gave to doing the research that preceded the writing of this book. Ginny isn't likely to follow in Dorothy Day's steps, but she knew in her heart, in her soul, some of the spiritual questions and yearnings Dorothy Day described to me. "There were times when I felt even my parents didn't understand me; but they'd come around if I pressed them — if need be, even bothered them. They'd say, 'All right, Dorothy, let's get to the bottom of this,' and we would. When I told my mother I'd had a dream about God — that I was taken to see Him, and He was living in a cabin in the woods, and looked pretty poor and tired, and had rags on, but served me warm soup — she took me seriously. I was thirteen or fourteen, I think, maybe younger. But now, I'm afraid, a 'modern mother' would wonder what this girl is 'going through'; and I'll bet a few of those dreams, and a child excited by them — I was! — would mean a visit to a doctor, your kind!

"I probably *am* being too gloomy. I know a lot of families are plenty religious, and take their children seriously when they are being religious. Maybe that's how it goes for most American families. I've strayed from a part of America I grew up knowing — my parents were conventional, middle-class Protestants, not too devout. People are always asking me about my conversion, but I guess I'd undergone a cultural conversion before my religious one!"

She stopped and took some tea and quietly listened, it seemed, to what she had told herself as well as me. When I have listened to children such as those I met in Lawrence, Massachusetts, I have remembered her. "Sometimes the simple faith of the poor puts me to shame," she once remarked. "The worst moments are when I realize how surprised and impressed and moved I am by the faith of the humble people I've met, the men or women who live every day with God, speaking to Him, letting Him enter their lives, *thinking* of Him — not because they want a favor, or some special help, but because He is a true companion for them, and they want to be with Him and learn from Him and be guided by Him. Why should I be so surprised? Because I've given up on people — at moments I have. I've forgotten that for people all over the world, thousands and thousands, the Lord is *there*, a big part of the 'contemplation' they do. We use the word 'contemplation.' We forget that others *do* their 'contemplation' — and don't write about it, and talk about it, and study it! I have always had this struggle: the poor, the people of faith, whom I admire — and me, part of another world, a writer, a reader of 'literature,' though the Church has helped me bridge these separate places in my head, maybe in my soul. I hope it has! Today, I doubt it has. All the years here in this [Catholic Worker] community — and here I am, still torn: 'them' and me! It's so much easier for me to criticize myself than to lift a finger of reproach against the people we serve here [in the soup kitchen], even when I know in my heart I'm a witness to wrongdoing!"

For a long time I wondered why she, of all people, who for years had celebrated the dignity and worth of the poor, the homeless, the down-and-out, she who gave her life to them, why she should have been so tough on herself that afternoon. But now I think I understand, thanks to those children in Lawrence. She was struggling hard to understand the complex nature of ordinary life — and felt inadequate to the task. She was turning herself into an outsider, as if she, too, didn't live her own kind of humble and ordinary life. She wanted to bow in awe toward others who, despite great odds, nevertheless manage to build a spiritual life for themselves — but she found it harder to take note of another side of their humanity: the warts and blemishes, the streaks of egoism or meanness.

Earlier in this chapter I offered some moments unforgettable to me — moments from that morning in a classroom of ten-year-old fifth-graders in an aging factory city and in a school that was old and inadequate. These were children whose parents worked in factories, automobile repair shops, stores — or had no jobs and instead collected a welfare check. These were Catholic, mostly, and Protestant children, many black or Spanish-speaking, some of Irish or French-Canadian ancestry. These were children with no great future ahead of them. They came from hard-pressed families, neighborhoods; they attended schools lacking in so many respects, and themselves had learned to set their sights modestly at best. At times, I must admit, I've regarded them as blameless victims of a social and economic system, or eager victims of the excesses of mass culture — television, the movies, rock music. From the same children who spoke of God and pilgrimage I've heard quite other sorts of language — curses and worse: offhand insensitivity, outright callousness, even cruelty, as one observes in children anywhere. Ginny, for instance, once gave the cold shoulder to a friend of hers who badly wanted and needed to talk with her, only to find out later — how remorseful she was! — that the friend's sister had just been killed by a hit-and-run driver. The girl had arrived at school with a new hair style a day before Ginny had intended to get a similar one. "I felt like a copycat," Ginny explained to me, "and so I changed my mind [about the hair style]."

Ginny and her Lawrence schoolmates need no sanctification,

but they do deserve a faithful accounting of what they said about themselves and their lives — the past as they remembered it, the present as they struggled to get through it, the future as they dreamt it might be. The longer I've known such children, the more readily I've noticed the abiding interest they have in reflecting about human nature,[2] about the reasons people behave as they do, about the mysteries of the universe as evinced in the earth, the sun, the moon, the stars. Sometimes the moral and spiritual power that certain children display can give me some release — help me learn about matters I might not want to acknowledge as part of what I choose to call psychological "reality."

How memorable, for instance, are the moments of Ginny's response to movies: "I haven't gone to a lot of serious movies. Sometimes I see them late, when they come out on the cassettes. I saw *Platoon*; that really upset me. My uncle was hurt bad, real bad, over there in Asia, in Vietnam. He's still nervous. He cries a lot. He smokes a lot. He gets depressed. I wish there'd never be a war again. God should stop all of the wars. I wonder how He must have felt, when all the people were killing each other over there in Vietnam. If my uncle cries now, God must have cried, too. He must have *wept*. Don't you think?" I nodded.

"I look forward to getting all grown up," Ginny continued, "and then, maybe, someday, I'll get a few whispers from God! My aunt says she prays so hard, she hears God's answer. I've never heard Him, but maybe He'll tell me something. You don't have to hear Him — just pray He gets you on the right track. My dad sits and thinks about life, and why he's the one he is, and so do I. I'll find out why I'm me one day — maybe just before I die, or just after. I'll wait until then, and I hope I'll get to meet Him then. It's far off, but we all get there! Right?"

I nodded again — though what was it that caused me to nod? A somewhat frightened girl whose anxieties had touched me? A fairly bright, imaginative, articulate girl whose intellectual vitality and imaginative resourcefulness I had come to respect, hence my nod? A child from a family of "marginal socioeconomic status" but not without ambition, hence my nod? A child prone to prayer and the consolations of heaven as a means of tolerating the lower rungs of the ladder, hence my nod? But what of this child's everyday life?

"I was walking home the other afternoon," Ginny told me, "and there was a lady I'd never met before, not far from our house. She was old, with white hair, and I went to her and asked her what's the trouble, because she was talking to herself, I thought. She didn't hear me at first, but then she did. I asked her again, 'Can I help you?' She said, 'Oh, little girl, if you could, that would be wonderful.' I didn't like her calling me 'little girl.' I'm *not* a 'little girl.' I'm not even 'little' for my age. I looked at her and I was going to tell her that she isn't any bigger than I am. Maybe an inch taller, no more. But then I thought: Ginny, you're being stupid — this old lady is lost, and she might be confused, the way old folks can be, and so just try to give her a hand; anyway, when she calls you 'little,' she just means you're a girl and she's an old lady, so she's got big years behind her, and you've only got a few of them, so they're 'little' compared to hers.

"No, I didn't think all of that, exactly — not the way I'm saying it now. But I sort of did; I mean, I calmed down and I tried to keep talking with her, and not feel huffy with her. You know what I mean? [Nod!] Then she told me she was trying to get to see her daughter; she's moved near here. But she'd taken a wrong turn. She showed me the directions, and I figured that out. I was going to tell her where she'd gone wrong, and I started to, but she couldn't get what I was telling her. I didn't know what to do. I had to be home; I had my chores to do. But I thought to myself: Hey, this right here is a chore you'd better do, and then you can go home. Besides, I really felt sorry for the lady. Besides, I thought: Ginny, the day will come — you know, I'll be there myself, and I'll need someone to help me, and if no one does, I might get into real trouble. That lady, she was in real trouble, I could see she was.

"I just made a snap decision. I told her, 'Missus, if you come with me, I'll get you to where you're going.' She wasn't sure I meant what I said! She kept clutching that piece of paper, and asking me where we were — even though I'd already told her. I decided not to argue with her. I decided to try to be nice to her. I just kept walking, and I gave her a tour — I told her about the stores and the short cuts and I told her where the phones are. I asked her where she lived, and pretty soon she was telling me everything. She'd lost her husband, and her son had been in Vietnam, just like my dad and my uncle. He got killed! Her daughter just moved to this part of town. Her [the daughter's] husband was a soldier over there, too. He came back and he had a job and everything was great, but then he got sick, and now he's in a hospital; he has some bad disease, and he's 'half paralyzed,' she said. She said it was terrible — that she can walk, and she's way older than he is. I didn't know what to say. I was going to say that it's like that, life, but I felt stupid telling *her* that; she already knew!

"We kept walking and I didn't need those directions, but she was afraid *I'd* get lost without them, so I pretended I was following them. I'd look at the piece of paper, and make her think I'd been saved by it! We got to be pretty good friends by the time we were there, where her daughter lives, and her grandchildren. She was tired. She was breathing heavy. I'd had to walk *so* slow; and I guess she'd been walking fast for her — to keep up with me. I felt bad for her. I tried to be 'considerate.' Mom says, 'Always try to be considerate.'

"Anyway, I said goodbye to her, and she said thank you so many times I thought she'd never stop! She grabbed my arm, and she said God sent me to her, and she'd pray to Him later, before she went to sleep, to thank Him for me, for having me be there. I didn't know what to say. I wasn't sure, at first, she was serious. But I looked at her, and she had tears in her eyes, so I knew she was. I was going to tell her it was an accident we'd met, but I decided not to. I just thanked her for saying such a nice thing to me. She gave me a kiss, and I left. On the way home I wondered if I'd live to be old like her, and if I might meet some kid then, and she'd be like me. Maybe God puts you here and He gives you these hints of what's ahead, and you should pay attention to them, because that's Him speaking to you."

To me, of course, the story was affecting — another occasion to nod. As I listened, though, the elderly woman took shape in my mind. This is what we do as we hear a storyteller speak: let our own imagination, our past experiences, our various passions and problems, help form images that accompany the words we're hearing. I caught myself picturing that elderly woman as looking like the older Dorothy Day I knew[3] — who also walked slowly, had a heart condition, had a daughter and grandchildren to go visit, and was not averse to finding in life's small moments evidence of the Lord's nearness to us. Dorothy Day's life had now, through the accidents of my life, connected with the life of this "little girl." The older woman's writing and speaking of her "pilgrimage" suddenly gave me help in understanding that girl: *her* pilgrimage, and that of children the world over who "march through life." So it is we connect with one another, move in and out of one another's lives, teach and heal and affirm one another, across space and time — all of us wanderers, explorers, adventurers, stragglers and ramblers, sometimes tramps or vagabonds, even fugitives, but now and then pilgrims: as children, as parents, as old ones about to take that final step, to enter that territory whose character none of us here ever knows. Yet how young we are when we start wondering about it all, the nature of the journey and of the final destination.

NOTES
INDEX

Notes

Introduction

1. Only in retrospect did I realize the importance of those years of hospital work, especially the time I spent with children afflicted with polio — the last epidemic before the Salk vaccine came into everyday use. To know children faced with paralysis, even the distinct possibility of death, is to begin to encounter the moral and spiritual struggles that even elementary school boys and girls can wage. I learned from Kenneth H. Beach, my psychoanalyst in New Orleans, the connection in my mind between that first hospital research I did up North and the later work I began in that Southern city: I was moving from an investigation of medical stress and jeopardy to a study of the social and racial kind. See "Neuropsychiatric Aspects of Acute Poliomyelitis" (with Jimmie C. B. Holland), *American Journal of Psychiatry* 114, no. 1 (July 1957).

2. I have described this professional transition in "Serpents and Doves," in *Youth: Change and Challenge*, ed. Erik H. Erikson (New York: Basic Books, 1963); and in *A Farewell to the South* (Boston: Little, Brown, 1972).

3. In the five volumes of *Children of Crisis* (Boston: Atlantic–Little, Brown, 1967, 1972, 1978) and in *The Moral Life of Children* and *The Political Life of Children* (Boston: Atlantic Monthly Press, 1986).

4. Those children had extraordinarily, culturally sanctioned mentors in their grandparents, as Alex Harris, a photographer who worked with me in New Mexico, and I gradually learned. See *The Old Ones of New Mexico* (Albuquerque: University of New Mexico Press, 1973). The same thing was true for the Eskimos Alex Harris and I came to know. See *The Last and First Eskimos* (New York: New York Graphic Society, 1978).

5. I have tried to do justice to these two extraordinary child analysts in *Erik H. Erikson: The Growth of His Work* (Boston: Atlantic–Little,

Brown, 1970); "The Achievement of Anna Freud," *Massachusetts Review* 7, no. 2 (Spring 1966); and "Children's Crusade," *The New Yorker,* September 23, 1972.

6. The T. B. Davie Memorial Lecture — an annual commemoration of the struggle a great university has waged on behalf of academic freedom, often in the face of severe statist interference.

7. Years later, as I look back and go over old transcripts, I realize that the children I met were eager indeed to speak of their religious and spiritual interests, concerns, worries, beliefs — but the doctor listening to them had his own agenda, some of it a consequence of a professional ideology all too well learned. See, in this regard, an essay I wrote in the early 1960s, "A Young Psychiatrist Looks at His Profession," *Atlantic Monthly,* July 1961, and, more recently, an essay on the first black American psychoanalyst, "A Doctor's Odyssey," *New Republic,* March 27, 1989.

8. I have tried to describe some of those personal confrontations — the tension between the modern agnosticism of contemporary psychoanalysis, familiar to me throughout my working life, and the spiritual concerns that some of us in my profession still find quite important. See *Harvard Diary: Reflections on the Sacred and the Secular* (New York: Crossroad Publishing Company, 1988).

1. *Psychoanalysis and Religion*

1. Rieff's work has been enormously helpful to those of us who want to balance a great respect for psychoanalytic work with serious reservations about what has emerged, intellectually and culturally, in its name these past decades. See his *Freud: The Mind of the Moralist* (New York: Viking, 1959). Also of help are Peter Gay's *Freud: A Life of Our Time* (New York: Norton, 1988) and *A Godless Jew: Freud, Atheism, and the Making of Psychoanalysis* (New Haven: Yale University Press, 1987).

2. This book of Dr. Rizzuto's is by no means the first effort by a psychoanalyst to examine the phenomenon of religious faith from the vantage point of psychoanalytic theory. Dr. Rizzuto's candid discussion calls upon two generations of revisionist speculations, which in turn were a response to Freud's own passionate interest in metapsychological matters and, not least, his interest in the hold faith has on so many people — not all of them, he had to realize, as gullible or superstitious as he sometimes would aver. His daughter Anna Freud remarked to me in 1979: "Yes, in *The Future of an Illusion* my father was hard, at times, on convinced believers. I know that he could also be quite respectful of those who hold to a faith with honesty and sincerity. I think of his exchanges with the Reverend Oskar Pfister, a good friend." Those exchanges, years of letters sent back and forth during a friendship of twenty-eight years, between Dr. Freud and the Swiss clergyman Pfister, are well worth reading: *Psychoanalysis and Faith: Dialogues Between Sig-*

mund Freud and Oskar Pfister (New York: Basic Books, 1963). I ought to
mention here, of course, Erik H. Erikson's important work, a challenge
to psychoanalytic reductionism with respect to religious faith and spiritual life: *Young Man Luther* (New York: Norton, 1958), and *Gandhi's
Truth* (New York: Norton, 1969). The entire body of his work is well
worth taking into consideration as a distinct psychoanalytic amplification
and emendation with respect to such matters. I have tried to do justice
to this friend and mentor in *Erik H. Erikson: The Growth of His Work*
(Boston: Atlantic–Little, Brown, 1970). Many of the important psychoanalytic pioneers of this century have, in fact, found their own ways
of considering religious, spiritual, and moral questions: Heinz Hart-
mann in *Psychoanalysis and Moral Values* (New York: International University Press, 1960); Bruno Bettelheim in *Freud and Man's Soul* (New
York: Knopf, 1982); Erich Fromm in so much of his sociological and
even political writing, and specifically in *The Dogma of Christ* (New York:
Holt, Rinehart and Winston, 1963); Jung, of course, in his Terry Lectures at Yale, published as *Psychology and Religion* (New Haven: Yale
University Press, 1938), and in *Essays on Contemporary Events* (London:
Kegan and Paul, 1947), and in *Modern Man in Search of a Soul* (New
York: Harcourt, Brace, 1933). Nor did Piaget and his colleagues fail to
address such matters in their own fashion. See the chapters "The Origin
of Night" and "The Concept of Life" in *Causal Thinking and the Child:
A Genetic and Experimental Approach* (New York: International University
Press, 1962).

3. The best avenue to D. W. Winnicott's many excellent medical,
pediatric, and psychoanalytic papers is his *Collected Papers: Through Pediatrics to Psychoanalysis* (London: Tavistock, 1958) and *The Maturational
Processes and the Facilitating Environment: Studies in the Theory of Emotional
Development* (London: Hogarth, 1965). Charles Rycroft's suggestive
books include *Imagination and Reality* (New York: International University Press, 1968), *The Innocence of Dreams* (London: Hogarth, 1979), and
Psychoanalysis and Beyond (London: Hogarth, 1985). H. Guntrip's *Psychoanalytic Theory, Therapy and the Self* (New York: Basic Books, 1971) is
of help in understanding Dr. Rizzuto's views. A valuable summary of
what those British theorists have offered contemporary psychoanalysis
can be found in *Reshaping the Psychoanalytic Domain*, by Judith M. Hughes
(Berkeley: University of California Press, 1989).

I have found the work of the Jesuit psychoanalyst William Meissner
quite helpful. See his *Life and Faith* (Washington: Georgetown Press,
1987) and his *Psychoanalysis and Religious Experience* (New Haven: Yale
University Press, 1984). A most provocative and suggestive book — a
tour de force, surely — is Paul Vitz's *Sigmund Freud's Christian Unconscious* (New York: Guilford, 1988). Dr. Vitz tries to indicate how intimately Freud lived with a particular and complex mix of religious
traditions, no matter his professed agnosticism.

2. Method

1. This chapter on method joins seven others I have written — for the five volumes of *Children of Crisis* (Boston: Atlantic Monthly Press, 1967, 1972, 1978) and for *The Moral Life of Children* and *The Political Life of Children* (Boston: Atlantic Monthly Press, 1986). I especially refer the interested reader to the chapter titled "Psychoanalysis and Moral Development" in *The Moral Life of Children,* including the notes for that chapter — it was an effort to connect the research I had done to psychoanalytic child psychiatry and to the observations of cognitive psychologists. I strongly recommend, as general background for the research presented in this book, a reading of Piaget's *Moral Judgment of the Child* (New York: Free Press, 1965), Lawrence Kohlberg's *Philosophy of Moral Development* (New York: Harper and Row, 1981), and Carol Gilligan's quite helpful and instructive *In a Different Voice* (Cambridge, Mass.: Harvard University Press, 1982). I also recommend the work of James Fowler: *Stages of Faith* (San Francisco: Harper and Row, 1981) and *Life Maps* (Minneapolis: Winston Press, 1978). I have no quarrel with the notion of "faith development," nor with efforts to learn, through cognitive analysis, how our reasoning life connects with our religious or spiritual life. I can only repeat here, more or less, what I wrote in *The Moral Life of Children* — that my work is *contextual,* that it aims to learn from children as they go about their lives: in the home, the playground, the classroom, the Hebrew school or Sunday school. It is important, and revealing, for children to be asked questions, presented with morally suggestive (or ambiguous) scenarios, asked to respond in a range of ways to inquiries aimed at elucidating the structure of their thinking, its values and assumptions. It may also be helpful for some of us to spend months or even years with children, watch them and listen to them as they struggle with their ongoing lives, and learn from them as they casually chat with each other and as they answer questions they themselves put to one another. I have tried to understand how particular children fit the religious traditions (or the secular ideals) of their family into their ordinary conversational life. If I have a rationale for the "methodology" I use, it is probably best explained in *The Call of Stories: Teaching and the Moral Imagination* (Boston: Houghton Mifflin, 1989). In a sense, the present book offers excerpts of a listener's long-term involvement with certain children — what children have said when asked about God, about the meaning of religion to them: said to one another, often enough, as well as to me alone.

2. Gabriel Moran's *Religious Education Development* (Minneapolis: Winston Press, 1983) offers a fine analysis of the various theoretical vantage points with respect to psychological studies of children. I am obviously less interested in analyzing the structure of the thought of the children I have come to know than in rendering for others what I have regarded as highlights in what I have been privileged to hear them

say. Perhaps we could call it documentary work — by someone who has learned to be a pediatrician and a child psychiatrist and thus has (he hopes and prays) some ability to spend time with children in such a way that they do, indeed, want to talk about a few matters. Perhaps it is not totally inappropriate that children be asked, now and then, to respond to the Bible as they will, out of their lives, out of their hearts. The Bible is not a theological text, a philosophical study, a write-up of a research project; it is a series of stories, of narratives, with moments, too, of lyrical poetry.

3. I might as well confess that as I have done this work I have taken major inspiration from Robert Alter's marvelous pair of books, *The Art of Biblical Narrative* and *The Art of Biblical Poetry* (New York: Basic Books, 1981 and 1985), and, as well, the exceptionally instructive *Literary Guide to the Bible* (Cambridge: Harvard University Press, 1987), which Mr. Alter and Frank Kermode edited; also Cynthia Ozick's *Metaphor and Memory* (New York: Knopf, 1989) and Dan Jacobson's *The Story of the Stories: The Chosen People and Its God* (New York: Harper and Row, 1982). As I have sat, sometimes, in a room and heard children — whether they are believers or agnostics — wrestle for life's meaning, I have thought of Robert Alter responding so finely and sensitively to those old-time stories, those exalted, lyrical moments of long ago, and of Dan Jacobson doing his own wrestling with a great people's great (and, at times, aggrieved, perilous) fate, and of Cynthia Ozick's powerful, compelling reinvigoration of the Hebrew spiritual and literary tradition.

Additional sources of encouragement, edification, even inspiration, include Gareth Matthews's extraordinary explorations, as given in *Philosophy and the Young Child* (Cambridge, Mass.: Harvard University Press, 1980), a revealing study of the moral sophistication children can bring to a particular observer; Richard Coe's *When the Grass Was Taller* (New Haven: Yale University Press, 1984), a fine analysis of the genre of childhood autobiographical statement; William Damon's *The Social World of the Child* (San Francisco: Jossey-Bass, 1977), which offers valuable sociological amplification of the cognitive psychology of Piaget, Kohlberg, and Gilligan; Peter Berger's *The Sacred Canopy: Elements of a Sociological Theory of Religion* (Garden City, N.J.: Doubleday, 1967), which, similarly, grounds religious life in particular social and cultural worlds; Jerome Kagan's *The Nature of the Child* (New York: Basic Books, 1989), especially the fine chapter "Establishing a Morality"; Reinhold Kuhn's *Corruption in Paradise: The Child in Western Literature* (Hanover, N.H.: University Press of New England, 1982), and in particular the chapter "The Heaven and Hell of Childhood"; an unusual historical study by Colleen McDonnell and Bernhard Land, *Heaven: A History* (New Haven: Yale University Press, 1988); another valuable historical work, *The Spiritual Self in Everyday Life* (Boston: Northeastern University Press, 1988), which deals with "personal religious experience" in nineteenth-century New England, by Richard Rabinowitz; and a sensitive study by John Allan of children's artistic work (he is a Jungian analyst): *Inscapes of the Child's World* (Dallas: Spring, 1988). I would like to make special mention as well of the William James classic *Varieties of Religious Experience* (Cambridge, Mass.: Harvard University Press, 1985), which I had read many years ago, in college, and read again while doing this research; and also David Heller's fine *The Children's God* (Chicago: University of Chicago Press, 1986), an excellent study of the manner in which a variety of children think of, represent, and in their minds address God.

4. I have described at some length the time I spent with Dr. Williams — an unforgettable privilege. See *William Carlos Williams: The Knack of Survival* (New Brunswick, N.J.: Rutgers University Press, 1975); *The Doctor Stories of William Carlos Williams* (New York: New Directions, 1984); *Rumors of Separate Worlds* (Iowa City: University of Iowa Press, 1989).

3. *The Face of God*

1. I suggest as background reading for this chapter Ann Belford Ulanov's *Picturing God* (Cambridge: Cowley Press, 1986) — a first-rate collection of essays, one of which takes up the manner in which various adults "see" God, a consequence, of course, of the nature of their own inner lives. I also found parts of Clifford Geertz's book *Local Knowledge* (New York: Basic Books, 1983) quite helpful — the chapters titled "Found in Translation: On the Social History of the Moral Imagination" and "Art as a Cultural System." The children I met were summoning visions, then setting them down — and I needed to be reminded, occasionally, that these were boys and girls who lived at a certain time and in a certain place: the sociology and anthropology of children's art, their visual life.

2. See *A Spectacle Unto the World: The Catholic Worker Movement* (New York: Viking, 1973) and *Dorothy Day: A Radical Devotion* (Boston: Addison-Wesley, 1987).

4. *The Voice of God*

1. As I heard these children tell me their stories — God's words part of them — I thought of and referred to Arthur Applebee's *The Child's Concept of Story* (Chicago: University of Chicago Press, 1978). I also remembered a moment from a class I took with Perry Miller when I was a college junior: "The Puritans spent their lives trying to hear God's voice." At the time I wasn't sure exactly what the professor meant — why he had put the matter in those words. He emphasized, later, the *hearing* of God among some of the Puritans — hard for me, then, to imagine. Now, so many years later, I think I understand what Perry Miller was trying to say — the Word becomes our own struggling words

as they seek expression of who He is, what He has to say to us.

2. See *The Moral Life of Children* and *The Political Life of Children* (Boston: Atlantic Monthly Press, 1986).

5. *Young Spirituality: Psychological Themes*

1. I hope someday to acknowledge further the considerable debt I owe to Anna Freud for the encouragement she gave me as I hesitated long and hard before taking on the research that enabled this book. Her letters, her willingness to sit with me and listen to some of the stories I was hearing from children, meant much to me. I expressed gratitude to her in *The Mind's Fate* (Boston: Atlantic–Little, Brown, 1975), but there is much more to say, I feel.

2. See, again, "Neuropsychiatric Aspects of Acute Poliomyelitis," *American Journal of Psychiatry* 114, no. 1 (July 1957). This work still comes to mind, decades later — my first attempt at clinical research done amid the great stresses of an epidemic. I have kept in touch with some of those patients through all these years, an education in itself. To quote from Miss Freud again: "Our patients are our professors!"

3. A most useful and illuminating light is cast on the fundamentalist world by Alan Peshkin in *God's Choice: The Total World of a Fundamentalist School* (Chicago: University of Chicago Press, 1986).

6. *Young Spirituality: Philosophical Reflections*

1. Sometimes these children's remarks threw me back to my college days with Perry Miller and the Kierkegaard assignments he kept pressing on us: *Fear and Trembling, Repetition, Either/Or.* Kierkegaard the abstract metaphysician had a way, also, of becoming Kierkegaard the shrewd observer of everyday mid-nineteenth-century bourgeois Copenhagen, including its "everydayness," even as these boys and girls, too, have stopped every now and then to try taking stock of life's meaning, its absurdities. An important moment for me, in so doing, was provided by my hope to do justice to the novelist Walker Percy's Kierkegaardian wisdom, as offered in a series of fictions and essays: *Walker Percy: An American Search* (Boston: Atlantic–Little, Brown, 1978).

7. *Young Spirituality: Visionary Moments*

1. See *Chicanos, Eskimos, Indians,* Volume IV of *Children of Crisis* (Boston: Atlantic–Little, Brown, 1978).

2. See *The South Goes North,* Volume III of *Children of Crisis* (Boston: Atlantic–Little, Brown, 1972).

8. Representations

1. Dr. Williams was no stranger to the opportunities artistic representation offers — and the obstacles in the artist's way. See *A Recognizable Image* (New York: New Directions, 1978), a collection of his essays on art and artists. See also *Poets on Painters,* ed. J. D. McClatchy (Berkeley: University of California Press, 1988). The children's drawings offered here may not be "art" in its most distinguished form, but those boys and girls have struggled, as writers and artists struggle all the time, not only to convey an idea to others but to render what is suggestive, provocative, satisfying, surprising.

2. Those interested may want to look at the References and Notes sections of the five volumes of *Children of Crisis* (Boston: Atlantic–Little, Brown, 1967, 1972, 1978), *The Moral Life of Children,* and *The Political Life of Children* (Boston: Atlantic Monthly Press, 1986), wherein there are suggestions for additional reading on the matter of children's artistic work, its meaning and usefulness for those of us who work with and try to understand children. As valuable as those social science books are, I sometimes turn to the artists themselves, such as Gauguin, who struggled with words to convey what he initially (and magnificently) offered representationally. See, in that respect, Wayne Andersen's *Gauguin's Paradise Lost* (New York: Viking, 1971), and of course van Gogh's letters (New York: Atheneum, 1963), so many of which reveal someone both artistically exalted and personally at the edge of things. I mention those two verbally expressive artists because so often, I have found, children are impelled to talk about what they have drawn or painted — often, I have to admit, when I need more time for silent contemplation of their work.

3. I recommend a discussion of Biblical leprosy by my Israeli friend Joseph Zias: "Leprosy in the Byzantine Monasteries of the Judean Desert," *Koroth* 9:242–248. Mr. Zias doubts that the disease leprosy, Hansen's Disease, as we know it today, existed in Biblical times; rather, "leprosy" then was a catchall name that referred to a number of clinical problems.

4. At times, as I watched children struggle artistically with Christ's life, with His birth or His miraculous deeds or His dying passion, I thought of the medieval and Renaissance art I studied in college, and more recently, have used in the art history course I have taught in a Cambridge elementary school (fourth grade). The boys and girls I know are in no danger of becoming great artists, yet Jesus has not rarely stirred them mightily, helped them surpass themselves as artists, as their teachers have noted. I have shown these children (and thought of, while working with them) Georges Duby's *History of Medieval Art* (New York: Skira, 1986) or Marvin Eisenberg's *Lorenzo Monaco* (Princeton, N.J.: Princeton University Press, 1989), and been struck by their unpretentious willingness to stare in awe at what others have managed to do, a

fixation that comes with an awareness of one's own shared aspiration: to give the word a "form" that is as "sacred" as one's aesthetic talent and spiritual energy make possible. Of related interest, certainly, is E. H. Gombrich's *Art and Illusion* (Princeton, N.J.: Princeton University Press, 1969), not to mention his review in *The New York Review of Books* (February 15, 1990) of David Freedberg's *The Power of Images* (Chicago: University of Chicago Press, 1990).

9. *Christian Salvation*

1. As I heard children talk of Christianity, I remembered moments in the New Testament, and, too, remembered not theology but the personal expressions of faith which autobiographies like Dorothy Day's *The Long Loneliness* (New York: Harper and Row, 1952) offer, or novels, which have their own way of suggesting what faith comes to ultimately: the everyday times of prayer and doubt, of commitment and skepticism — as given us in the Christian tradition of this century by Graham Greene, Georges Bernanos, Ignazio Silone, Walker Percy, François Mauriac. For several years I taught (with Robert Kiely) a course at Harvard titled "A Literature of Christian Reflection." We worked hard to draw on Luther and Calvin, on St. Francis and St. Benedict, on George Herbert, on Pascal and Kierkegaard, on Emily Dickinson and Robert Frost and Philip Larkin, on Flannery O'Connor and Simone Weil and Thomas Merton — the struggle of all sorts of men and women for a vision of God and His meaning to us. I thought of those writers, of Tolstoy, too, of James Agee's youth in *Morning Watch* as I heard these children give voice to their struggles and worries, their doubts and hopes.

2. Let me mention a mélange of books I found helpful as I tried to connect what I heard from these children to what some of their elders, living and dead, have had to say: James J. Thompson's *Christian Classics Revisited* (San Francisco: Ignatius Press, 1983); *Writers Revealed* (New York: Peter Bednick, 1989), in which contemporary novelists such as Iris Murdoch and Anthony Burgess "talk about faith, religion and God"; *Children in Amish Society*, by John Hostetler and Gertrude Huntington (New York: Holt, Rinehart and Winston, 1971), a look at an especially committed segment of young Christian life; *Evangelicalism: The Coming Generation*, by James Davison Hunter (Chicago: University of Chicago Press, 1987), an incisive and brilliant look at what is happening — and why — among some of America's most strenuous Christian believers; and three delightful and touching collections of brief responses on the part of children to God as a felt or putative presence — *The Child Is Superior to the Man: Children's Experiences with God in the Public School Classroom*, by Samuel Silverstein (Hicksville: Exposition Press, 1980), a lovely series of descriptions by a wonderfully observant teacher; *Children's Letters to God*, compiled by Eric Marshall and Stuart Hample (New York: Simon and Schuster, 1975); and *Mister God, This Is Anna*, by an

author who goes under the name of Flynn (New York: Ballantine, 1974), an account — a memoir, really — of a particular girl's intensely introspective religious life. What all these children possess is a passion of sorts, not unlike, I sometimes think, the passion Pascal felt as he worked his way from one *pensée* to the next, the mind at work, surely, but the soul's energy being expended, on occasion rather furiously — salvation itself at stake.

10. *Islamic Surrender*

1. I am, first of all, enormously grateful to Heidi Larson, a young, energetic, and gifted anthropologist who worked in London for a number of years with Pakistani children, and who tactfully and graciously introduced two of my sons, Danny and Mike, to those children — giving us all a start with young Islamic people (1986). Heidi Larson's doctoral thesis, "Culture at Play: Pakistani Children, British Childhood" (University of California at Berkeley, 1989), is an extraordinary document, an original mix of splendid photographs and highly literate, at times lyrical text. Her documentary work has been enormously helpful to my own. In many conversations she has patiently given me the benefit of her wisdom, based on fieldwork with Pakistani, Arab, and Jewish children in England, in Asia, in Israel.

2. As I listened to these Islamic children, I tried to learn of their religion. I read parts of the Koran, in the translation of A. J. Arberry (New York: Macmillan, 1955). I read Frederick Mathewson Denny's *An Introduction to Islam* (New York: Macmillan, 1985). I read Raphael Patai's *The Arab Mind* (New York: Scribners, 1983). I read Mohammad Zia Ullah's *Islamic Concept of God* (London: Kegan Paul International, 1984). I read *Islam: Beliefs and Teaching* by Ghulam Sarwar (London: Muslim Educational Trust, 1980). I read Paul Rabinow's fascinating *Reflections on Fieldwork in Morocco* (Berkeley: University of California Press, 1977). With great pleasure, I read some "Muslim Nursery Rhymes" and some "Sayings of Mohammad" given me by the children I worked with, wonderful and very helpful pamphlets they eagerly offered me and then refused to accept back. I am especially indebted to my friend Asif Sumal for his copy of "Love Your Brother, Love Your Neighbor" — a reminder to this Westerner of how much we all share, morally and spiritually, across continents and cultures. As more and more children gave me more and more to read, I began to balk, wonder what they were telling me, what they were saying about my ignorance. Finally, I took a tenet of their Islamic faith seriously and told them I could never know what they know as they know it — whereupon young Asif, who appears first in this chapter, joked with me: "Then you surrender!" "Yes, I surrender," I offered. "That is good," he replied — and added, tersely, enigmatically, "You are learning." He went no further, and I only smiled and said, "I hope so."

11. Jewish Righteousness

1. I read a number of books as I talked with Jewish children, one or two at their suggestion, courtesy of their parents: *What Is Judaism*, by Emil Fackenheim (New York: Macmillan, 1987), and Paul Johnson's long and accessible *A History of the Jews* (New York: Harper and Row, 1987). I also went back to Martin Buber and Gerschom Sholem, to Abraham Heschel's *The Prophets* (New York: Harper and Row, 1962), which I'd read while living in the South during the civil rights era, when I heard so much mention of Isaiah and Jeremiah and Amos and Micah from black children enduring mobs, threats, and violence in order to attend hitherto all-white schools. I read Max Kadushin's *Worship and Ethics: A Study in Rabbinic Judaism* (Chicago: Northwestern University Press, 1964), and Elie Wiesel's extraordinary *Four Hasidic Masters* (South Bend, Ind.: University of Notre Dame Press, 1964). I went back to Job, with the help of my friend Stephen Mitchell — *The Book of Job* (San Francisco: North Point Press, 1979) — and I read Freema Gottlieb's extraordinary *The Lamp of God: A Jewish Book of Light* (Northvale, N.Y.: Aronson, 1989), an examination of the history of the metaphor of light in Jewish writing. In Jerusalem, at Yad Vashem, I remembered my childhood, remembered the darkness Hitler cast on the world, looked at *The Children We Remember* by Chana Abells (New York: Greenwillow, 1983) with several of the children I knew in Jerusalem — the book's pictures bring back the young world the Nazis tried to extinguish. I read Dan Bar-On's *Legacy of Silence*, an Israeli's encounter with children of those Nazis (Cambridge, Mass.: Harvard University Press, 1989). I read *A Modern Jew in Search of a Soul*, a collection of personal essays by Drs. Marvin Spiegelman and Abraham Jacobson (Phoenix: Falcon Press, 1986). All of the above were of some help, brought me closer to a world I very much needed to understand through the eyes of children, yes, but also with the help of the above writers. The most helpful book, though, turned out to be *Congregation*, ed. David Rosenberg (New York: Harcourt Brace Jovanovich, 1987), a remarkable series of "readings" (interpretive essays) of the Jewish Bible by American writers. I told the children I was reading that book, told them of particular favorites in it, brought the book to our meetings, read passages — and heard the responses of those boys and girls, the "righteousness of the words being shared," the way one of the children described our discussions of *Congregation*, taking pains to credit his Hebrew school teacher for the phrase.

12. Secular Soul Searching

1. Reinhold Niebuhr was, of course, a Christian theologian, but he knew our twentieth-century secular world inside out — and his many

books are as good a moral introduction to that world's values and assumptions as any I know. I audited a course of his while a medical student, and went out of my way many times to hear him speak — an encounter with a prophetic tradition still alive, I used to think (and feel). See "Reinhold Niebuhr's Nature and Destiny of Man," *Daedalus,* Winter 1974.

2. I think I was first made aware of how intensely certain children from agnostic homes ask themselves essentially religious and spiritual questions when I worked with boys and girls from quite well-to-do families in New Orleans and in Boston during the 1970s. See *Privileged Ones,* Volume V of *Children of Crisis* (Boston: Atlantic–Little, Brown, 1978).

3. I tried to straddle the secular and the religious worlds in my thoughts as I did so in the interviews with these children. See *Harvard Diary: Reflections on the Sacred and the Secular* (New York: Crossroads, 1988). The book draws on columns I wrote for *The New Oxford Review,* a monthly magazine much interested in religious questions. I first wrote on spirituality in children in that magazine: several essays entitled "The Spiritual Life of Children" (*New Oxford Review,* November 1985, December 1985, January–February 1986). I also tried to respond in those columns to the strong moral introspection I often met with in children who never went to synagogue or church, but who had their own way of asking why and whither, their own way, even, of looking beyond themselves in order to address the question of life's meaning and purpose.

13. *The Child as Pilgrim*

1. Any of us who think about childhood in this century ought to keep close at hand Philippe Ariès's *Centuries of Childhood* (New York: Vintage, 1962) as a reminder of what boys and girls in earlier centuries were and were not, did and did not do. I rather suspect, if we make it as a species through this approaching third millennium, a social historian of childhood centuries from now will be writing about our times as Ariès did about centuries long since gone — a kind of life that was once taken for granted eventually ceases to be. On the other hand, we will always be finite — we're here out of nowhere, and gone soon enough, hence the constant theme of life as a journey, if not a pilgrimage, that I have noted (in children as well as adults) across barriers of race and class and nationality and religious persuasion or commitment. Gabriel Marcel's *Homo Viator* (Chicago: H. Regnery Company, 1951) explores the idea of man as a traveler, an itinerant — an appealing notion precisely because it connects with what boys and girls utterly unaware of religious existentialism nevertheless keep saying. Sometimes, as a matter of fact, children who are being observed for reasons utterly unconnected to their religious or spiritual life can still make

clear their reflective side in the things they say and do, as is evident in *Childhood's Domain* (London: Croom Helm, 1986), a study of "play and place in child development," a study of where children go and how they play when outdoors, by Robin Moore. It shows children walking and running and poking about the world, but at times stopping and wondering about "things," their moral meaning, as we all do.

2. Children, too, can summon narrative, can look at time and see themselves "in it" and eventually "out of it," as I have heard them put it, referring to a life lived over a span of years, and a life that ceases to be. What Jerome Bruner and Donald Spence have postulated for adults holds for boys and girls, too: they, too, think of their lives narratively. That is not quite the same as abstract propositional thinking — hence the view of life as a journey, as the unfolding of a story, a drama. See Bruner's *Actual Minds, Possible Worlds* (Cambridge, Mass.: Harvard University Press, 1986) and Spence's *Narrative Truth and Historical Truth* (New York: Norton, 1982). See also John Shelton Reed's "On Narrative and Sociology," *Social Forces*, September 1989.

3. Dorothy Day often pointed out to me that at the very start of the Bible — and, indeed, of the world as the Bible presents its beginnings — there was a mixture of thought and action, of word and deed, of symbol and substance. God spoke, said "Let there be light," but He also acted, breathed life into the dust; and so it goes to this day for children, too, as they hustle their way through space and time, doing and doing and doing, but also stopping and asking and wondering, and in their own fashion declaring and affirming.

Index